A Colour Atlas of Dermato-Immunohistocytology

EDITED BY
Hiroaki Ueki M.D.
Professor and Chairman of Dermatology
Kawasaki Medical School
Kurashiki, Okayama, JAPAN

Hideo Yaoita M.D.
Professor and Chairman of Dermatology
Jichi Medical School
Minamikouchi-machi, Tochigi, JAPAN

IN COLLABORATION WITH
Shojiro Nakagawa M.D.
Associate Professor of Dermatology
Kawasaki Medical School
Kurashiki, Okayama, JAPAN

Yasuo Kitajima M.D.
Associate Professor of Dermatology
Jichi Medical School
Minamikouchi-machi, Tochigi, JAPAN

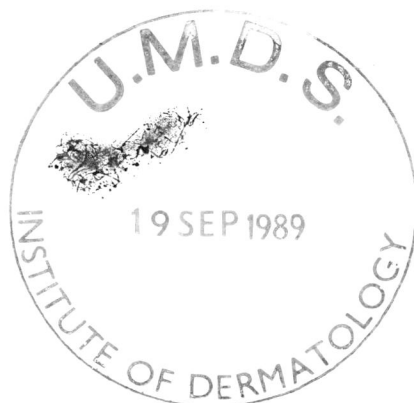

Wolfe Medical Publications Ltd

Copyright © H. Ueki, H. Yaoita, 1989
Published 1989 by Wolfe Medical Publications Ltd
ISBN 0 7234 1584 6

First published by Nankodo Co Ltd, 42–6 Hongo 3-Chome,
Bunkyo-Ku, Tokyo 113, Japan.

A CIP catalogue record for this book is available from the British Library.

This book is one of the titles in the series of Wolfe Medical Atlases, a series that
brings together the world's largest systematic published collection of diagnostic
colour photographs.

For a full list of Atlases in the series, plus forthcoming titles and details of our
surgical, dental and veterinary Atlases, please write to Wolfe Medical
Publications Ltd, 2–16 Torrington Place, London WC1E 7LT, England.

Contributors

Setsuya AIBA:
Department of Dermatology, Tohoku University
School of Medicine

Yutaka AKUTSU:
Department of Dermatology, Sapporo Medical
College

Tatsuyoshi ARAO:
Department of Dermatology, Kumamoto University
Medical School

Toru BABA:
Department of Dermatology, Institute of Clinical
Medicine, University of Tsukuba

Kiichiro DANNO:
Department of Dermatology, Faculty of Medicine,
Kyoto University

Hikaru ETO:
Department of Dermatology, School of Medicine,
Kitasato University

Hatsumi FUJII:
Department of Dermatology, Nagoya University
School of Medicine

Masutaka FURUE:
Department of Dermatology, Faculty of Medicine,
University of Tokyo

Hiroshi HACHISUKA:
Department of Dermatology, Kurume University
School of Medicine

Toshio HAMADA:
Department of Dermatology, Osaka City University,
Medical School

Takashi HASHIMOTO:
Department of Dermatology, School of Medicine, Keio
University

Tsutomu HIRAMOTO:
Department of Dermatology, Jichi Medical School

Yuji HORIGUCHI:
Department of Dermatology, Faculty of Medicine,
Kyoto University

Ryoichi IGARASHI:
Division of Dermatology, Niigata Prefectural Central
Hospital

Masafumi IIJIMA:
Department of Dermatology, Showa University,
School of Medicine

Hajime IIZUKA:
Department of Dermatology, Asahikawa Medical
College

Sadao IMAMURA:
Department of Dermatology, Faculty of Medicine,
Kyoto University

Yasunori INAGAKI:
Department of Dermatology, Kawasaki Medical
School

Shunichiro INOUE:
Department of Dermatology, Jichi Medical School

Masamitsu ISHII:
Department of Dermatology, Osaka City University,
Medical School

Hidekazu ISHIKAWA:
Department of Dermatology, Gunma University
School of Medicine

Fumiyuki ITO:
Department of Dermatology, First Hospital of Nippon
Medical School

Masaaki ITO:
Department of Dermatology, Niigata University,
School of Medicine

Kowichi JIMBOW:
Division of Dermatology and Cutaneous Science,
Faculty of Medicine, The University of Alberta,
CANADA

Toshiro KAGESHITA:
Department of Dermatology, Kumamoto University
Medical School

Kazuya KANAZAWA:
Department of Dermatology, Jichi Medical School

Fumio KANEKO:
Department of Dermatology, Fukushima Medical
College

Tamotsu KANZAKI:
Department of Dermatology, Nagoya City University
Medical School

Hiroshi KATAYAMA:
Department of Dermatology, Jichi Medical School

Masato KITABATAKE:
Department of Dermatology, Gunma University
School of Medicine

Yasuo KITAJIMA:
Department of Dermatology, Jichi Medical School

Yukio KITANO:
Department of Dermatology, Osaka University
Medical School

Akira KOHCHIYAMA:
Department of Dermatology, Kawasaki Medical
School

Mamoru KOHDA:
Department of Dermatology, Kawasaki Medical
School

Hiromi KUMON:
Department of Urology, Okayama University Medical
School

Takeshi KURATA:
Department of Pathology, National Institute of
Health, Tokyo

Kaori MAEDA:
Department of Dermatology, Sapporo Medical
College

Kazuo MAEDA:
Department of Dermatology, Sapporo Medical
College

Yoshihiro MAEKAWA:
Department of Dermatology, Kumamoto University
Medical School

Okitaka MAIE:
Department of Dermatology, Akita University School
of Medicine

Mikio MASUZAWA:
Department of Dermatology, School of Medicine,
Kitasato University

Tadahiko MATSUMOTO:
Department of Dermatology, Faculty of Medicine,
Kyushu University

Yoshiki MIYACHI:
Department of Dermatology, Faculty of Medicine,
Kyoto University

Sachiko MIYAGAWA:
Department of Dermatology, Nara Medical University

Kaoru MIYOSHI:
Department of Dermatology, Kawasaki Hospital,
Kawasaki Medical School

Toshihiro MIZUMOTO:
Department of Dermatology, Asahikawa Medical
College

Shunji MORI:
Department of Dermatology, School of Medicine, Gifu
University

Yutaka NAGAI:
Department of Tissue Physiology, Medical Research
Institute, Tokyo Medical and Dental University

Hiroyuki NAGATA:
Department of Dermatology, Kawasaki Medical
School

Hiroshi NAGURA:
Laboratory of Germfree Life Research Institute for
Disease Mechanism and Control, Nagoya University
School of Medicine

Shojiro NAKAGAWA:
Department of Dermatology, Kawasaki Medical
School

Shin-ichi NAKAMURA:
Department of Dermatology, First Hospital of Nippon
Medical School

Michihito NIIMURA:
Department of Dermatology, The Jikei University
School of Medicine

Takeji NISHIKAWA:
Department of Dermatology, School of Medicine, Keio
University

Shigeo NISHIYAMA:
Department of Dermatology, Kitasato University,
School of Medicine

Toshitatsu NOGITA:
Department of Dermatology, Faculty of Medicine,
University of Tokyo

Tadashi NOHARA:
Department of Dermatology, Nihon University,
School of Medicine

Shigeru NOMOTO:
Department of Dermatology, Faculty of Medicine,
Kagoshima University

Shigeo NONAKA:
Department of Dermatology, Nagasaki University,
School of Medicine

Hideoki OGAWA: Department of Dermatology, Juntendo University, School of Medicine

Daisuke OKA:
Department of Dermatology, Kawasaki Medical School

Natsuko OKADA:
Department of Dermatology, Osaka University Medical School

Masaru OOHASHI:
Department of Dermatology, Nagoya University, School of Medicine

Akira OOSHIMA:
Department of Pathology, Wakayama Medical College

Ryuzo SAITO:
Department of Dermatology, School of Medicine, Kitasato University

Mariko SAKUMA:
Department of Dermatology, Institute Clinical Medicine, University of Tsukuba

Yoichiro SASAI:
Department of Dermatology, Kurume University, School of Medicine

Yumiko SEZAI:
Department of Dermatology, Nihon University, School of Medicine

Tetsuo SHIOHARA:
Department of Dermatology, Kyorin University, School of Medicine

Shigenori SUDO:
Department of Dermatology, Toyama Medical and Pharmaceutical University, Faculty of Medicine

Hiroyuki SUZUKI:
Department of Dermatology, Nihon University, School of Medicine

Masayuki SUZUKI:
Department of Dermatology, Jichi Medical School

Shinya TAKAHASHI:
Department of Dermatology, Akita University School of Medicine

Yoshimasa TAKAHASHI:
Department of Dermatology, Hokkaido University, School of Medicine

Yoji TAKEI:
Department of Dermatology, Kawasaki Medical School

Shinichiro TAKEZAKI:
Department of Dermatology, School of Medicine, Kitasato University

Masahiro TAKIGAWA:
Department of Dermatology, Hamamatsu University School of Medicine

Kunihiko TAMAKI:
Department of Dermatology, Faculty of Medicine University of Tokyo, Tokyo University Branch Hospital

Akihiko TAMURA:
Department of Dermatology, Kyorin University, School of Medicine

Masaaki TASHIRO:
Department of Dermatology, Faculty of Medicine, Kagoshima University

Toshio TAZAWA:
Department of Dermatology, Niigata University, School of Medicine

Yasushi TOMITA:
Department of Dermatology, Tohoku University, School of Medicine

Masami UEHARA:
Department of Dermatology, Shiga University of Medical Science

Ayako UEKI:
Department of Hygiene, Kawasaki Medical School

Hiroaki UEKI:
Department of Dermatology, Kawasaki Medical School

Kaori YAMANA:
Department of Dermatology, Sapporo Medical College

Yuuichiro YAMASAKI:
Division of Dermatology, The 2nd Tokyo National Hospital

Makoto YANAGIHARA:
Department of Dermatology, School of Medicine, Gifu University

Hideo YAOITA:
Department of Dermatology, Jichi Medical School

Takashi YASUE:
Department of Dermatology, Nagoya University,
School of Medicine

Kunio YONEMASU:
Department of Bacteriology, Nara Medical University

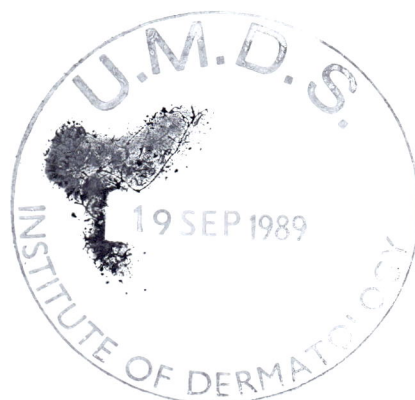

Preface

Skin is one of the most accessible and fascinating organs in the body and has attracted much social, aesthetic, scientific and clinical attention. Delicate but spectacular dramas are acted out on the macroscopical, microscopical, and ultramicroscopical levels, intermingled with morphological, chemical, immunological and molecular phenomena. It has long been the dream of dermatologists and pathologists to observe such dramas; now the introduction and development of the immunofluorescent technique by Coons has enabled us to realize that dream.

More than a quarter of a century has passed since the first application of the immunofluorescent technique to dermatological studies. This technique has shed light on previously unresolved problems concerning the skin and its disorders.

Microorganisms, antigens and antibodies, complement and enzyme have been dramatically observed in intracellular and extracellular tissues. The successful use of this technique in studies of infectious diseases, bullous dermatoses, collagen diseases and allergic vasculitis has resulted in exciting discoveries which have appeared in numerous journals throughout the world.

In addition, the establishment of the enzyme-labelled antibody method by Nakane *et al.* has made it possible to extend our researches to the ultrastructural levels. Markers for antibodies such as ferritin, horseradish peroxidase, gold, silver, radioisotopes and T4-phages have been introduced and applied in many studies. The experimental use of monoclonal antibodies has led to the detection of various components of the skin and dermatoses. From the studies carried out using these techniques during the past thirty years, we can now appreciate exciting areas of the immuno-histocytological art.

The purpose of this book is to collect and preserve the most outstanding examples of these studies together with the most impressive photographs to accompany these researches. The authors believe this collection will be of significant and educational value.

Hiroaki Ueki, M.D.
Hideo Yaoita, M.D.

Contents

Findings in Various Dermatoses

Introduction

Since 1941, when Coons *et al.*[1,2] developed the immunofluorescence technique, it became possible for us to observe microscopically antigens, antibodies and their related substances on tissue sections or on cell smears.

Initially, most efforts were made in the purification of specific antibodies, the choice of ideal labelling markers, the preparation of thin frozen sections, the improvement of fluorescent microscopic quality and the sensitivity of photographic films.

This technique has been improved continuously over the last few decades due to the progress in modern immunochemical procedures. The chemical synthesis of high quality markers such as fluorescein isothiocyanate (FITC)[3], tetramethyl-rhodamine isothiocyanate (TRITC)[4], and phycoerythrin (PE)[5], and the appearance of well-defined cryostats and fluorescence microscopes of both transmission and epi-illumination (incident) systems[6,7] have contributed to the development of immunofluorescence techniques.

In 1967 the enzyme-labelled antibody technique was described by Nakane and Pierce[8], and by Avrameas[9]. Paraffin sections were widely available for the studies using this technique and it also became possible to detect the markers by electron microscopy.

Several kinds of labelling markers, such as horseradish peroxidase (HRP), ferritin, gold[10], silver[11], radioisotopes[12] and T4-phage[13] proved applicable for transmission and scanning electron microscope studies.

HRP is the most stable and reliable marker. The sensitivity of the technique greatly increased with the introduction of various methods, such as the PAP method (peroxidase-anti-peroxidase complex)[14], the avidin-biotin-complex method[15], and the protein A-binding method.

In the field of dermatology, the immunofluorescence technique has been applied to the detection of micro-organisms[16,17], to viral particles[18–20] in tissues or cells, and subsequently to the examination of circulating antibodies against *micrococcus* and *treponema* in patient sera. The FTA (fluorescent treponemal antibody) test[21] is an example of this application. Prior to 1970, anti-nuclear factors (ANF)[22,23] and anti-pemphigus antibodies[24,25] were demonstrated in sera of patients with SLE and pemphigus, respectively. As the immunochemical techniques quickly progressed, many types of purified antibodies, antigens and related substances became commercially available and were applied to immunohistological studies. Thus, the immunofluorescence or enzyme-labelled antibody technique became a very popular method.

From 1970 to the present, exciting and crucial discoveries have accumulated in the fields of autoimmune diseases, collagen diseases[26,27], vasculitis[28,29], immune complexes[30], allergic disorders, infectious disorders, and tumours[31], through the use of immunohistochemical techniques.

Recently, cellular and subcellular components of cutaneous structure in physiological and pathological conditions have been studied employing this technique – similarly, their origins. Studies of the cytoskeleton[32], laminin[33], fibronectin[34], collagen[35], immunoglobulin, complement, fibrin, plasminogen, factor VIII RAg[36], and S-100 protein[37] have resulted.

Since the establishment of techniques to produce monoclonal antibodies[38] against cellular or subcellular components, it has become possible to investigate the maturation steps of many types of cells and to identify the nature and origin of malignant tumours.

The application of monoclonal antibodies to lymphocytes[39,40] or macrophages has also made it possible to identify and classify the subsets of infiltrating lymphocytes in various dermatoses and to comprehend the nature of these diseases better.

Now the immunohistocytological technique is one of the most important and widely-used procedures for the clarification of cutaneous diseases. This method is a very delicate one, however, with certain limitations in its application. It is necessary to consider the advantages and disadvantages. Only a carefully-executed study will provide impressive and reliable information.

The first part of this atlas describes the principles of immunohistochemical techniques, material preparation procedures and the application of monoclonal antibodies. In the second part, the immunohistological detection of skin components in normal and abnormal states is introduced, using the most recent and conclusive findings. The third part comprises the accumulated evidence from clinical applications, with special reference to technical notes, to enable readers to understand thoroughly the diagnoses, results and outcome of specific diseases.

We hope this atlas will be of benefit to readers throughout the world.

Hiroaki Ueki, M.D.

Foreword I

Dermatology represents one of the most fascinating disciplines in medicine as there are only very few diseases which do not show skin manifestations. In addition, the skin allows easy access to biopsy material and as such is a very suitable system for the study of the pathogenesis of disease processes. Morphology has always been of the greatest importance for dermatological research, on both the macroscopical and the microscopical level. Histological procedures have been supplemented by electron-microscopy and also by histochemical identification of various biochemical constituents. Furthermore, increasing knowledge has enabled the preparation of highly specific polyclonal and monoclonal antibodies, which can be used to detect antigenic determinants in frozen and paraffin-embedded sections. This technique has been applied to the identification of circulating antibodies in the serum of patients with autoimmune diseases, e.g. bullous diseases, lupus erythematosus, scleroderma and vasculitis. The use of antibodies directed against defined proteins has additionally enabled the identification of the origin of various tumour cells in primary lesions as well as in metastases. Moreover, microorganisms can be easily detected in infectious diseases with the help of immunohistochemical procedures. Now, using enzyme or other labelled antibodies in direct or indirect techniques, the methods can also be applied to the ultrastructure level, providing new insights into the pathogenesis of many disease processes, as well as being employed in the understanding of basic biological events. In addition to dermatology, these techniques are commonly used in most scientific disciplines, and probably represent the most exciting example that the combination of modern biochemical and immunochemical techniques with classic morphological procedures can lead to new discoveries in basic and clinical research.

I hope that this book will not only enthuse with its marvellous pictures, but will demonstrate that similar approaches — for example, the use of molecular biology techniques with *in situ* hybridization—will have major implications for dermatological research in the future.

I wish this book great success!

Dr. h.c. Otto Braun-Falco, M.D.
Professor of Dermatology
Chairman of the Department of Dermatology
Ludwig Maximilian University
Frauenlobstr. 9-11
8000 München 2
Federal Republic of Germany

Foreword II

Over 25 years ago, Cormane, Beutner and Jordon altered the course of dermatological practice with their discoveries — arrived at by use of direct immunofluorescence — which demonstrated that immunoreactants were present in the skin of patients suffering from lupus erythematosus, pemphigus, and bullous pemphigoid. Since those discoveries, our approach to the diagnosis, treatment and prognosis of these and many other diseases has changed, with immunofluorescence microscopy assuming a crucial role. Furthermore, as a consequence of the numerous important immunofluorescence studies, other immunological approaches, such as immunoelectron microscopy, immunoblotting and immunoprecipitation, now make an important contribution to the achievement of a definitive diagnosis. The autoantibodies found in the sera and in the skin of patients presenting with numerous of these diseases have become useful probes in the identification and characterization of cellular and extracellular components within the skin. In fact, such studies over the past quarter of a century have enhanced our knowledge of the cell biology of skin enormously.

In this highly illustrated, full-colour atlas, Professors Ueki and Yaoita have very effectively depicted the morphological advances in dermatology that have been achieved using immunohistochemical techniques; the atlas also concerns itself with the identification of many of the interesting cell biological processes which are found within the skin. Finally, in addition to the distinguished co-authors, outstanding investigators from all parts of Japan have contributed to this book.

Stephen I. Katz, M.D., Ph.D.
Chief, Dermatology Branch
National Cancer Institute
Bethesda
Maryland 20892
U.S.A.

TECHNICAL PROCEDURES IN IMMUNOHISTOCYTOLOGY

A   Immunofluorescence technique

Synopsis

The immunofluorescence technique enables us to observe intracellular and extracellular antigens, antibodies and related substances by fluorescence microscopy, using a fluorochrome-labelled antigen or antibody. One of the most reliable characteristics of this technique is the combination of immunological specificity and sensitivity with morphological localization. This method has been widely applied to dermatological studies, both clinical and basic research.

Principles and methods

PRINCIPLES:

In immunofluorescence techniques, antigens, antibodies or their complexes can be viewed under a microscope, using the corresponding antibodies coupled to fluorochrome. Several methods, such as direct, indirect, complement, and membrane immunofluorescence, or several modified tests, can be implemented (1). For the membrane immunofluorescence figure 1 method, usually unfixed, viable cells are used.

CHARACTERISTICS

The immunofluorescence technique consists of a specific, delicate, *in vitro* immunological reaction on the glass slide. Every procedure, therefore, should be carried out carefully to preserve immunological nature and specificity. A specific antigen-antibody reaction can easily be influenced by several factors such as incubation time, temperature, pH, ionic strength or concentration of the solution, fixation and preservation of the cells or tissues, contamination from related antigens or antibodies, or infected microorganisms etc.[41–43]. Specific reactivity may thus be lost through these factors.

One advantage of the immunofluorescence technique is the short procedure time. The complete technique, including the preparation of the sections, staining and observation can be performed in one to three hours.

Another characteristic is its sensitivity. The sensitivity of the direct method seems to correspond to that of the classical complement fixation test. It may be impossible to determine precise sensitivity because specific fluorescence cannot be examined quantitatively. Generally, the sensitivity of the indirect or the complement method is estimated to be between five and ten times higher than that of the direct one. At least 5,000 to 10,000 molecules of immunoglobulins are necessary for the detection of surface immunoglobulins on B-lymphocytes by the membrane immunofluorescence method.

PREPARATION OF ANTIGENS

To obtain adequate results, it is essential to preserve the antigenic nature of the cells, tissues or organs. Firstly, it is necessary to perform the section preparation at a cool temperature (4–10°C) before fixation.

This applies not only to the target antigens; the surrounding cells and tissue background should also be kept carefully for immunological reactions. If the cells or tissues are not well preserved, it may be very difficult to detect or interpret the findings correctly. Bacteria and cultured cells can be smeared directly onto the glass slide, while frozen tissues must be arranged in sections in a cryostat. Any biopsy specimen should be frozen immediately at −80°C – using liquid nitrogen – and cut into sections within a few weeks. The paraffin-embedded sections can also be used for this method in some cases.

PREPARATION OF LABELLED ANTIBODIES

The specific antibody, fractionated IgG molecules or the F(ab) portion can be labelled with certain tracers, such as fluorescein isothiocyanate (FITC)[44], tetramethylrhodamine isothiocyanate (TRITC)[45] or phycoerythrin (PE)[46]. It has been reported that these fluorescent markers can be tagged with antibody molecules without losing specificity[41–43]. The first of these tracers emits a yellow-green fluorescence, while the latter two show red fluorescence under UV excitation. PE has an excitation wave similar to that of FITC and a stronger red fluorescence than TRITC. In double-staining sections FITC-labelled antibody and PE-labelled antibody can be used under the same excitation system. The following important factors should be taken into consideration when choosing an ideal conjugate.

F:P (fluorescein/protein) molar ratio. The ideal F:P molar ratio is 1:2. Higher molar ratios of conjugate may yield a non-specific reaction, due to the free non-tagged fluorochrome, laden with a strong negative charge, reacting non-immunologically with positively-charged cells or tissues.

Concentration of the conjugate solution. An adequate antibody or protein concentration for the conjugate is estimated to be 25–50µg/ml or $\frac{1}{8}$ to $\frac{1}{4}$ units/ml at the final dilution. Other unrelated proteins or contaminants should be avoided. Labelled F(ab') fragments of the specific antibody, monoclonal or polyclonal, are recommended as the most suitable conjugates. All conjugates should be absorbed at least three times with tissue powders, such as acetone liver powder, just before use to rid the stored conjugates of possible undesirable factors such as free fluorochromes, denatured conjugates, etc. The specificity and cross-reactivity of the conjugate should always be carefully checked before use.

Storage of the conjugates. The purified conjugates can be stored for up to a year at −80° or 4°C in 0.1% sodium-azide after sterilization by millipore-filtration. The frozen conjugates should be carefully stored in a proper place which prevents repeated thawing and refreezing[41–43]. The temperature should be constant, and the conjugate solution should not be shaken or bubbled, as these will also result in an unsatisfactory reaction.

STAINING PROCEDURES

The immunofluorescence technique is based on a delicate immune reaction, not merely a staining method. The staining procedures should be carefully carried out in a moist chamber. The diluted conjugates can be incubated at 37°C for 30 to 60 minutes, at room temperature for two to three hours, or overnight at 4°C. There are four principal staining methods: direct, indirect, complement and membrane immunofluorescence. Additionally, there are the following special variations: double staining, counterstaining, *in vivo* staining, protein A binding and avidin-biotin complex methods.

(III)
antiC
(II)
antiAb
(I)
Ab
Ag
C
Ab
Ag
Ag
Ab
tissue. cell

*:   fluorochrome   (I)   direct method
Ag: antigenic determinants   (II)   indirect method
Ab: antibody   (III) complement method
C: complement

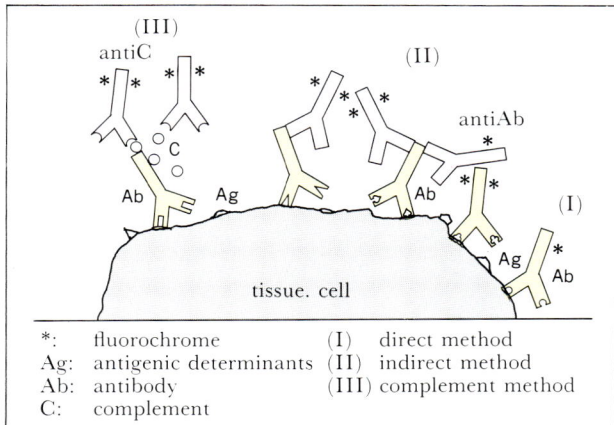

Fig. 1. The principle of immunofluorescence techniques.

1. Basic procedures
section . . . fixed or unfixed
   wash in gently stirring PBS
   3 times, for 15 minutes
staining the conjugate
   incubate for 30 minutes
in a moist chamber
   wash in PBS,
   3 times for 15 minutes
Place a drop on the glass slide
   Mount in PBS glycerol
Observe under fluorescence microscope

2. Control study
a. Control test of the conjugate section
   Stain in the unrelated conjugate
   Observe . . . specific fluorescence (−)
b. Inhibition test (I)
   Section
   Stain the specific antibody
   Observe . . . specific fluorescence (−)
c. Inhibition test (II)
   Section
   Stain the specific conjugate previously absorbed in the
   specific antigen
   Observe . . . specific fluorescence (−)

Fig. 2. Technical procedure of the direct method.

antibody   fluorochrome   specific conjugate

antigen   specific   specific fluorescence (+)
                conjugate

antigen   unrelated   specific fluorescence (−)   (control study)
                conjugate

antigen   antibody   (antigen-antibody   specific   specific fluorescence (−)
                      complex)   conjugate   (inhibition test)

Fig. 3. The direct method.

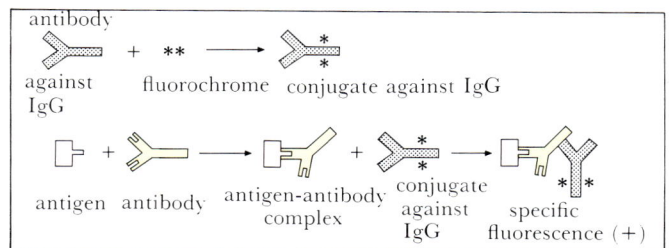

antibody
against   fluorochrome   conjugate against IgG
IgG

antigen   antibody   antigen-antibody   conjugate   specific
                      complex   against IgG fluorescence (+)

Fig. 4. The indirect method.

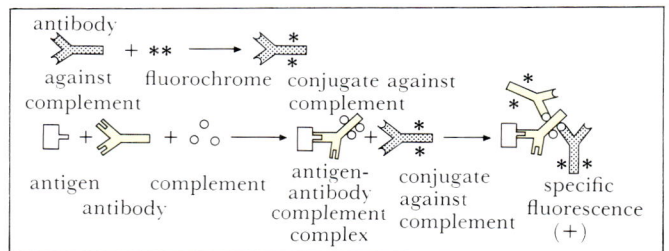

antibody
against   fluorochrome   conjugate against
complement   complement

antigen   complement   antigen-   conjugate   specific
          antibody   antibody   against   fluorescence
                         complement   complement   (+)
                         complex

Fig. 5. The complement method.

The pre-treatment of the samples. For samples containing antigens, adequate fixatives must be selected. Antigens may be on the cell surface of the tissue or within the cells. Unfixed cells or frozen tissues are often available. Usually 95% ethanol, 10% formalin or acetone is used as the fixative. A cryostat is recommended. In addition to the target antigen, surrounding cells or tissues should also be carefully treated and adequately fixed.

The direct method. The pre-treated sections or cells are covered directly with the prepared conjugates in a moist chamber, as shown schematically in figures 2 and 3. It is necessary to perform the control test and the specific blocking test on the serial sections and they should be negative. The direct method is simple and very specific, but not as sensitive as the other methods.

The indirect method. The principle of the indirect method is shown in figure 4. Sections or smears are incubated with the optimally diluted, non-labelled primary antibody, washed with PBS, and then incubated with the fluorochrome-labelled secondary antibody. By this method, antigens in sections or antibodies in sera can be indirectly examined. The sensitivity is higher than that of the direct method, but some undesirable non-specific reactions may occur. Antinuclear titre are examples of this application. Controls must always be included with this method.

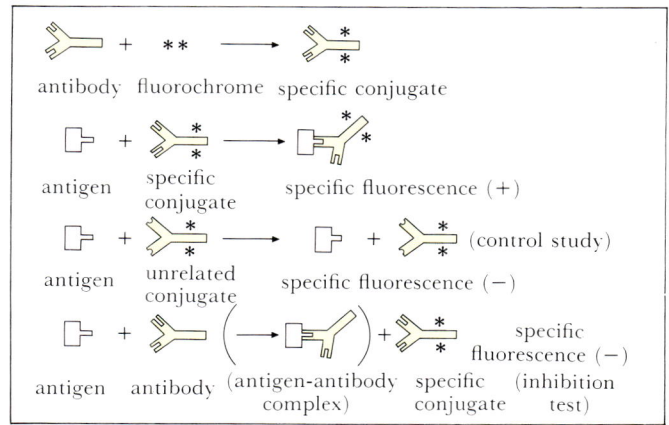

The complement method. This is a modification of the indirect method, as described in figure 5. The complement activation or binding capacity of the primary antibody can be monitored with this method.

Membrane immunofluorescence. The antigenic determinants on the surface of viable cells can be directly or indirectly incubated with conjugates in test tubes. This method is generally used for the differentiation of lymphocytes, and the detection of surface globulins on B-lymphocytes, or immune complexes on Raji cells. In order to prevent 'capping' of the cell membrane, all the procedures should be carried out at 4°C, or an inhibitor such as 0.02M NaN$_3$ should be added to reagents.

OBSERVATION AND PHOTOMICROGRAPHY

Two types of fluorescent microscopes are now available; transmitted light and incident light illumination. With regard to fluorescence excitation systems, the UV or BV excitation filter system and interference filter system are widely used[42, 47]. Fluorochromes emit different fluorescence under different excitation filters. For example, FITC emits a yellow-green fluorescence, while TRITC and PE emit brilliant red or orange. The fluorescence-emitting materials can be photographed using highly-sensitive colour films. Several materials or tissues in the dermis emit natural autofluorescence when irradiated with UV or BV visible rays. The collagen fibres fluoresce white-blue, the elastic fibres yellow-white, the epidermal granular cell layers or the lipofuscin in the eccrine glands, yellow-orange[48, 49]. Strongly-charged cells or tissues may react non-specifically with conjugates. As demonstrated in figure 6, eosinophilic leucocytes may often display a non-specific reaction. Some of the autofluorescence can be blocked with specific absorptive filters.

Important notes for specific reactions and some examples of technical pitfalls

Immunofluorescence techniques are based upon a very delicate and specific immune reaction. All of the necessary materials must be carefully prepared. As the possibility of non-specific reactions is always present, the blocking test and good control studies are essential. Figures 7 and 8 show complete non-specific reactions, because free non-coupled FITC solutions were incubated with frozen human tissue sections. FITC in PBS has a strong negative charge, and thus easily reacts non-immunologically with the tissues. This means that the presence of free FITC in the conjugates may cause non-specific reaction.

Figures 9, 10 and 11 show bound IgG deposits in frozen unfixed sections from lesion tissue of SLE by the direct method, using various conjugates and section pre-treatment. Figures 9 and 10 show the presence of non-specific reactions, while figure 11 reveals ideally stained specific granular IgG deposits on the dermo-epidermal junction. In figure 9, an unadsorbed conjugate with a high F:P molar ratio was applied to 95% ethanol-fixed frozen section. The same conjugate was used for non-fixed and washed sections of the same specimen in figure 10.

Figures 12 and 13 also show human IgG deposits in erythematous tissue of SLE. Figure 12 is an example of the non-specific reactions of anti-IgG, due to the unabsorbed conjugate. In figure 13, the properly diluted and absorbed conjugate was used on serial, non-fixed, frozen sections of that used in figure 12. The granular specific deposits are found in the dermo-epidermal junction and also in the dermis. Figure 14 reveals granular immune complexes on the surface of viable Raji cells under an incident light illumination system, using membrane immunofluorescence. An example of the double staining method is shown in epidermal cell suspensions from DNCB (dinitrochloro-benzene)-painted mouse skin in figure 15. In this study, FITC-labelled anti-DNP antibody and PE-labelled avidin and biotin-labelled anti-Thy-1, 2 monoclonal antibody solutions were applied. Most keratinocytes are positive for the presence of DNP-antigens and thus emit green fluorescence, while Thy-1-positive cells emit red fluorescence.

Once again, the immunofluorescence technique is based on a delicate immune reaction. In all the procedures, careful examination and selection of materials and conjugates, ideal pre-treatment of cells or tissues, and skilful observation and judgement must be made under adequate optical systems with accompanying proper control studies in order to produce the specific reactions which result in useful and valuable findings.

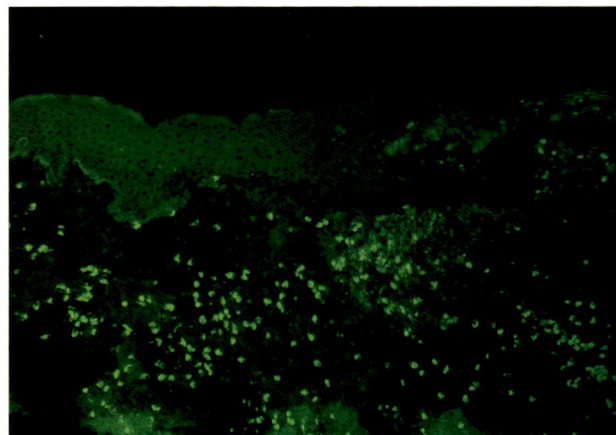

Fig. 6. Eosinophilic leucocytes in the dermis show non-specific reactivity against the free non-tagged FITC solution (0.3 μg/ml) (× 200). (Courtesy of H. Yaoita, M.D.)

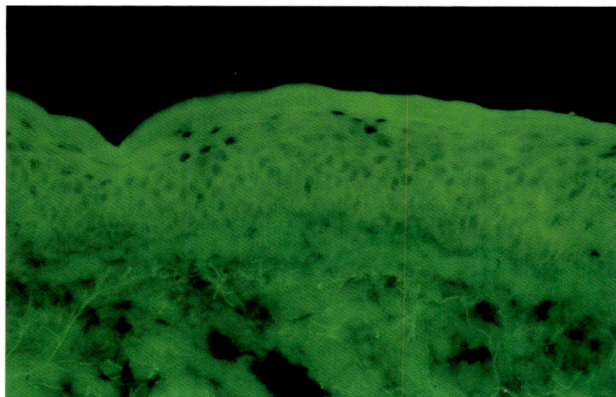

Fig. 7. Human frozen tissue section incubated with FITC solution (1 μg/ml) for twenty minutes. Conspicuous non-specific reaction throughout the section. (× 600)

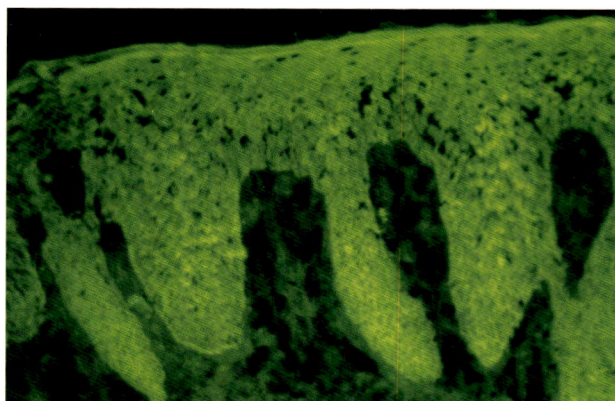

Fig. 8. After washing in PBS, the cutaneous section was incubated with FITC solution (1 μg/ml) for 40 minutes. Non-specific staining is evident in the epidermis. (× 400)[27]

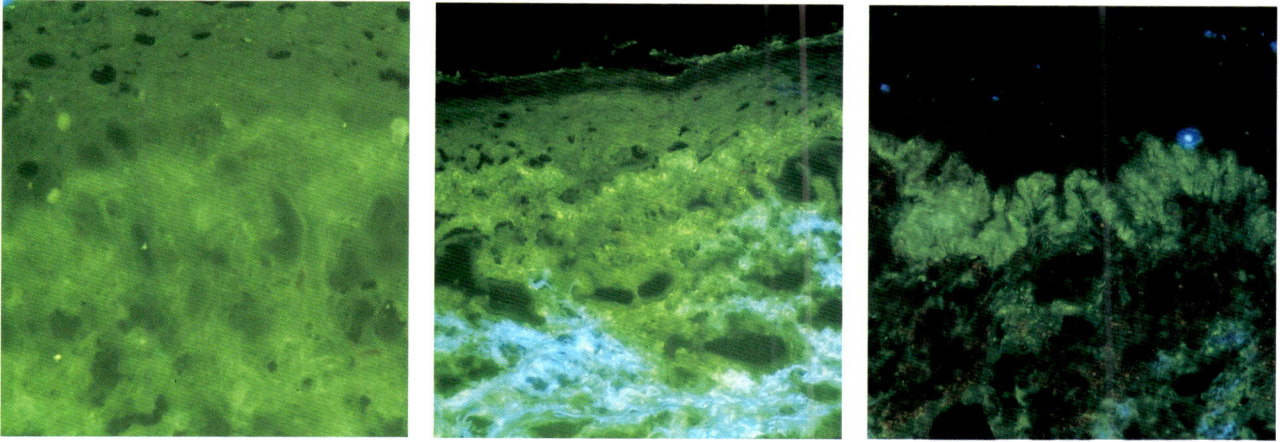

Fig. 9. The direct method for human IgG deposits in a section from butterfly erythema of SLE. The frozen, 95% ethanol-fixed section is incubated with non-absorbed anti-IgG conjugate at a 2.5 F:P molar ratio. The strong non-specific fluorescence is seen throughout the skin. ($\times$ 600)

Fig. 10. Serial section from the same specimen as Fig. 9, and incubated with the same conjugate. The frozen unfixed section was washed in PBS before incubation. The non-specific reaction was relatively diminished. ($\times$ 400)

Fig. 11. Serial section from the same specimen as Fig. 9, incubated with absorbed anti-IgG conjugate at a 1.8 F:P molar ratio. The specific granular fluorescence of IgG is observed on the dermo-epidermal junction and along the collagen fibres. The non-specific reaction of the epidermis completely disappeared. ($\times$ 400)

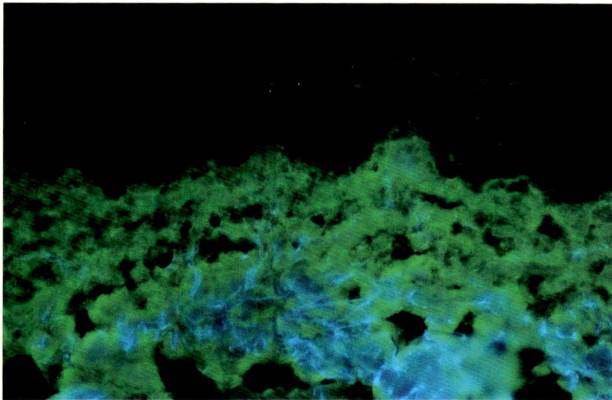

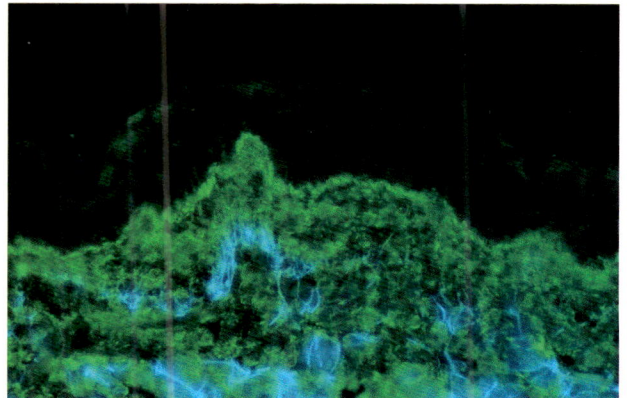

Fig. 12. The direct method was used for IgG deposits in tissue from SLE. The non-fixed, frozen section was incubated with unabsorbed anti-IgG conjugate at a 1.8 F:P molar ratio. Diffuse non-specific fluorescence is seen throughout the dermis. ($\times$ 400)

Fig. 13. The direct method was used for IgG deposits in the same serial section as Fig. 12, incubated with absorbed conjugate. The specific fluorescence is seen on the junction and the upper dermis. ($\times$ 400)[27]

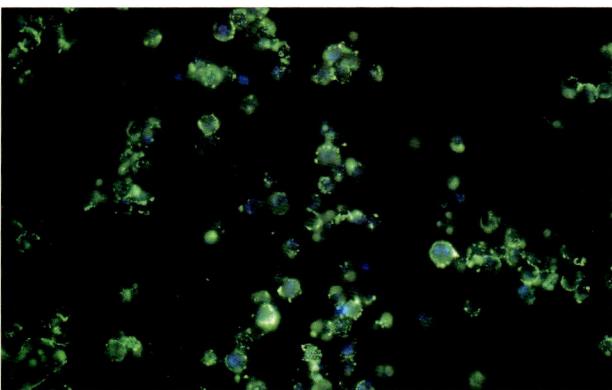

Fig. 14. The indirect method was used for immune complexes on the surface of viable Raji cells, incubated primarily with SLE sera and subsequently with absorbed anti-IgG conjugate. Granular fluorescent areas are seen on the cell surface under epi-illumination. ($\times$ 600)

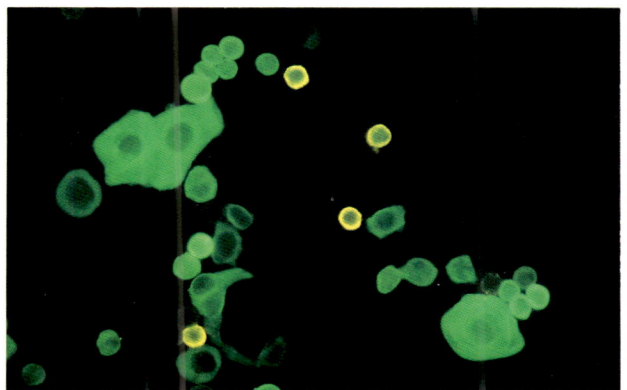

Fig. 15. Double staining for DNP-determinants with the FITC-labelled anti-DNP conjugate and for Thy-1 antigen with PE-labelled avidin plus biotin-labelled anti-Thy-1, 2 monoclonal antibody on epidermal cell suspensions from DNCB-painted C3H mouse skin. ($\times$ 400)

B   Enzyme-labelled antibody method

The enzyme-labelled antibody method is one of many immuno-histopathological techniques. In this method, the enzyme itself cannot be seen but reaction products can be seen. The advantages and disadvantages are shown in Table I.

Peroxidase, cytochrome, and acid phosphatase are examples of the enzymes available for labelling[50–52]. Horseradish peroxidase is the most commonly used enzyme for labelling.

There are two methods for labelling the enzyme to the antibody. One is a chemical reaction[50], and the other is an immunological reaction[51], called the peroxidase-antiperoxidase method. The advantages and disadvantages of each method are described in Tables I and II.

Materials and methods

LABELLING METHODS (1)
Chemical reaction[50]
Immunological reaction[53, 54]
  i. soluble peroxidase-antiperoxidase complex method[53]
  ii. peroxidase-antiperoxidase bridge method[54]
Avidin-biotin-peroxidase complex method[55, 56]
The peroxidase-antiperoxidase bridge method is much more widely used than the soluble peroxidase-antiperoxidase complex method, due to better penetration. Good penetration is particularly essential for the demonstration of bullous pemphigoid antigen or linear IgA antigen at lamina lucida.

TISSUE PREPARATION PRIOR TO STAINING
It is necessary to treat tissue to retain antigenicity and structure. Unfortunately, in the attempt to retain the structure, some antigenicity may be lost and vice versa. So the most suitable tissue preparation prior to staining should be chosen from among the following:

1. 10% glycerin (10% DMSO)[54]
2. agar[57]
3. Mclean's fixative (PLP)[51]
4. Zamboni's fixatives[50]
5. Lawicryl[58]

However, there is no standardized technique yet.

The most suitable tissue thickness and manner of tissue slicing depend on the method of tissue preparation, thus each of the above procedures should be carefully and completely followed. However, these can be modified according to your purpose.

STAINING PROCEDURE
Due to the shortage of space, we cannot describe each procedure here. Please refer to the following references for each procedure.

1. peroxidase labelled antibody method[50, 51]
2. peroxidase-antiperoxidase bridge method (PAP)[54, 57]
3. soluble peroxidase-antiperoxidase complex method[53]
4. avidin-biotin-peroxidase complex method[55, 56]

NOTE
Identification of non-specific reactions and staining methods is described in figures 2–5. There are two kinds of non-specific reaction; 1, the reaction which comes from the native peroxidase in the neutrophil, and 2, non-specific deposits of peroxidase or DAB (3, 3' diaminobenzidine) in the tissue. Na-azide treatment is effective to avoid the native peroxidase reaction[51] (**5**). To avoid the latter reaction, normal animal serum (usually 10% PBS) is thought to be the most effective (**4**)[54]. Neuraminidase can also be used for non-specific staining in the epidermis (**3**).

Figures 2–5 are the controls for figure 6.

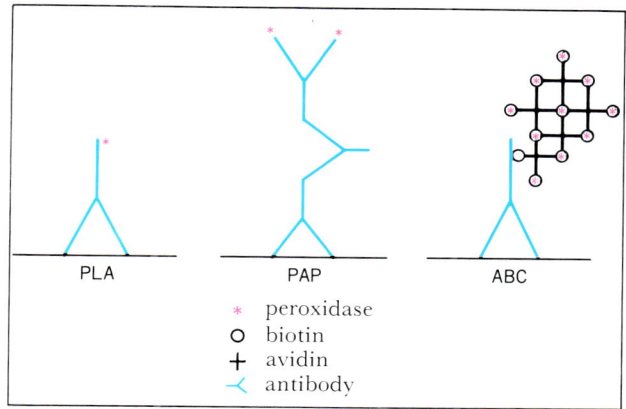

Fig. 1. Horseradish peroxidase methods (PLA: peroxidase-labelled antibody method, PAP: peroxidase-antiperoxidase bridge method, ABC: avidin-biotin complex method).

TABLE I   COMPARISON OF THE IMMUNO-ENZYME METHOD AND THE IMMUNOFLUORESCENCE METHOD

IMMUNO-ENZYME METHOD	IMMUNOFLUORESCENCE METHOD
Advantages: • good stain preservation • easy to see tissue structure • more sensitive • easy to apply to immunoelectron microscopy	Advantages: • better contrast • easy to see small subjects • immediately visible after immuno-reaction • simple procedure
Disadvantages: • more complicated procedure • labelled enzyme cannot be seen, the reaction products can be seen • bad contrast	Disadvantages: • fluorescence decreases immediately • tissue structures are barely visible

TABLE II   ADVANTAGES AND DISADVANTAGES OF PEROXIDASE METHODS

	ADVANTAGES	DISADVANTAGES
peroxidase-antiperoxidase bridge method	• good penetration • good antibody activity • label enzyme to antibody	• lengthy procedure
peroxidase-labelled Fab	• good penetration • simple procedure	• unstable antibody activity • higher background
long incubation time with whole peroxidase-labelled antibodies	• simple procedure	• bad penetration • lengthy procedure (14 hours) • bad tissue structure • bad antigen-antibody reaction
avidin-biotin-peroxidase complex	• high sensitivity	• poor penetration

9

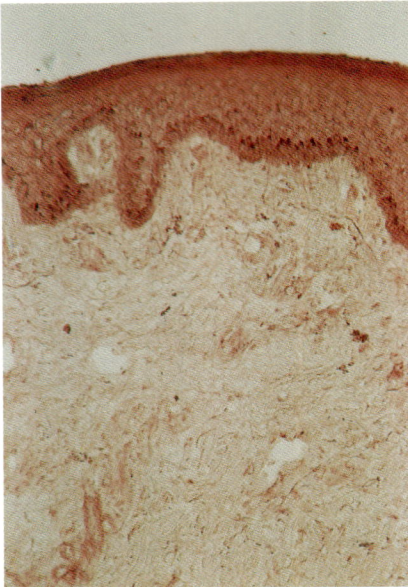

TABLE III   ABC PROCEDURE

tissue
↓
3% normal nonimmune serum
                    for 20 min
    ↓ blot excess serum from sections
primary antiserum for 30 min
    ↓ wash with Tris buffer
biotin-labelled secondary antibody
                    for 30 min
    ↓ wash with Tris buffer
avidin-biotin-peroxidase complex
                    for 30-60 min
    ↓ wash with Tris buffer
DAB solution for 5 min
    ↓ wash with water
counterstain, clean and mount

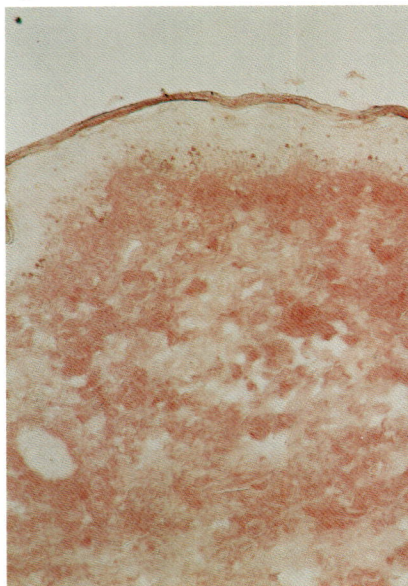

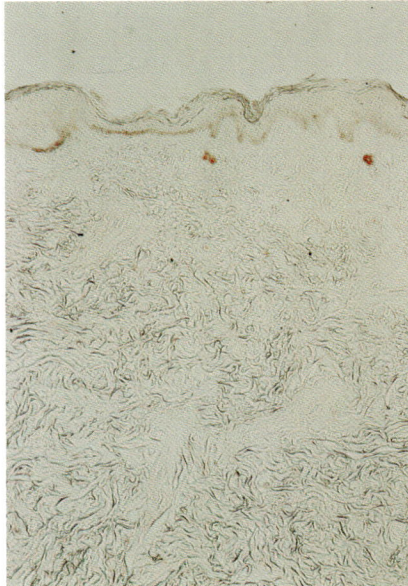

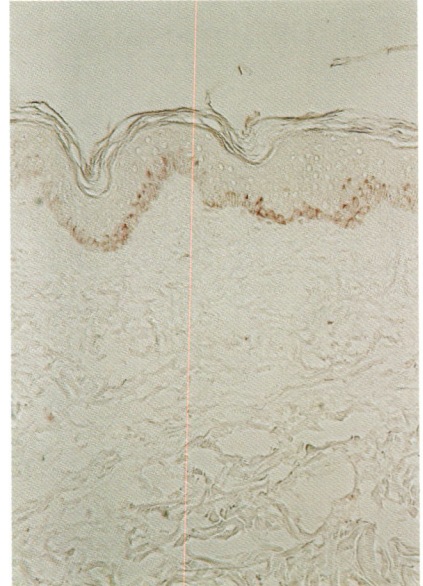

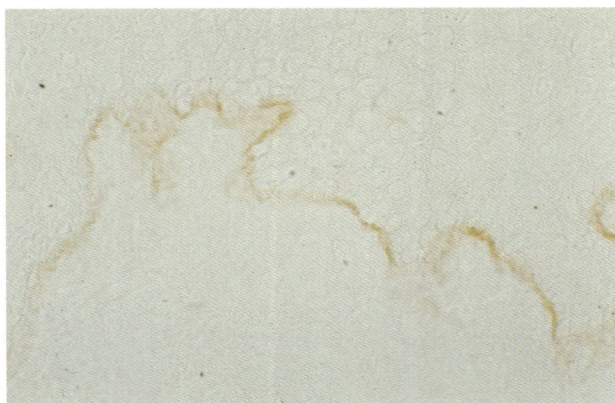

Fig. 2. Non-treated normal skin tissue (PAP), diffuse brown background (non-specific deposition and reaction). (× 100)

Fig. 3. Normal skin tissue treated with neuraminidase (PAP). Non-specific staining decreased in epidermis. (× 100)

Fig. 4. Normal skin tissue treated with normal animal serum (PAP). Only inherent peroxidase reaction can be seen in the upper dermis. (× 100)

Fig. 5. Normal skin tissue treated with normal animal serum and peroxidase blocker (PAP). All non-specific staining disappeared. (× 100)

Fig. 6. Herpes gestationis skin tissue treated in the same way as Fig. 5. Linear brown deposits at the dermal-epidermal junction are indicative of C3. (× 200)

C Immunoelectron microscopy

Horseradish peroxidase-labelled method

Sensitivity of this method is influenced by: 1, antigenicity; 2, antibody activity; 3, enzyme activity, and 4, visibility of reaction products.

The antigenicity of tissue decreases with fixatives. The antibody activity decreases due to the modification of antibodies needed to obtain good penetration. The main advantage of this method compared to the Ferritin or gold-labelled antibody method is better penetration (Table I). Many other kinds of enzymes are used for antibody labelling, as described in the previous chapter. With the exception of peroxidase[59], these enzymes are not used in the dermatological field due to the many disadvantages[60].

Non-specific staining of background mainly comes from: 1, inherent peroxidase (neutrophil etc.), and 2, non-specific deposits of enzymes, DAB or osmium.

The method for removal of the native peroxidase reaction is described in the previous chapter. To identify the positive reaction from non-specific deposits of reaction products, good control steps should be taken[59]. Specimens should be observed without counter-staining, as it is much easier to see the reaction products (1–3). The results of our studies on the bullous diseases are shown in Table II.

TABLE I CHARACTERISTICS OF IEM

LABELS	ADVANTAGE	DISADVANTAGE	APPLICATION
radio-isotope	good penetration	needs specific treatment	cell structure
ferritin	well established staining, simple procedure	bad penetration	well exposed area
gold	different sizes of gold particles can be used	bad penetration	multiple staining
PLA	simple procedure	penetration not so good due to decrease in antibody activity	PLA Fab can be widely used
PAP (IB)	good penetration	false negative	widely used
ABC	high sensitivity	bad penetration	well exposed area

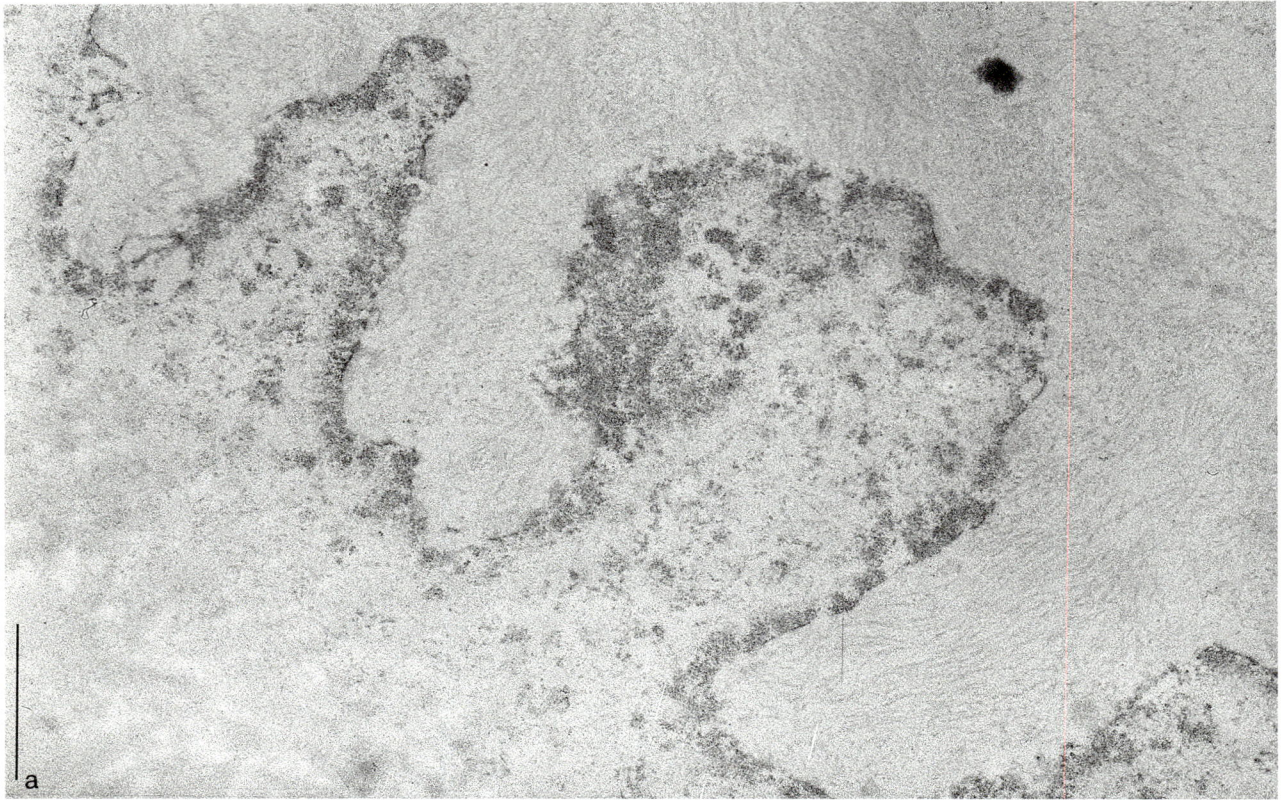

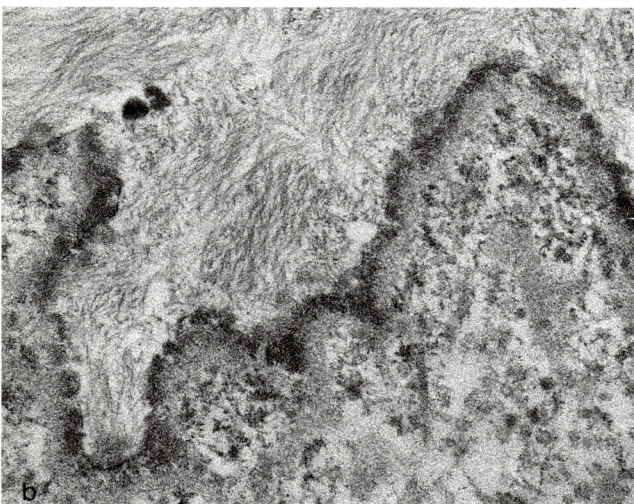

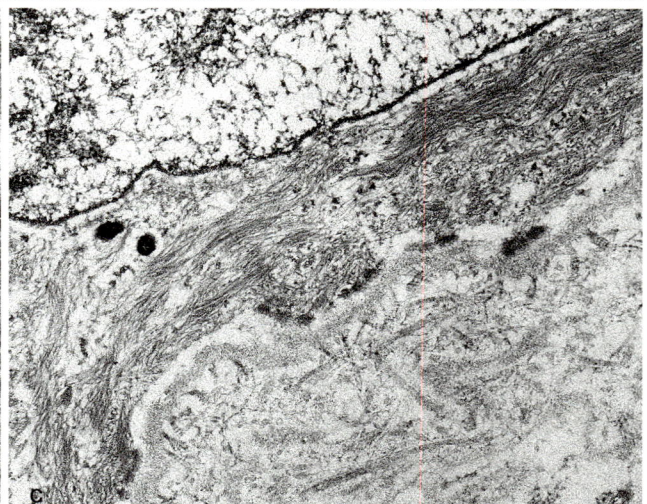

Fig. 1a. Horseradish peroxidase-labelled antibody method without counter-staining. (Skin of patients with herpes gestationis (HG skin)). Linear dark granular reaction products indicate C3 deposits.

Fig. 1b. The specimen used in Fig. 1a counter-stained with lead citrate and uranyl acetate[54].

Fig. 1c. Normal human skin[54].

The specimen was stained by the same method as in Fig. 1b.

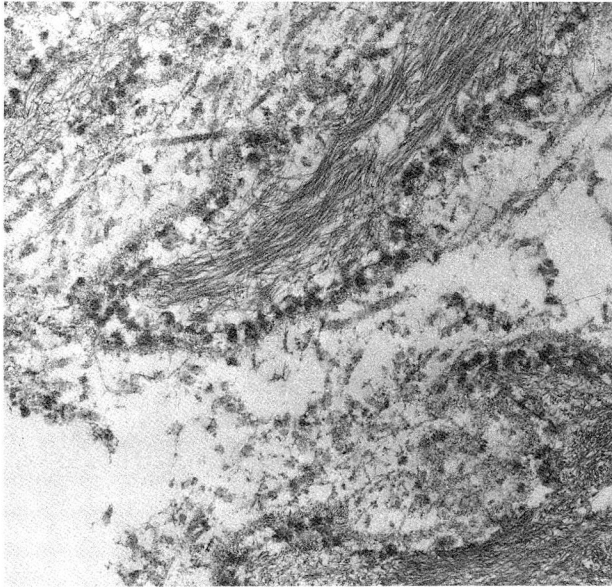

Fig. 2. The tissue (HG skin) was not incubated with cryoprotector before staining. (Same staining method as in Fig. 1b.)[54]

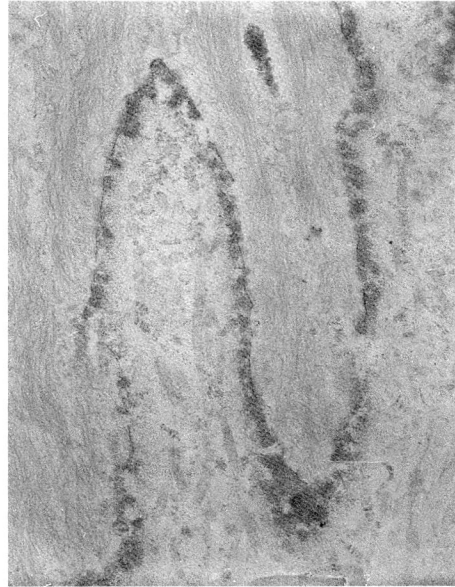

Fig. 3. The tissue was stored for 4 months at −40°C. (Same staining method as in Fig. 1a.)

TABLE II   THE SUMMARY OF THE RESULTS OF IEM ON BULLOUS DISEASE

LESION	DIAGNOSIS	DIF Ig	COMPLEMENT
epidermis	pemphigus	IgG	+
	bullous pemphigoid	IgG	+
	cicatricial pemphigoid	IgG	+
epidermal-dermal junction	(BMP, Brunsting-Perry)		
	herpes gestationis	(IgG)	+C3
	lamina lucida type IgA bullous disease	IgA	+
	sub-basal lamina	IgG	+
	type bullous disease	IgA	+
dermis	dermatitis herpetiformis	IgA	+
	epidermolysis bullosa acquisita	IgG (IgM)	+

LESION	DIAGNOSIS	IIF Ig	COMPLEMENT
epidermis	pemphigus	IgG	+
	bullous pemphigoid	IgG	+
	cicatricial pemphigoid	IgG	+
epidermal-dermal junction	(BMP, Brunsting-Perry)		
	herpes gestationis	HGF (IgG)	+C3
	lamina lucida type IgA bullous disease	IgA	+
	sub-basal lamina	IgG	+
	type bullous disease	IgA	+
dermis	dermatitis herpetiformis	−	−
	epidermolysis bullosa acquisita	IgG	+

LESION	DIAGNOSIS	IEM
epidermis	pemphigus	intercellular
	bullous pemphigoid	lamina lucida
	cicatricial pemphigoid	lamina lucida
epidermal-dermal junction	(BMP, Brunsting-Perry)	
	herpes gestationis	lamina lucida
	lamina lucida type IgA bullous disease	lamina lucida
	sub-basal lamina	sub-basal lamina
	type bullous disease	anchoring fibril system
dermis	dermatitis herpetiformis	elastic fibre system
	epidermolysis bullosa acquisita	dermis

Immunoferritin electron microscopic method

INTRODUCTION

Ferritin (F) is a protein containing more than 20% iron. F molecules can be seen as electron-opaque particles having an approximate diameter of 5 nm by electron microscopy. Thus, F-conjugated antibody can be successfully used as a tracer to localize specific antigens and receptors. The advantage of this method is the ease with which each F molecular particle can be recognized. This allows semi-quantitation of antigen doses under certain conditions. On the other hand, due to the large molecular size, manipulation is necessary for F to penetrate into the tissue or the cell cytoplasm, in which antigens are localized[61]. Recently, a method has been developed in which F-antibody is applied directly to ultracryosections.

PREPARATION OF F-ANTIBODY

F is further purified by cadmium sulphate recrystallization and ultracentrifugation. The conjugation is performed according to the method by Kishida *et al*[62]. Sucrose density gradient and affinity chromatography are employed for the purification of conjugates. The titre of the conjugate is determined by passive haemagglutination. Purification is also necessary for commercial conjugate.

EXPERIMENTAL PROCEDURE

The conjugate is easily accessible to antigens present on the surface of isolated and cultured cells and cells lining the lumen of the tubular structure. In the direct method, cells are reacted with the F-conjugate. In the indirect method, cells are incubated first with the specific antibody and then with the F-labelled second antibody. The specimen is fixed and embedded for electron microscopic observation. Ultra-thin sections are destained or counter-stained with uranylate which makes F easily discernible against background granularity. The figure shows an electron micrograph of a Langerhans cell in isolated guinea pig epidermal cells treated with F-concanavalin A (Con A) to show the cell surface distribution of Con A binding sites. To avoid non-specific binding, the F-conjugate should be absorbed with the appropriate materials before use.

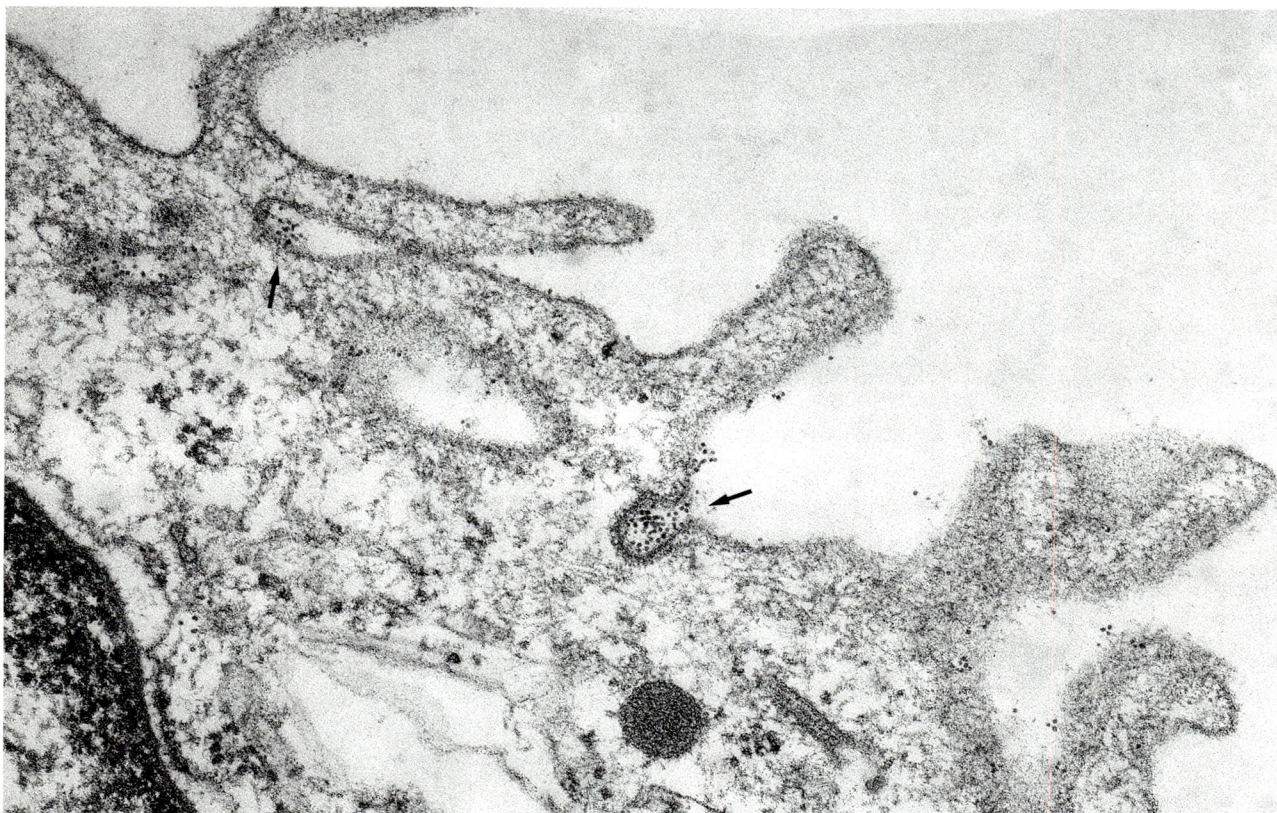

Fig. 1. Distribution of Con A binding substance on a Langerhans cell. Isolated guinea pig epidermal cells were reacted with F-Con A at 37°C for five minutes. F particles are observed in a coated pit as well as on the cell surface. ($\times$ 70,000)[64]

14

Colloidal gold-labelled antibody method

Immunoelectron microscopy using colloidal gold-labelled antibody was first introduced by Faulk *et al.* in 1971[65]. Colloidal gold can be recognized easily and, by simply changing the size of the gold particles, double staining can be performed[66, 69].

The freeze-fracture method is also an excellent technique, which splits the lipid bilayer of the membrane allowing the membrane plane with the intramembranous fine structures – including desmosomes, tight junctions and gap junctions – to be visualised.

The label-fracture method introduced by Pinto da Silva and Kan in 1985[67], is shown in this section.

LABEL-FRACTURE

The dispersed cells, labelled with colloidal gold, are suspended, frozen and fractured. The cell in the middle of figure 1 was fractured and revealed its E-face (exoplasmic membrane face). The electron beam of the electron microscope passes through the lipid membrane and the image of the E-face is visualized with the shadows of the labelled gold[67].

METHOD

Dispersed human keratinocytes were obtained by treatment with dispase (5,000 U/ml, Hank's solution, 15 minutes) and trypsinization (0.02%, PBS (−), EDTA (−), 10 minutes). The cells were incubated with the serum of a patient with pemphigus foliaceus for one hour at room temperature and labelled with colloidal gold-labelled antihuman IgG. The

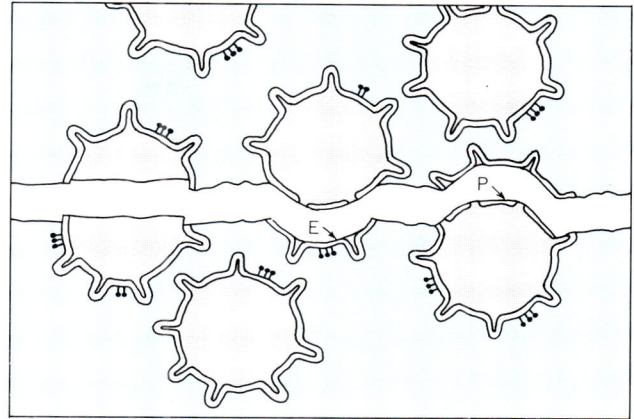

Fig. 1. Label-fracture schema

labelled cells were fixed with 1%-glutaraldehyde, suspended in buffer solution, frozen, fractured, shadowed with platinum evaporation and replicated with carbon evaporation (**2**)[68].

FINDINGS

The lipid membrane is seen as a plane and the intramembranous particles as convex dots. Desmosomes are recognized as macules of particles. The black dots, labelled colloidal gold, represent the desmosomal areas.

POTENTIAL

Protein A may be used with the colloidal gold-labelling method[66, 69]. The label-fracture method has potential for investigating the correlation of intramembranous antibodies and receptors of the intramembranous fine structures.

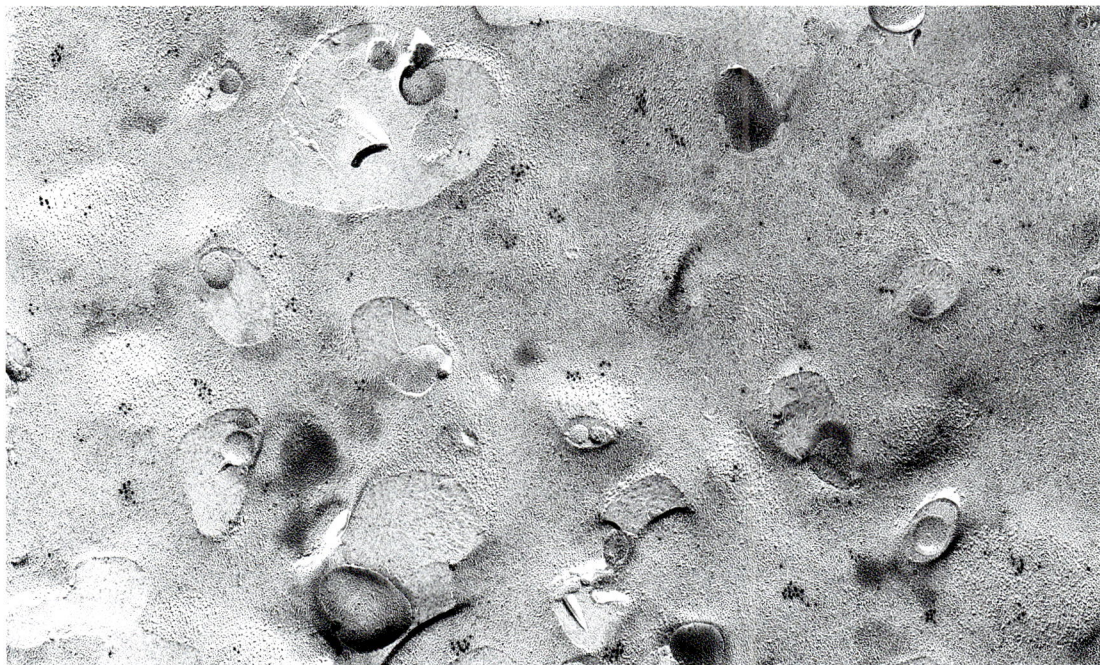

Fig. 2. Label-fracture image (× 10,000)

Scanning immunoelectron microscopy

The topographical three-dimensional distribution of specific molecules on the cell surface can be studied best by scanning immunoelectron microscopy[70,71]. In principle, the labelling methods are identical to those of immuno-fluorescent microscopy and transmission immunoelectron microscopy. The only significant difference resides in the choice of visual markers which must be recognizable by scanning electron microscopy (SEM).

SELECTION AND PREPARATION OF SEM MARKERS

As shown in Table I, synthetic polymers, macromolecular proteins and viruses have been used as visual markers for SEM. However, they vary in size, shape, surface property and stability and the most suitable marker for each experimental system must be selected. Methods of preparation of immunomarker conjugates may be roughly classified into the non-covalent absorption method (polystyrene latex, colloidal gold, etc.) and the covalent conjugation method using crosslinking reagents (synthetic polymer having functional groups, macromolecular protein, virus, etc.). Glutaraldehyde has been most commonly used as the bifunctional crosslinking reagent to couple amino groups of antibodies to amino groups of markers. As in other immuno-histochemical techniques, a direct and an indirect method are employed in labelling, and when using a relatively large marker such as T4 bacteriophage (T4), the indirect method has a higher labelling sensitivity and brings about better results[72]. Special labelling methods, such as the hapten-sandwich method or hybrid-antibody method are known, but they are not generally applied.

APPLICATIONS FOR DERMATOLOGY

In the field of dermatology, no reports on this technique could be found in our literature search, other than our papers[73,74,75]. An outline of our method using T4 is as follows. T4 and its host bacterium *E. coli* are grown in nutrient broth and the lysate is prepared by conventional methods. The purified T4 can be obtained only by differential centrifugation of the lysate. T4 (4–6 mg/ml) and the target antibody (IgG, 10–20 mg/ml) are mixed at a protein ratio of 2 to 1, and 0.5% glutaraldehyde is added for a final concentration of 0.05%. After one hour of conjugation, glycine is added to render inactive the remaining aldehyde groups and the T4-IgG conjugate is collected by differential centrifugation. The resulting T4-IgG can be stored for at least six months at 4°C or twelve months at −70°C. As a general rule, cells are prefixed with 1% glutaraldehyde at 4°C for ten minutes and treated with glycine. Then the cells are labelled with T4-IgG using the indirect method. Regarding the labelling of cell suspensions, the cells are first adhered to the coverslip coated with poly-L-lysine and then brought into the reaction.

In conclusion, a marker of about 100 nm, such as T4, is the most suitable for the analysis of wide surface areas and simultaneous observation of many cells, as well as for tissue analysis[76]. The characteristic shape of T4, consisting of a hexagonal head and tail, makes it possible to survey the cell surface at relatively low magnification and to examine the site specificity at high magnification (**1, 2**).

SPECIAL FEATURES

● Commercial latex can be used

● Conjugation with antibody by using surface functional groups ($-NH_2$, $-OH$, or $-COOH$)

● Has functional amino group

● Conjugation with antibody by its surface negative charge, suitable for backscatter electron mode

● Various labelling methods can be used as in TEM

● Morphological features similar to TMV

● Common features of bacterial and plant viruses: easy purification in a large quantity, characteristic shape and uniformity

● Labelling by the difference in brightness

TABLE I VISUAL MARKERS FOR SEM

	MARKER	SHAPE	SIZE (nm)
Synthetic polymer	Polystyrene latex	spherical	200–1000
	Polymethacrylate latex	spherical	500–1000
	Carboxylated polystyrene sphere	spherical	220–325
	Copolymer microsphere	spherical	30–340
	Silica sphere	spherical	13.5–20
	Gold granule	spherical	5–150
Macromolecular protein	Ferritin	spherical	12–15
	Hemocyanin	spherical	35 × 50
	Pyosin R	rod-like	15 × 110
Virus	OX174	spherical	25–30
	Bacteriophage T4	hexagonal head and tail	85 × 115 / 19 × 95
	Bushy stunt virus	spherical	30
	Tobacco mosaic virus	rod-like	18 × 300
Others	Fluorescein	not uniform	–
	Peroxidase-diaminobenzidine	not uniform (or roughly (20–30) spherical)	–

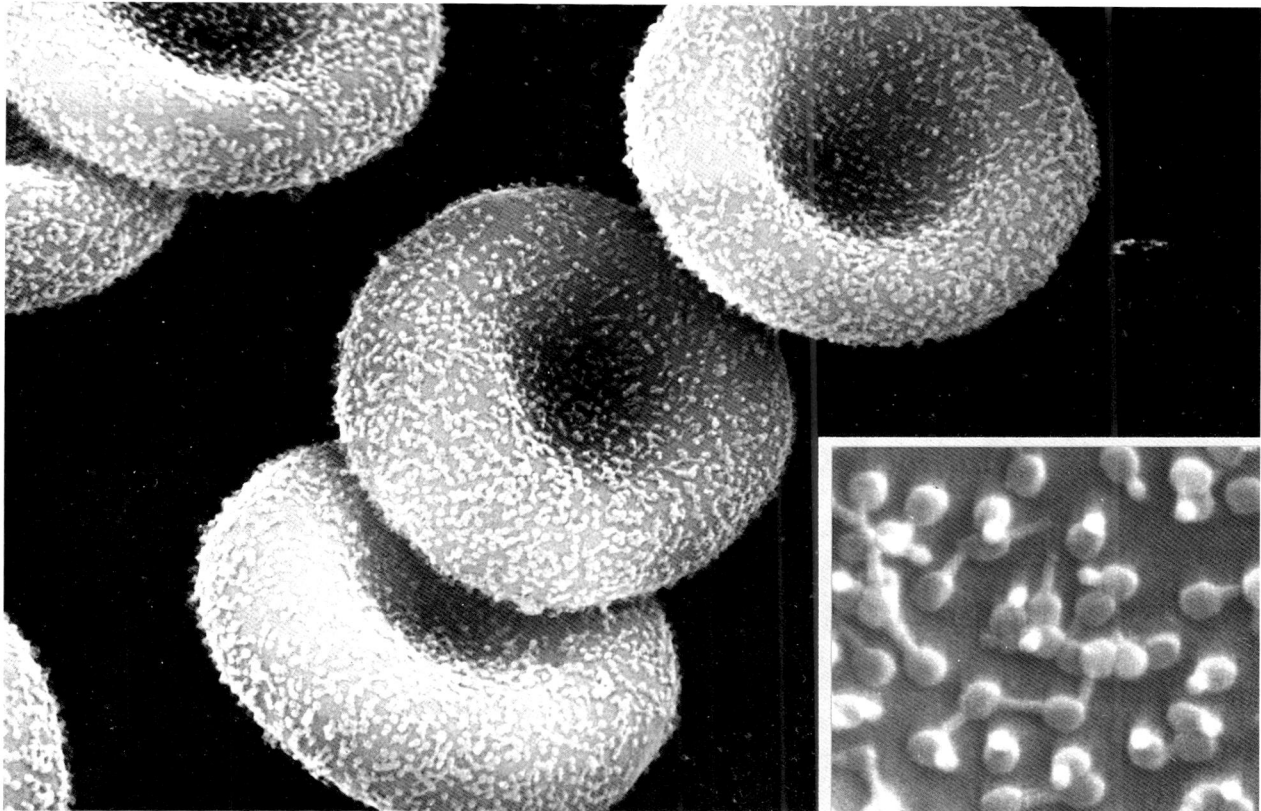

Fig. 1. Blood group A antigens on human RBC labelled with T4-IgG. T4-IgG is evenly distributed over the cell (× 10,000). The characteristic shape of each T4 can be clearly resolved at a high magnification. (× 60,000)

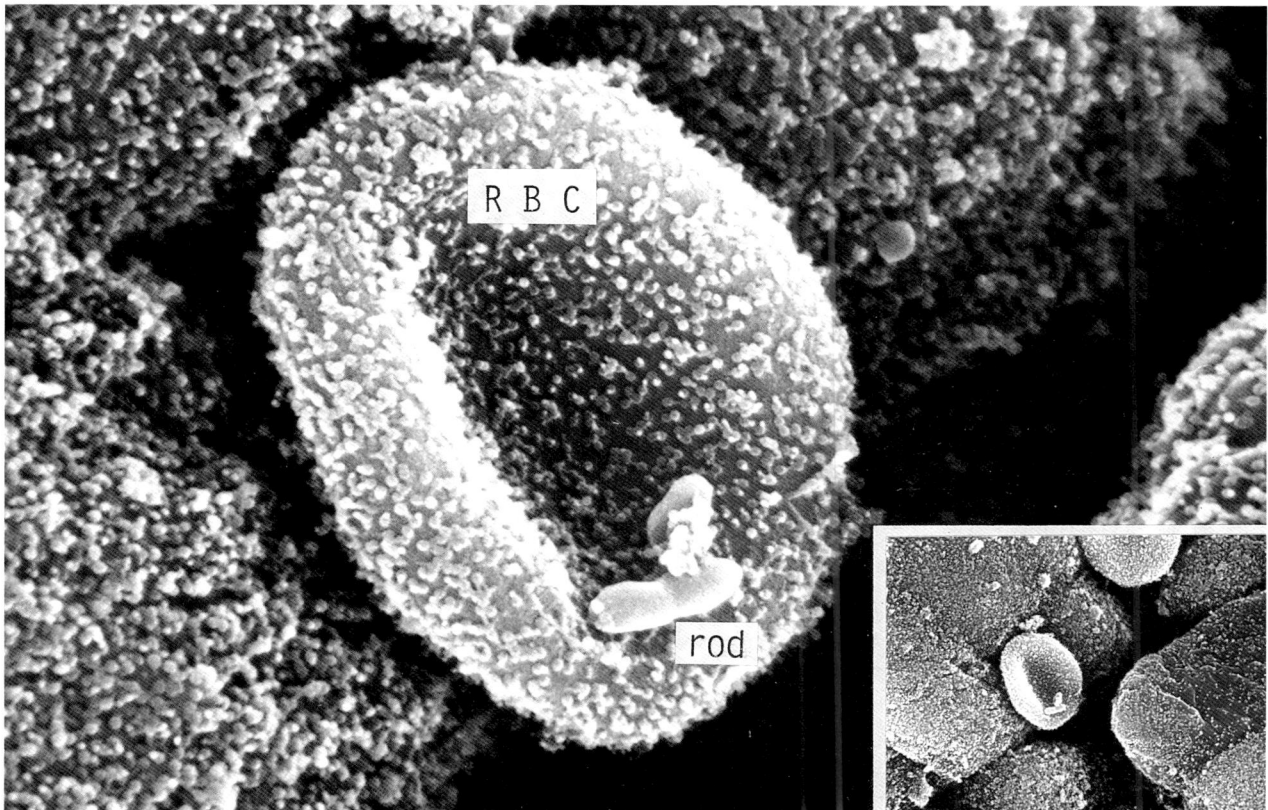

RBC

rod

Fig. 2. Blood group A antigens on human bladder epithelial cells labelled with T4-IgG. RBC and rods are seen in the same observation field due to the presence of infection. The antigens which are present on the RBC are also distributed densely on the epithelial cells. (× 14,000)

D Application of monoclonal antibodies

INTRODUCTION

The purpose of immunohistocytology is to identify various components or cells in the tissue, by use of antibodies as probes. There is no doubt that antibodies are required to attain high specificity. In this context, monoclonal antibodies (MoAb), produced by hybridoma technology, are becoming an extremely potent tool in this field.

In this chapter, the characteristics of MoAb and suggestions for the application of MoAb to immunohistocytological study (particularly immuno enzymatic staining) are generally discussed.

Characteristics of MoAb

SPECIFICITY

MoAb is a kind of myeloma protein which is secreted from a clonal growth of hybridoma cells. Hybridoma is usually established in a murine system by fusing (1) a cultured murine myeloma cell and (2) a murine B lymphocyte which was pre-defined to make a specific antibody against a single antigenic determinant[77]. Therefore, MoAb can be considered as a 'pure reagent,' having homogeneity, purity and specificity. Furthermore, the same MoAb can be supplied in unlimited quantities and continuously, in theory, by cultivating the hybridoma cell line. This capacity to reproduce specificity and the fact that there is no need for the time-consuming absorption procedure to render specificity are the advantages of MoAb over conventional (polyclonal) hetero antisera.

The characteristics of MoAb when applied to immuno-histocytology are summarized in Table I. In general, MoAb have a high affinity due to their homogeneity, and also high specificity from the reactivity to a single antigenic determinant. However, an intensification procedure is sometimes necessary, in case the antigenic determinant is expressed in very small quantities in the tissue. Since conventional antisera are a mixture of antibodies against various antigenic determinants on the immunizing molecule, there are instances where conventional antisera are superior to MoAb. Another

drawback in the application of MoAb to immunohistocytology is that their reactivity is easily lost in formalin-fixed-paraffin-embedded specimens. This is due to the precise binding between MoAb and antigen molecules via the antigen binding site on MoAb and the three-dimensional structure of the antigenic determinant. If this structure is altered or denatured during fixation or tissue processing, MoAb can no longer recognize the antigen. Therefore, cryostat sections are usually recommended for MoAb. Whereas, in the case of conventional antisera, reactivity is preserved if they contain antibody against an antigenic determinant which is resistant to those procedures.

CROSS REACTION

As mentioned above, MoAb bind to the uniquely structured antigenic determinant. However, they may even bind to non-antigenic molecules if the molecules share the same antigenic determinant as the immunizing molecule. And this type of cross reactivity can not be removed by absorption. An example of such cross reactivity has been reported[78]. In other words, even though MoAb have defined specificities for each antigenic determinant, they may not be molecule-specific, or cell-specific. If these MoAb drawbacks are not recognized, it is possible to misinterpret the results of the immunohistocytological study. It should be noted that later introduction of MoAb does not reduce the value of appropriately absorbed, conventional hetero antisera of proved specificities.

OTHER CHARACTERISTICS

It should also be stressed that MoAb are somewhat peculiar immunoglobulin, which are produced by artificial cells (hybridoma). Therefore, they are known to behave in unexpected ways in some immune reactions (i.e. MoAb of the IgG subclass, but which are not reactive with anti-IgG or protein A). For this reason, it is essential to pay attention to the matching of MoAb and second antibodies.

TABLE I   PROPERTIES OF MoAb AND CONVENTIONAL ANTISERA

	MoAbs	CONVENTIONAL ANTISERA
composition:	monoclonal immunoglobulin	mixture of polyclonal immunoglobulins
bind to:	one antigenic determinant of one immunizing molecule	several antigenic determinants of immunizing molecule
reproducibility:	no scatter	vary between batches
tissue processing:	usually not available on formalin-fixed, paraffin-embedded sections. Cryostat sections recommended	usually available on formalin-fixed, paraffin-embedded sections
cross reaction:	usually absent, but complete if antigenic determinant is common	usually present; appropriate absorption procedure is required
physical properties of immunoglobulin:	sometimes peculiar; may not work in conventional immunological procedures	typical

18

TABLE II   SPECIFICITIES OF 5 MoAb RAISED AGAINST MALIGNANT TRICHILEMMOMA

MoAb	3D6	5C6	2B6	4B2	4A5
trichilemmoma	+	+	+	+	+
keratinocytes	+ (horny layer)	+ (granular layer)	+ (prickled cell layer)	+ (granular layer)	+ (basal layer)
fibroblasts	−	−	−	−	−
dermal components	+ (arrector pili muscle)	−	−	+ (elastic fibre?)	−
hair follicle	+ (hair, internal root sheath)	+ (internal root sheath)	+ (external root sheath)	−	+ (basal layer)
sweat glands	−	+ (myoepi- thelium)	+	−	+ (basal layer)

TABLE III   TECHNICAL SUGGESTIONS FOR IMMUNOHISTOLOGICAL STAINING USING MoAb

1. Start with cryostat sections from specimens which were embedded in OCT compound, frozen in liquid nitrogen immediately after surgery or biopsy and kept frozen at −80°C. Cryostat sections can be preserved for several weeks if they are snap fixed in acetone and kept at −80°C.

2. Control sera (positive and negative) are essential. MoAb with proven reactivity to any component in the tissue serve as the positive control (we usually use anti-HLA MoAb on human specimens) and pre-immune mouse sera or culture supernatant of parental myeloma cell line serve as the negative control.

3. Avoid section drying at all stages of immunohistocytological staining.

4. Care should be taken when matching the MoAb and the second antibody, especially if the MoAb is unfamiliar.

5. When blocking the endogeneous peroxidase activity, be careful not to lose antigenicity. When blocking is not essential, positive peroxidase activity in infiltrating mono-histiocytic cells determines whether the substrate solution is appropriate or not.

Application of MoAb

The details of various immunohistocytological methods can be found in the several good reviews already published[79, 80]. Essentially, there is no fundamental difference between the methodology employed with hetero antisera and that with MoAbs. From our experience, simple indirect staining (indirect immunofluorescence staining or indirect immuno-enzyme staining) gives good results, and positive findings can never be overlooked. However, when immunohisto-cytological staining is done routinely using commercially available MoAb, the avidin-biotin (ABC) method or PAP method will become the choice to reduce the cost of expensive MoAb. Intensification techniques are also required when the antigen is known to be present in small quantities in the tissue.

Figures 1–4 depict examples of indirect immunoenzyme staining of normal skin using MoAb which were raised in our laboratory against human malignant trichilemmoma cell line. The MoAb react with various components of normal skin and the specificities are shown in Table II[81].

Recently, several 'staining kits' have been made commercially available with MoAb against lymphocyte subsets and others. 'Universal kits,' which come with all the reagents necessary except the first MoAb, are now available. These kits also give satisfactory results. Figures 5–8 show examples of immunoenzyme staining lymphocyte subsets.

An example of clinical application, a case (Japanese male) with an ulcerated forearm tumour, is shown in figures 9–13.

Immunohistocytological studies were performed to characterize the nature of the tumour cells. The tumour cells were positive to anti-LCA (leucocyte common antigen) but negative to anti-EMA (epithelial membrane antigen). OKT antibodies were applied to elucidate further the lineage of the tumour cells. The final diagnosis of cutaneous T cell lymphoma (non-epidermotrophic type) was made upon revealing the helper/inducer T cell phenotype of the tumour cells.

Finally, practical suggestions for immunohistocytological staining using MoAb are summarized in Table III.

The potential of MoAb in immunohistocytology

In the area of immunohistocytology, MoAb which are scientifically significant (i.e. MoAb against functional molecules of the cells or MoAb against oncogene products) will be selected among the flood of newly-developed MoAb. On a practical level, MoAb which can be used on formalin-fixed paraffin-embedded sections, which would enable retrospective immunohistocytological studies of the vast number of specimens from the past, are anticipated.

In the field of autoimmune diseases or tumour immunology, human MoAb from human-human hybridoma which reflect the recognition pattern of the human immune system will be more valuable to analysis of the immune response *in vivo*, than mouse MoAb which are based on the murine immune system.

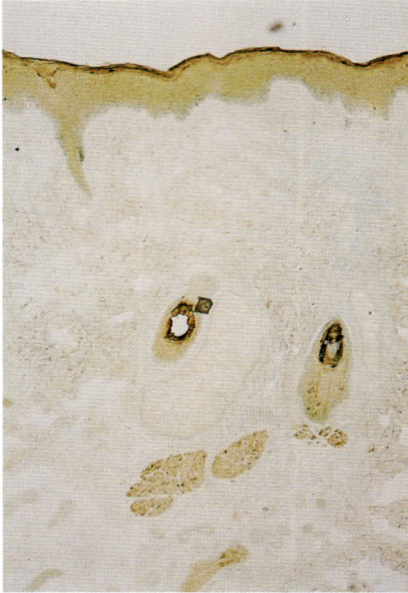

Fig. 1. MoAb 3D6 reacts with horny layer, hair, internal root sheath and arrector pili muscle. (× 20)

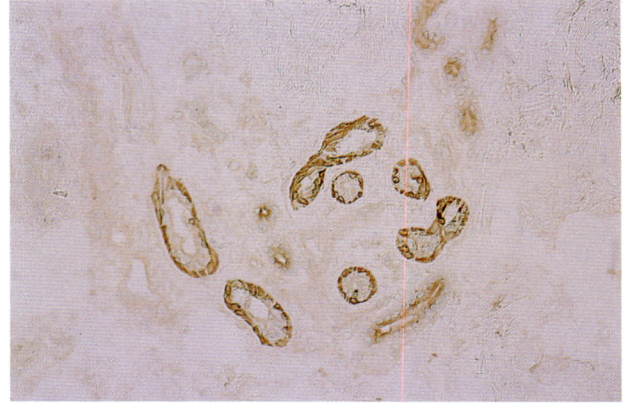

Fig. 2. MoAb 5C6 reacts with myoepithelium of eccrine glands. (× 100)

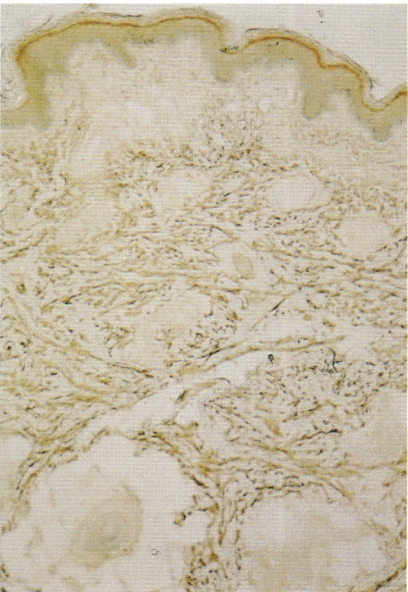

Fig. 3. MoAb 4B5 reacts with dermal fibrus components (presumably elastic fibre). (× 20)

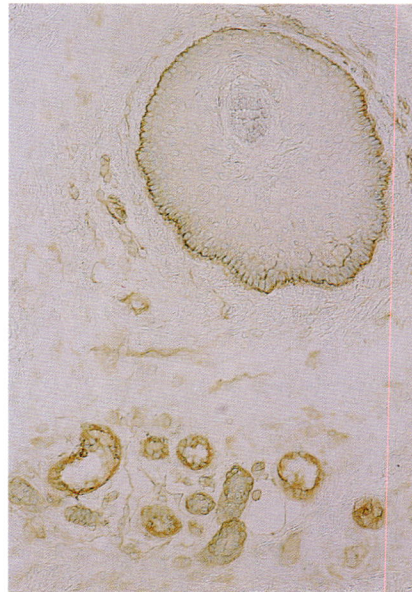

Fig. 4. MoAb 4A5 reacts with basal layer of hair follicles and eccrine glands. (× 100)

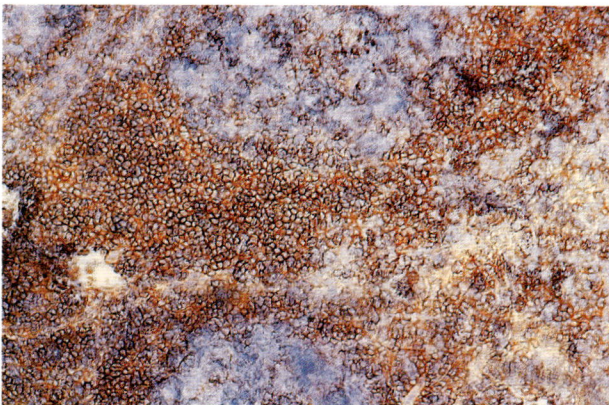

Fig. 5. OKT4 on human tonsil. Majority of perifollicular lymphocytes are positively stained. (× 100)

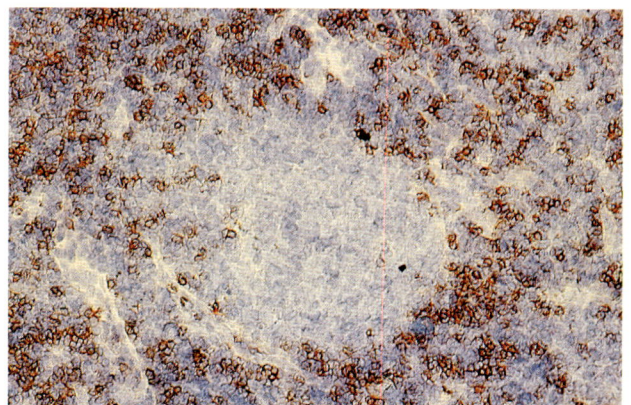

Fig. 6. OKT8 on human tonsil. Some of the perifollicular lymphocytes are positively stained. (× 100)

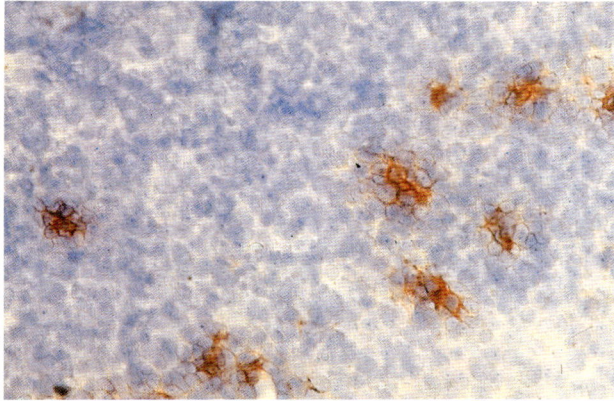

Fig. 7. Interdigitating reticulum cells of tonsilar T cell zone are stained by OKT6. (× 200)

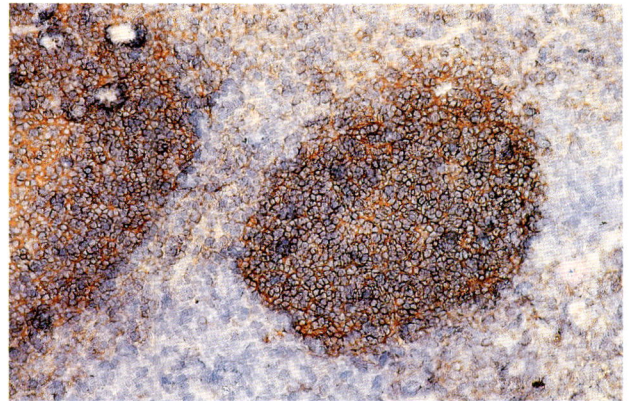

Fig. 8. OKT7 (anti-pan B MoAb) strongly reacts with follicular B-lymphocytes. (× 200)

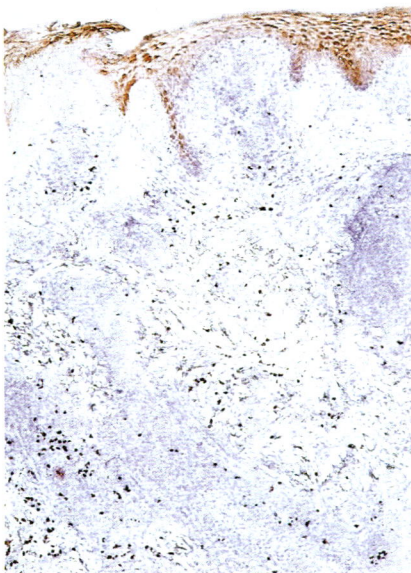

Fig. 9. A case of cutaneous T cell lymphoma. Tumour cells in the dermis do not react with anti-EMA (epithelial membrane antigen). (× 20)

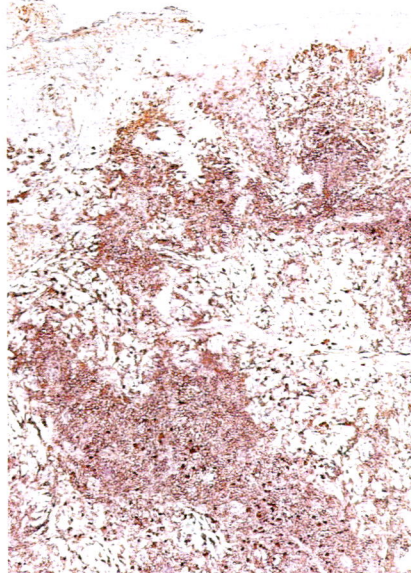

Fig. 10. Tumour cells and infiltrating cells are positive to anti-LCA (leucocyte common antigen). (× 40)

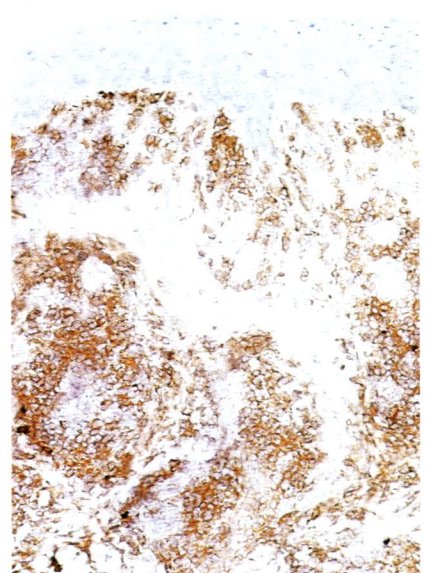

Fig. 11. Tumour cells are OKT11(+), revealing T lymphocyte phenotype. The cells do not invade the epidermis. (× 100)

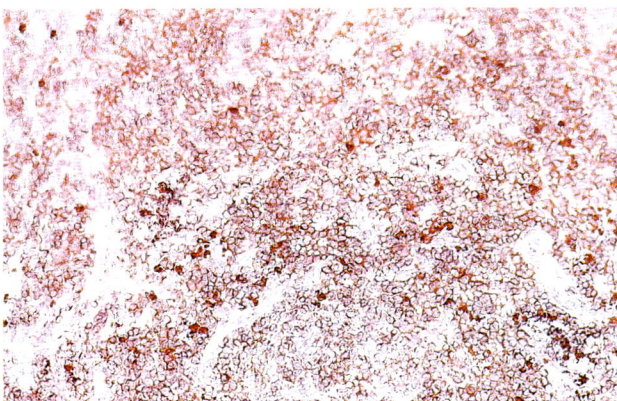

Fig. 12. OKT4. Most of the tumour cells are also OKT4(+). (× 100)

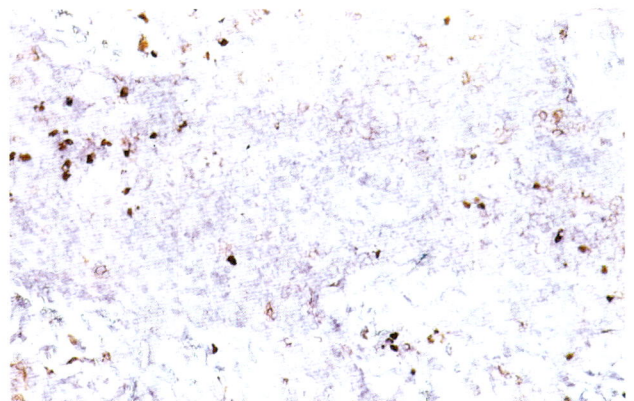

Fig. 13. OKT8. Tumour cells are OKT8(−). Scattered positive cells are mono-histiocytic cells with endogenous peroxidase activity. (× 100)

21

CELLULAR AND EXTRACELLULAR COMPONENTS IN NORMAL SKIN

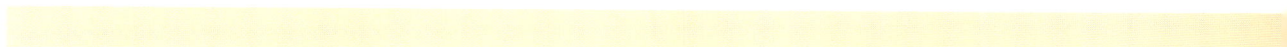

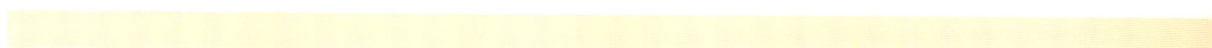

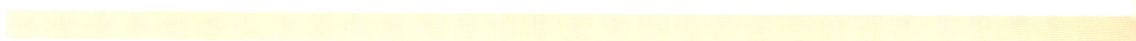

Keratinocytes

1.1 Cytoskeleton

INTRODUCTION

Cytoskeletons are protein filaments forming networks in the cytoplasm. Three classes of ultrastructurally and chemically distinct fibrillar structures have been recognized in the cytoplasm of eukaryotic cells: microfilaments of 6-nm diameter, biochemically composed mainly of actin with a molecular weight of $42–43 \times 10^3$ daltons (d); microtubules, composed of A-tubulin with a molecular weight of 56×10^3 d; and B-tubulin with a molecular weight of 42×10^3d. Intermediate filaments (IFs) can be divided into five major classes by means of their cell type specificity and subunit structures[82]. These classes are keratin IFs found in epithelial cells, desmin IFs in muscle cells, vimentin IFs in mesenchymal cells, glial filaments in glial cells, and neurofilaments in neurons. Cytoskeletons of keratinocytes, since they are epithelial cells, consist of microfilaments, microtubules and keratin IFs.

IMPORTANT FINDINGS

Normal cultured keratinocytes. Fine cytoskeleton network cannot be visualized in sections of epidermal tissues because the sections are too thick. Therefore, cells grown on glass coverslips are usually used for the observation of cytoskeletal networks.

Microfilaments do not usually form stress fibres in keratinocytes. By immunofluorescence microscopy, individual filaments or their bundles cannot be recognized, but fluorescence of microfilaments appears homogeneous in the cytoplasm, and brighter in the centre of the cell and at the cell periphery than in other intracellular spaces[83] (**1a**).

Microtubules (**2a**) form juxtanuclear dense networks and radiating filament bundles from the central networks. The ends of these radiating filaments are not bound to the adjacent cells, while keratin IFs appear to be connected to those of adjacent cells (**1b, 2b**)[84, 85]. Keratin IFs also compose central dense networks and radiating bundles of filaments.

Desmosomes can be recognized as black, unstained spots at the end of the radiating bundles of keratin IFs, to which those of the next cells are bound. These keratin bundles, connected with desmosomes of two adjacent cells, appear to have a common tension of fibres. These cytoskeletons show a dynamic rearrangement during mitosis[85].

Normal skin. Epidermal cells are well stained with anti-actin, anti-tubulin and anti-keratin by the immunofluorescence method. Since there is nothing in particular to describe regarding the results of anti-actin and anti-tubulin in epidermis, the observations of keratin IF staining will mainly be described here. The keratin filaments represent the most complicated class of IFs, consisting of many polypeptides with molecular weights ranging from 40×10^3d to 68×10^3d and with isoelectric values between ph 5 and 8. They are divided into nineteen subunits, each of which is called keratin. Keratin IFs in the epidermis are mainly composed of four of these nineteen keratins. They are two acidic keratins – Type I keratins (with molecular weights of 56.5×10^3d and 50×10^3d); and two neutral-basic keratins – Type II keratins (with molecular weights of $65–68 \times 10^3$d and 50×10^3d). Sun *et al.* have developed specific monoclonal antibodies: AE_1 against Type I, AE_3 against Type II and AE_2 against both types of keratins expressed only in suprabasal cells[85, 86]. The specific reactivity of these antibodies is confirmed by immunoblotting. AE_1 reacts immunohistologically with basal cells of epidermis. AE_2 and polyclonal antibodies against 67×10^3 d-keratins react with suprabasal cells[87]. From the results of their studies using these monoclonal antibodies, it has been shown that 56.5×10^3 d-(Type I)/$65–68 \times 10^3$ keratins (Type II) are markers for keratinization; 48×10^3 d-(Type I) $\times 56 \times 10^3$ d-keratins (Type II) are markers for proliferation/non-differentiation; and 50×10^3 d-(Type I)/58×10^3 d-keratins (Type II) are permanent markers for keratinocytes[86]

Diseased skin. Although there have been no reports on abnormal organization of cytoskeletons in diseased epidermal cells, the abnormal expressions of subunit keratins have been studied in several skin diseases (Weiss[88]).

SIGNIFICANCE FOR DERMATOLOGY

Since a large number of monoclonal antibodies to keratins have been developed recently, they can be utilized for diagnosis and experimental studies as markers of keratinocyte differentiation and non-differentiation[89]. The non-immunofluorescence observation of keratin IF organization can be employed for the study of the mechanism of cell-to-cell detachment, since the retraction of keratin IFs sensitively reflects the loss of desmosomal contacts (**3**)[90]

TECHNICAL POINTS

In order to obtain good resolution of immunofluorescence micrographs, cells must be grown on glass coverslips and fixed with $-20°C$ methanol (for 7–10 minutes), followed by treatment with 0.5% Triton X-100. The cells on the glass coverslips must then be subjected to immunological staining procedures.

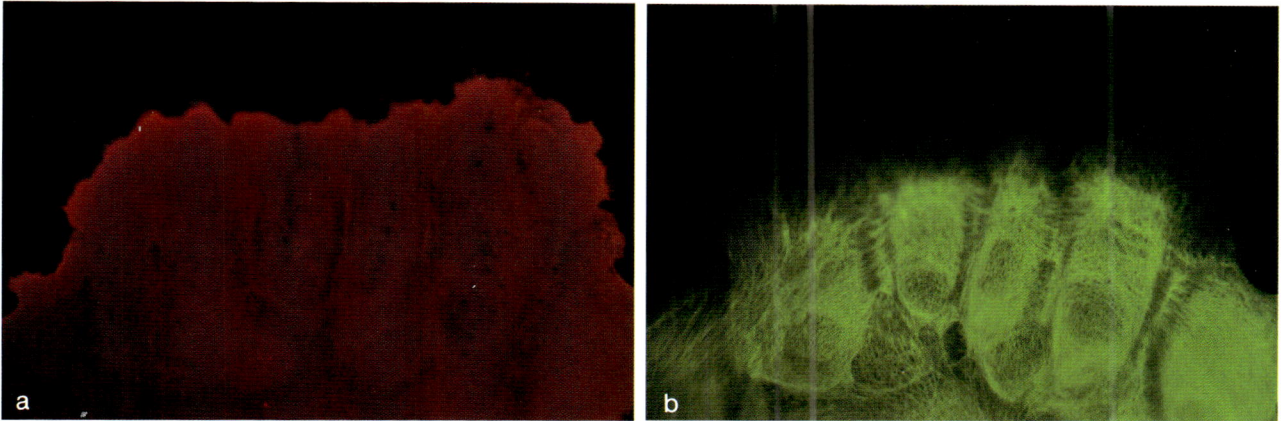

Fig. 1. Cultured human keratinocytes simultaneously stained with anti-actin (rhodamine, a) and anti-keratin (FITC, b).

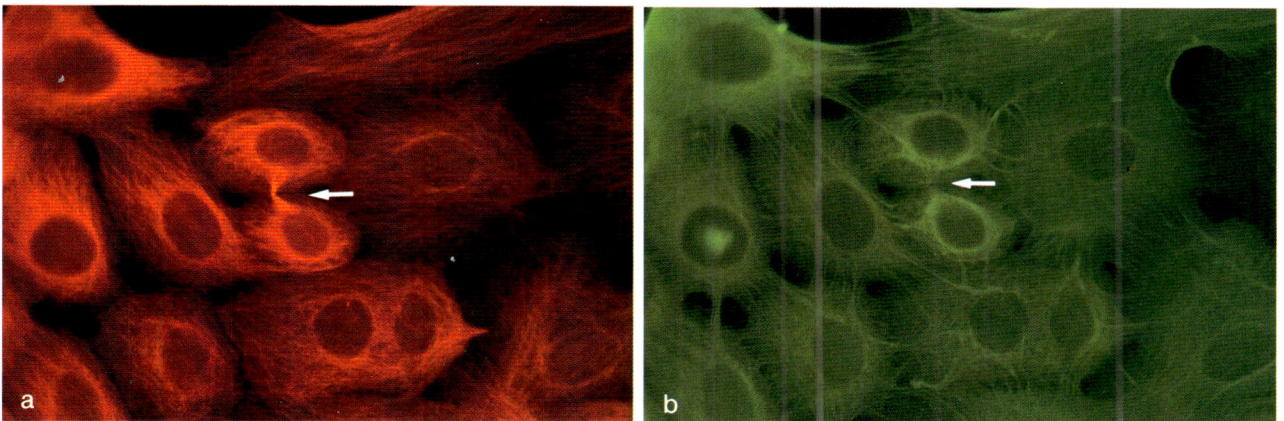

Fig. 2. Cultured human keratinocytes simultaneously stained with anti-tubulin (rhodamine, a) and anti-keratin (FITC, b). The cells in the centre are in mitotic phase (telophase) and are still connected to the bundles of microtubules (midbody). Bundles of keratin IFs are connected to those of the adjacent cells. The microtubules are independent of those of the adjacent cell in interphase.

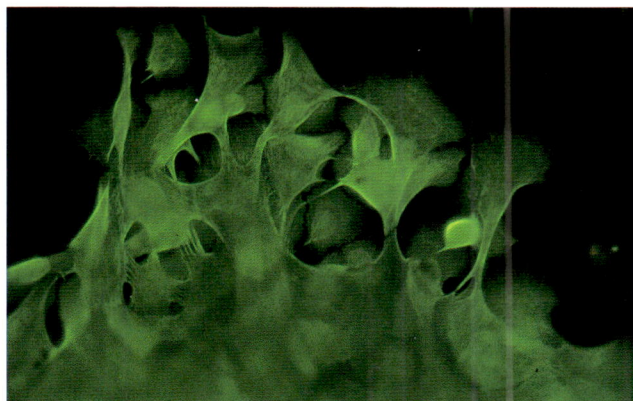

Fig. 3. Loss of cell-to-cell contact induced by the addition of pemphigus serum. The retraction of keratin IFs from cell periphery indicates the loss of cell contacts.

1.2 Hair keratin

ORIGIN AND CHARACTERISTICS

Hair keratin is composed of fibrous proteins (FP) and matrix proteins (MP). Using urea and 2-mercaptoethanol, FP and MP are extracted from hair as low and high sulphur fractions, respectively. During the extraction, alkylation of these proteins is necessary; hair FP are obtained as S-carboxymethyl keratin[91]. Hair FP are different from epidermal FP, as alkylation is not necessary for epidermal FP extraction. It is considered that hair FP form tonofilaments or keratin filaments which are one of the main structures in the cells of the hair shaft. Hair FP have been analysed by one- and two-dimensional gel electrophoresis and separated into several polypeptide bands or spots; by such electrophoreses, it is known that hair FP are different in molecular composition from epidermal and nail[92,93]. An immunological survey using anti-keratin polyclonal antibodies has suggested that there is no immunological cross-reactivity between hair and epidermal FP[92]. However, this concept should be modified, as anti-hair keratin monoclonal antibodies which have recently been produced against human hair FP and designated as HKN-2, -4, -5, -6 and 7, display various patterns of immunohistochemical reactivity with human tissues[94,95]. By immunoblot analysis, HKN-2, and HKN-4 positively react with some of the electrophoretic bands of either hair or epidermal FP, whereas HKN-5, -6 and -7 stain only hair FP bands[94,95].

IMMUNOHISTOCHEMICAL FINDINGS IN NORMAL HUMAN TISSUES

Immunohistochemically, HKN-5, -6 and -7 are specific for hair; HKN-6 and HKN-7 positively react only with cells in the hair medulla, cortex, cuticle and inner root sheath layers in the keratogenous zone (1)[94]. HKN-5 further stains the innermost cell (IMC) layer of the outer root sheath (ORS) (2)[95]. The IMC layer ultrastructurally shows a unique cell differentiation which differs from that of other cells of the ORS[96]. On the other hand, there is HKN-2, other ORS cells, epidermis (3a), sebaceous glands and sweat glands including myoepithelial cells on these hair layers, although the basal cells of the ORS and epidermis (3a) and the secretory cells of the sweat glands show no positivity to HKN-2. The reaction sites of these monoclonal antibodies are limited to areas within skin epithelial tissues, whereas HKN-4 reacts with cells in all skin epithelial tissues including whole epidermal layers (3b), hepatocytes and bile duct cells in the liver, epithelial cells of convoluted segments and parietal cells of Bowman's capsule in the kidney, and intestinal epithelial cells. HKN-4 is thought to recognize one of the antigenic determinants in FP molecules commonly present in the epithelial cells in various human organs. None of these monoclonal antibodies reacts with cells in neural, muscular, or vascular tissues or other mesenchymal components.

SIGNIFICANCE FOR DERMATOLOGY

These anti-hair keratin monoclonal antibodies seem to be very useful for the investigation of cell differentiation in normal human hair layers as described above, or to study the hair cycle in animals, since they also react with animal epithelial cells (unpublished data). Monoclonal antibodies specific for one or some parts of each cutaneous appendage, such as the present anti-hair keratin monoclonal antibodies, HKN-5, -6 and -7, will be beneficial to obtain more precise information of appendage differentiation of various skin epithelial tumours and to study the biological behaviour of various types of skin epithelial cells both *in vivo* and *in vitro*.

POINTS FOR STAINING

For both the immunofluorescence and immunoperoxidase method, unfixed, frozen tissues are necessary; any fixation reduces the intensity of positive reactions of the anti-hair keratin monoclonal antibodies. One cannot deny that there are false-negative reactions, if a fixed tissue is used. There is only a minimum reduction in intensity when tissues are fixed in alcohol.

All monoclonal antibodies, HKN-2, -4, -5, -6 and -7, are in the subclass of mouse IgG_1.

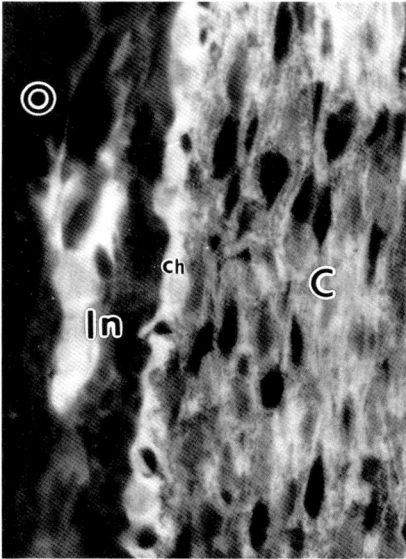

Fig. 1. Immunohistochemical findings of hair keratogenous zone stained with HKN-6. C, hair cortex; ch, hair cuticle; In, inner root sheath; O, outer root sheath. (× 220)

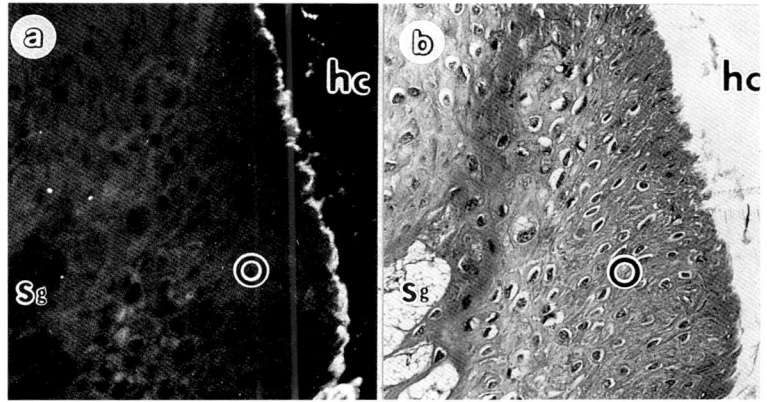

Fig. 2. a, Immunohistochemical findings of follicular epithelium stained with HKN-5. b, The same section stained with haematoxylin and eosin. Note the linear immunofluorescence on the surface of the outer root sheath (O) undergoing trichilemmal keratinization toward the hair canal (hc). Sg, sebaceous gland. (× 220)

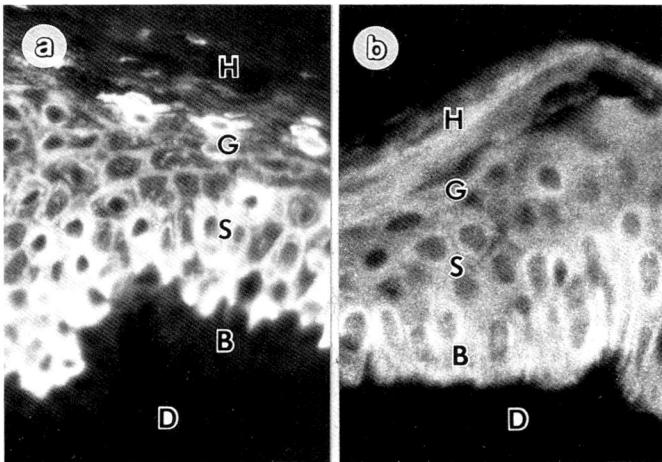

Fig. 3. Immunohistochemical findings of epidermis, a, HKN-2 staining. b, HKN-4 staining. B, basal layer; D, dermis; G, granular layer; H, horny layer; S, spinous layer. (× 300)

1.3 Desmosome

ORIGIN AND CHARACTERISTICS OF ANTI-DESMOSOME ANTIBODY

Desmosome, one of the intercellular junction structures, is widely distributed between epithelial cells and myocardial cells. Desmosomes are well developed, especially in the epidermis, and by light microscopy their location as intercellular bridges can be seen mainly in the spinous layer. The cell membranes of two adjacent cells run closely parallel to each other and if, by transmission electron microscopy, a desmosome is cut through a plane vertical to the cell membrane, a highly electron-dense linear structure, the intercellular contact layer, is seen between the two cell membranes. A highly electron-dense plaque, the attachment plaque, adheres to the inner surface of each cell membrane and a large number of tonofilaments accumulate and attach to the plaque (1).

Freeze-fracture electron microscopy of the epidermis indicates that the desmosome area of the cell membrane is oval-shaped and 0.3 to 0.7 μm long. One or two desmosomes are distributed per two μm^2 area of the cell membrane. An increased number of intramembranous particles are present in the desmosome area[97]. When epidermal cells are cultured, the desmosome formation by the cells depends on the calcium concentration of the culture medium; as the concentration of calcium increases, more desmosomes appear between the cultured cells[98].

Desmosome components have been biochemically analyzed; desmoplakin I and II are desmosomal polypeptides extracted from bovine epidermis with a molecular weight of 250,000 and 215,000, respectively. Polyclonal antibodies react immunohistochemically with both the desmosomes and the hemidesmosomes of epithelial cells and myocardial cells in bovines, humans, chicken and rodents, and cytochemically with the attachment plaque areas[99]. On the other hand, two glycoproteins with molecular weights of 115,000 and 100,000 dalton called desmocollins, are reported to be located in the intercellular spaces of desmosomes, and to be involved in the adhesive function of desmosomes[100].

An anti-desmosome monoclonal antibody, HK-1, a mouse monoclonal antibody produced against low sulphur proteins extracted from human hair, specifically reacts with desmosomes in various epithelial cells and myocardial cells. By the electron microscopic immunoperoxidase method, HK-1 decorates attachment plaque areas of desmosomes; this monoclonal antibody seems to recognize an attachment plaque-related substance, which may be different from the desmoplakins described above, since HK-1 does not stain hemidesmosomes[101].

IMMUNOHISTOCHEMICAL FINDINGS WITH HK-1

Normal human skin. Immunohistochemically, HK-1 weakly stains the intercellular borders between the basal cells and strongly stains the membranous parts of the spinous layer of granular cells. The immunofluorescence appears dotted in the lower layers and linear in the upper layers (2a). The dermal-epidermal junction and the horny layer show no positivity to HK-1 (2a). The cell peripheries of the inner cells of sweat ducts are also strongly decorated by HK-1, while those of the duct outer cells (2b) and secretory cells of sweat glands show only weakly positive reactions to this antibody. In hair tissues, the cell peripheries of the outer root sheath cells clearly reveal a dotted immunofluorescence

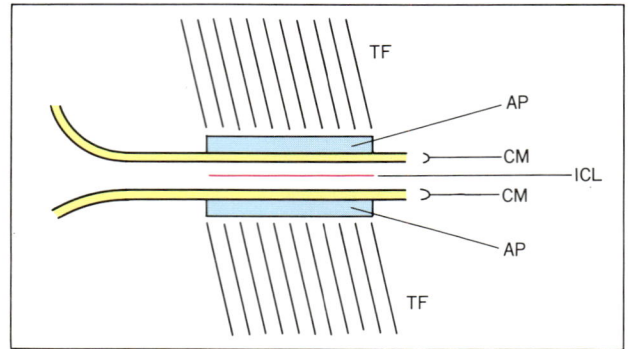

Fig. 1. Electron microscopic schema of desmosome. AP, attachment plaque; CM, cell membrane; ICL, intercellular contact layer; TF, tonofilaments.

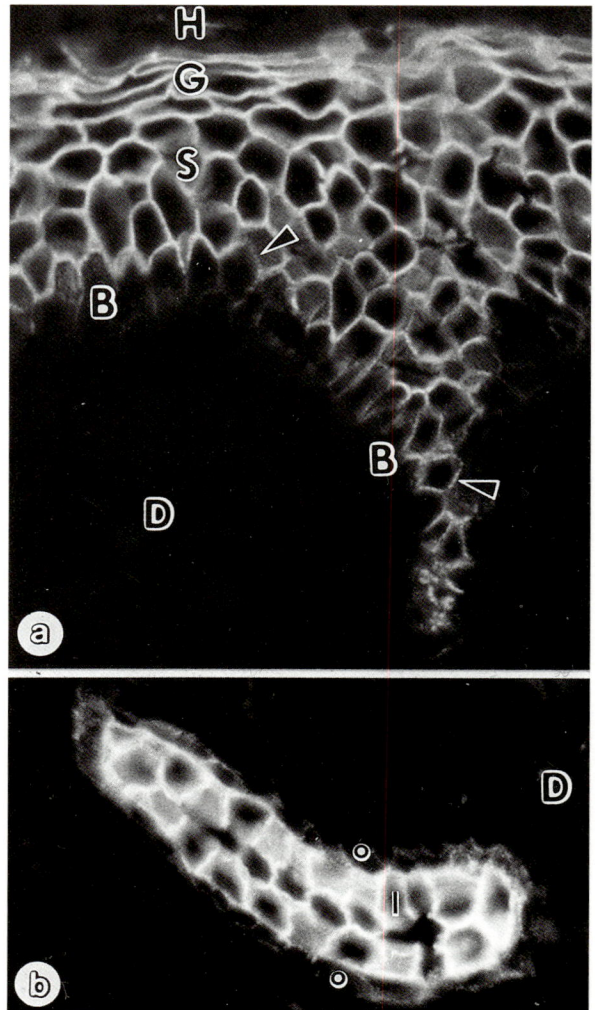

Fig. 2. Immunohistochemical findings by HK-1. a, Normal epidermis. b, normal eccrine duct. B, basal layer; D, dermis; G, granular layer; H, horny layer; I, inner cells; O, outer cells; S, spinous layer; asterisk, dotted immunofluorescence. (× 340)

with HK-1 (**3a**). Hair matrix (germinative) cells show almost no positive staining; however, as the hair cells differentiate upwards, the cell borders gradually become immunofluorescent. In the keratogenous zone, moderate linear immunofluorescence with HK-1 is observed at the cell peripheries of the hair cells and strong linear immunofluorescence at those of inner root sheath cells just before keratinization (**3b**). Keratinized hair cells show no reactivity with HK-1. In the sebaceous glands, peripheral (germinative) cells and differentiating cells show moderate and weak staining from HK-1, respectively. Mesenchymal tissues such as pilar muscles, nerves, vessels, fibroblasts, infiltrated cells and collagen and elastic fibres show no positive reaction with HK-1.

Pathologic skin. Although there have been a few immunohistochemical studies on skin disorders using anti-desmosome polyclonal or monoclonal antibodies, the findings in acantholytic skin diseases using HK-1 are of great interest. The acantholytic epidermal cells in pemphigus vulgaris show a dotted immunofluorescence at the cell periphery similar to that of normal epidermal cells; whereas in Darier's disease

and Hailey-Hailey's disease the cytoplasm of the acantholytic cells is diffusely stained by HK-1 (**4**). These findings indicate that there may be an abnormality in the intracellular distribution of attachment plaque-related substance of desmosomes in the latter diseases[102].

SIGNIFICANCE FOR DERMATOLOGY
Anti-desmosome monoclonal antibody, HK-1, seems very useful as a marker for epithelial cells, and for the investigation of skin tumours and cultured cells. Such antibodies against desmosome components will further make the progress in bio-chemical and immunohistochemical studies of desmosomes.

POINTS FOR STAINING
For either the immunofluorescence or immunoperoxidase method with HK-1, unfixed, frozen tissue materials are the most appropriate, as any fixative reduces the intensity of positive reactions.

HK-1 monoclonal antibody is in the subclass of mouse IgG_1.

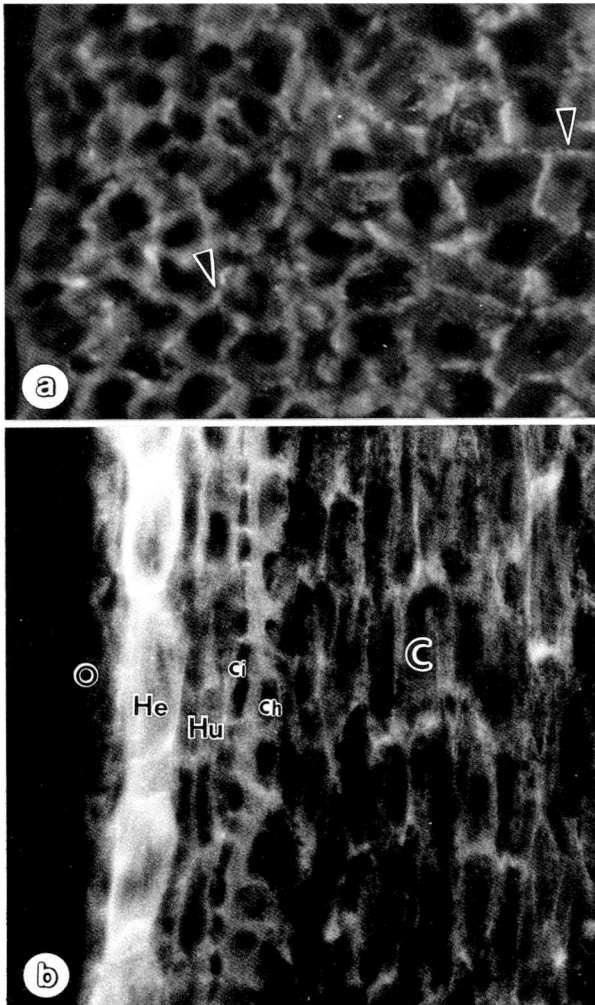

Fig. 3. Immunohistochemical findings by HK-1. a, follicular outer root sheath in isthmus portion. b, hair keratogenous zone. C, hair cortex; ch, hair cuticle; ci, cuticle of inner root sheath; He, Henle's layer; Hu, Huxley's layer; O, outer root sheath; arrowhead, dotted immunofluorescence. (× 340)

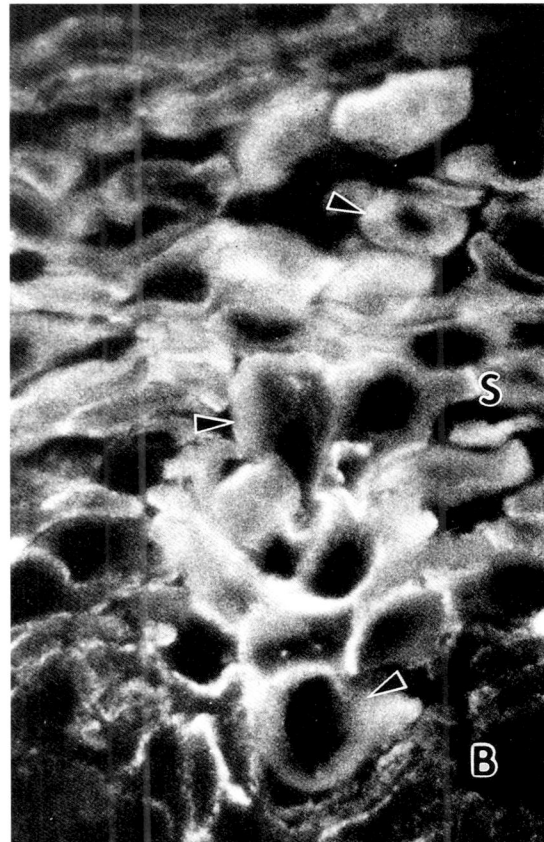

Fig. 4. HK-1 staining in Darier's disease. Note the diffuse immunofluorescence (arrowheads) in the cytoplasm of acantholytic cells in the spinous layer (S). B, basal layer. (× 520)

29

1.4 Lysozyme

THE BIOLOGICAL SIGNIFICANCE OF LYSOZYME AND ITS DISTRIBUTION IN SKIN

In 1922, Alexander Fleming discovered a human bacteriolytic substance by accident and six years later made his famous discovery of penicillin. Speculating that this substance might be an enzyme, he gave it the name of lysozyme. It is well known that numerous exogenous bactericidal substances (antibiotics) have been developed since the discovery of penicillin; on the other hand, biological studies on endogenous antibacterial substances such as lysozyme were not performed until the systematic studies on lysozyme distribution in humans made by Jollès and his colleagues in the 1960's. They found a high content of lysozyme in milk[103], tears[103], plasma[103] and leucocytes[104]. In 1971, Ogawa, *et al.* isolated, purified and crystallized human skin lysozyme[105]. This was the first purified enzyme protein from human skin. Regarding the biochemical and immunological characterization of this enzyme, there is species specificity but not organ specificity[106]. Furthermore, using FITC-conjugated anti-human milk lysozyme antibody, the localization in human skin was studied. Consequently, lysozyme was localized in epidermal cytoplasm, particularly in the granular layer (**1**)[107]. Lysozyme alone lysed two out of four straphylococcal species and 16 out of 22 streptococcal species from the human body. Coexistence with antibodies, complement and other enzymes proved lysis to all species. These results suggest that lysozyme plays an important role in the skin defence mechanism against infection.

BEHAVIOUR OF LYSOZYME IN SKIN DISEASES

Lysozyme activities are increased in sera of infectious diseases and in skin lesions of inflammatory diseases. As the lysozyme content is high in phagocytic cells such as in microphage and macrophage[108], the histochemical and cytochemical study of lysozyme is a valuable tool for the detection and identification of tumour cells in myelocytic or monocytic leukaemia (**2**). Futhermore, measurement of lysozyme activity in serum and urine facilitates the differentiation of leukaemias and determination of the disease activity or the therapeutic effect[109]. Since epitheloid cells of sarcoidosis have a high lysozyme content, lysozyme analysis in sarcoidosis can be diagnostically applied.

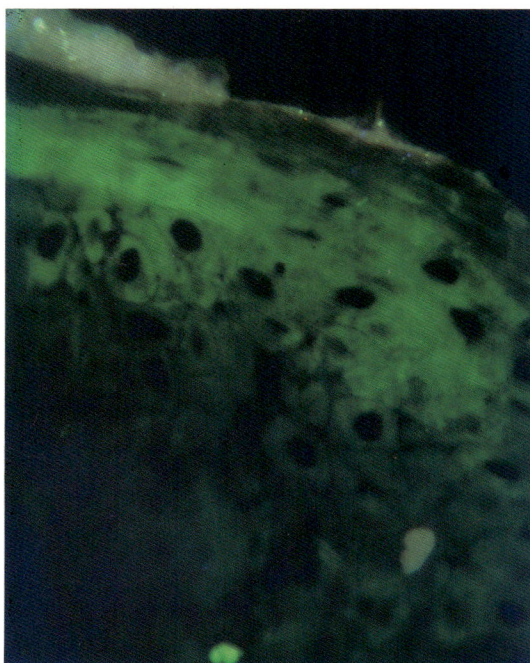

Fig. 1. Distribution of lysozyme in human epidermis.

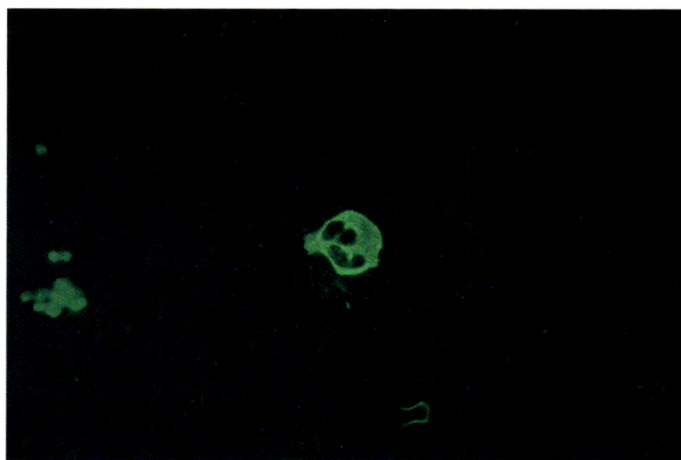

Fig. 2. Specific staining pattern of lysozyme in human polymorphonucleocytes.

1.5 Cyclic AMP

SOURCE AND PROPERTY

Cyclic adenosine 3′, 5′-monophosphate (cAMP) is an intracellular second messenger of various extrinsic signals. cAMP synthesis is carried out in a wide variety of cells via membrane-bound adenylate cyclase in the presence of a divalent cation (Mg^{++} or Mn^{++}) and ATP as the substrate. Since cAMP plays a pivotal role in multiple cell functions, such as cell proliferation and differentiation, as well as in various enzyme systems, it is of interest to know the cellular cAMP-localization in pathologic hyperproliferative conditions such as psoriasis, compared to normal epidermal keratinocytes.

Detection of cAMP localized in the epidermal keratinocytes was performed using the immunofluorescence technique as previously described[110], with an antibody against cAMP (Yamasa Shoyu Co., Tokyo). In addition to the immunofluorescence technique, the enzyme-labelled antibody technique was also performed using horseradish peroxidase-conjugated antiserum rather than FITC-conjugated antiserum. It has been reported by several investigators[111, 112] that this method gives more precise cAMP histotopography in various tissues or cells.

Normal epidermis. In normal epidermis, the major portion of cAMP deposition was cytoplasmic in most epidermal keratinocytes. In the upper epidermis, including the granular cell layer, positive findings were also observed within the nuclei in addition to the cytoplasm (**1**).

cAMP was detected in the cytoplasm and plasma membrane of the entire prickle cell layer showing a fine granular pattern, and also in nuclei of the granular cell layer as coarse granular deposits (**2**).

Epidermis in hyperproliferative condition. In the psoriatic epidermis, the localization of cAMP was essentially the same as that of normal epidermis. Intranuclear deposits of cAMP were more striking in the granular cell layer and the neighbouring prickle cell layer of the psoriatic epidermis than in that of normal epidermis (**3**). The cAMP content was similar in the psoriatic epidermis and the normal epidermis, as had been previously suggested[113].

SIGNIFICANCE FOR THE DERMATOLOGICAL FIELD

The epidermis contains at least four independent receptor adenylate cyclase systems (adrenergic, prostaglandin E, adenosine and histamine). The decreased adrenergic and protaglandin E response in hyperproliferative psoriatic epidermis has been well documented. The significance of the altered intracellular distribution pattern of cAMP in terms of keratinocyte proliferation or differentiation remains unknown.

As the cAMP content of cells and tissues easily fluctuates due to the ischaemic effect[114], skin samples must be frozen immediately with liquid N_2, mounted on ice, and then stored until use at $-80°C$. Pre-treatment of the biopsy sites with liquid N_2 is recommended whenever possible. If skin samples are taken with local anaesthesia, the use of epinephrine must be avoided.

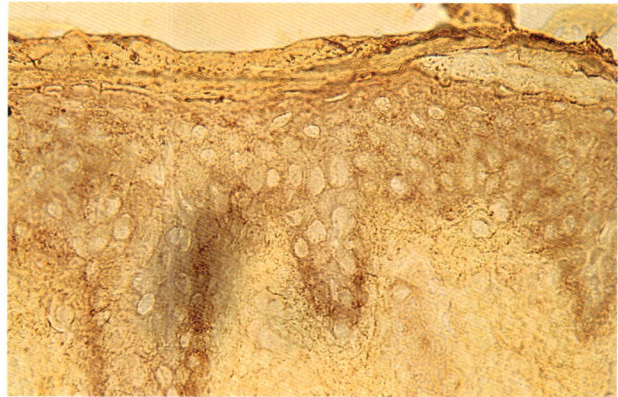

Fig. 2. The immunoperoxidase technique used to study the localization of cAMP in normal epidermis. Cyclic cAMP is detected in the cytoplasm and plasma membrane of the entire prickle cell layer showing a fine granular pattern, and also in nuclei of the granular cell layer as coarse granular deposits. ($\times$ 400)

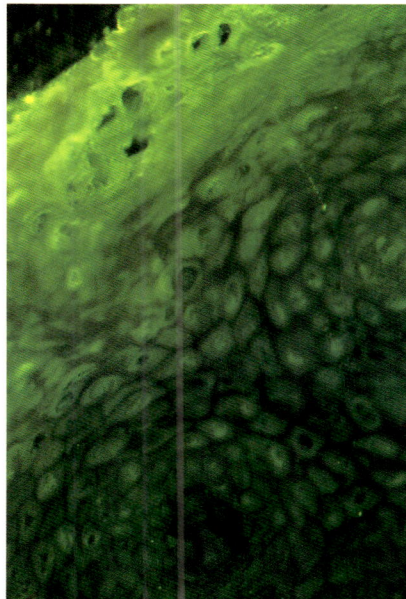

Fig. 1. Immunofluorescence technique applied to the study of the localization of cAMP in normal epidermis. The cAMP deposit is observed predominantly in the cytoplasm and plasma membrane of almost all epidermal keratinocytes, and also within the nuclei in the upper portion of the epidermis. ($\times$ 200)

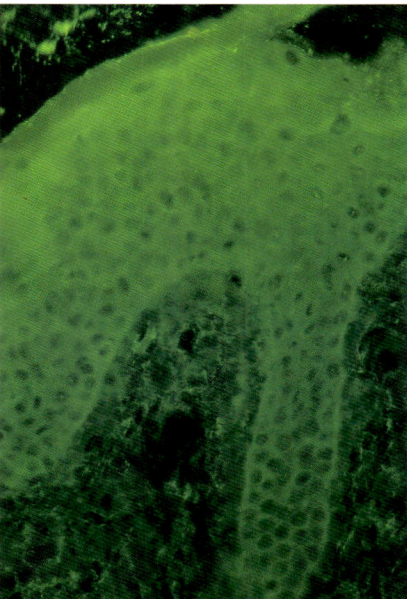

Fig. 3. The immunofluorescence technique used to determine the localization of cAMP in psoriatic epidermis. Intranuclear deposits of cAMP are more striking in upper epidermal keratinocytes. ($\times$ 200)

1.6 DNase I and RNase A

ORIGIN AND NATURE OF DNase I AND RNase A
DNase I (deoxyribonuclease I), isolated from bovine pancreas, has a molecular weight of about 31,000. DNase I hydrolyzes highly-polymerized DNA by splitting the phosphodiester linkages, preferentially adjacent to a pyrimidine nucleotide. RNase A (ribonuclease A) was isolated from bovine pancreas.

OBSERVATIONS:
DNase I
NORMAL SKIN
Light microscopy. DNase I immunoreactivity is clearly observed in most cell nuclei of human, bovine, rat and guinea pig skin[115,116,117]. In the epidermis, the intensity of the reaction in the epidermal keratinocyte nuclei changes during keratinization. The epidermal keratinocyte nuclei at the basal layer and the lower portion of the spinous cell layer show a moderately positive reaction[115,117]. At the upper part of the spinous cell layer and granular layer, the nuclei of the epidermal cells are strongly positive. The strongest reactivity for DNase I is seen in the nuclei of the uppermost cells of the granular layer[115,117]; however, DNA in the epidermal keratinocyte nuclei gradually decreases, as the cells keratinize[118]. DNase I is seen even in the cornified cells, whereas the nuclei disappear in the horny layer[116].

Electron microscopy. Reaction products of various sizes are present in the karyoplasm and seem to be distributed in the euchromatin area of the nuclei[117]. Reaction products are present in a large mass in the flattened cornified cell, while the nuclei disappear[116].

ABNORMAL HUMAN SKIN AND EXPERIMENTAL SPECIMENS
Light microscopy. In psoriatic skin[119], staining for DNase I shows a positive reactivity in the epidermal cell nuclei cases examined, and for DNase I etretinate in the parakeratotic cells. There are variations in intensity between the effective and non-effective cases of therapy with PUVA, etretinate and steroid ointments. Before the treatment, the immuno-reactivity for DNase I was stronger in the effective cases than in the non-effective cases. Staining for DNase I was enhanced in the non-effective cases after the therapy. On the other hand, in the non-effective cases, the intensity of staining before the therapy was very weak and enhancement of staining was very slight after the treatment.

Between 48 and 72 hours after UVB irradiation, the nuclei of the epidermal keratinocytes revealed a very weakly positive reaction in guinea pig skin[117].

Electron microscopy. After UVB exposure of guinea pig skin, DNA is dispersed throughout the karyoplasm[120], and the immunoreactive production of DNase I is scattered in the nuclei in small clusters[117].

RNase A
Staining for RNase A is seen in most nuclei of the cells in the skin[115]. Positive reactivity is also seen in the cytoplasm. Immunoreactivity of RNase A in the nuclei of the epidermal keratinocytes changes during keratinization in human epidermis as does the immunoreactivity of DNase I[115].

SIGNIFICANCE FOR THE DERMATOLOGICAL FIELDS
Immunostaining for DNase I and RNase A is useful for studies of the nucleic acid hydrolytic enzymes in the cells and tissues, in particular the examination of the nuclear DNase and RNase changes[115,116,117,119]. Clinically, DNase I staining seems to be a good indication of the effectiveness of various therapies for psoriasis[119].

TECHNICAL POINTS
Freeze sections 8 μm thick should be used. Prior to the immunostaining, these sections are fixed in Zamboni solution for between 30 and 120 minutes at 4°C. For electron microscopy, the specimens are postfixed with osmium tetroxide following the immunostaining.

Fig. 1. DNase I. Immunoreactivity is shown in the nuclei of epidermal keratinocytes. The strongest reactivity is observed in the upper granular layer. Guinea pig skin. (× 570)

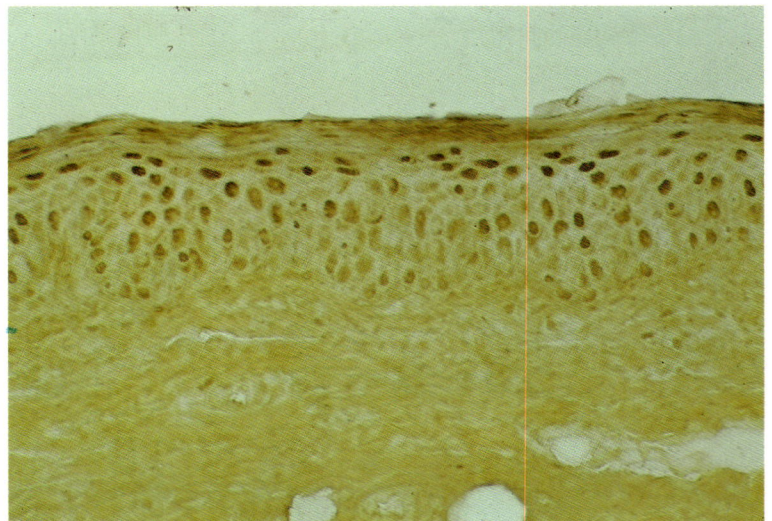

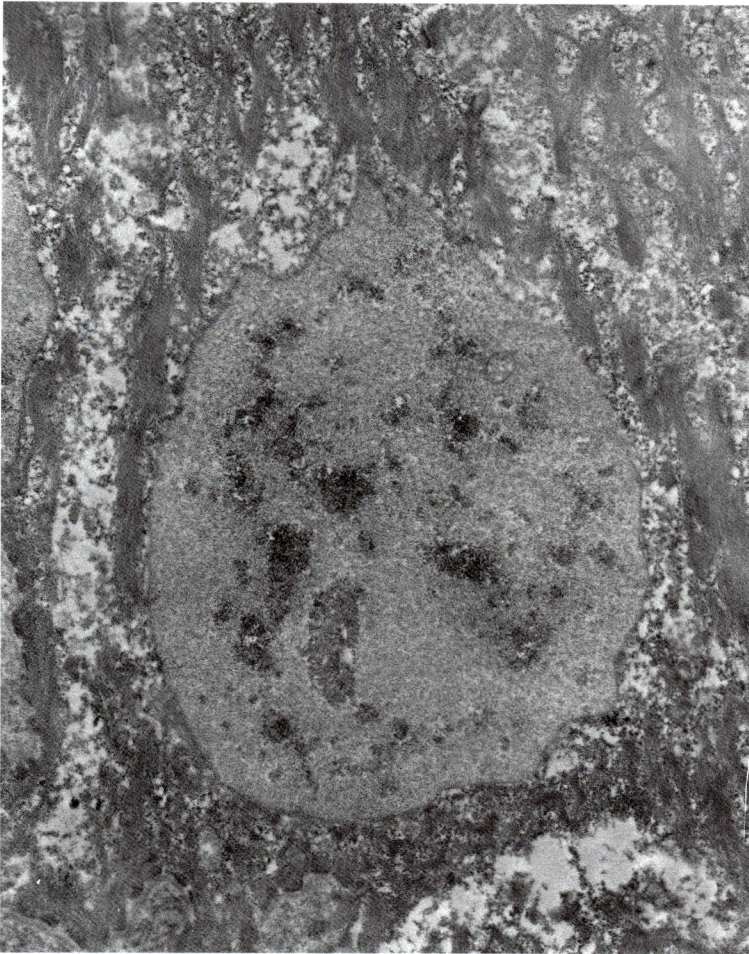

Fig. 2. DNase I. Reaction products are seen in the karyoplasm in small masses. Basal cells in guinea pig epidermis. (× 22,000)

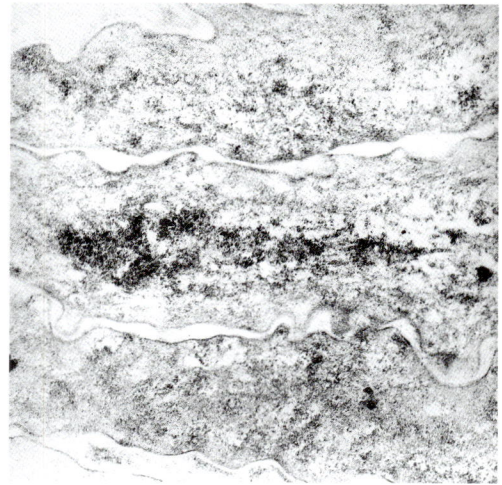

Fig. 3. DNase I in the cornified cell. Human epidermis (vertical section). (× 8,400)

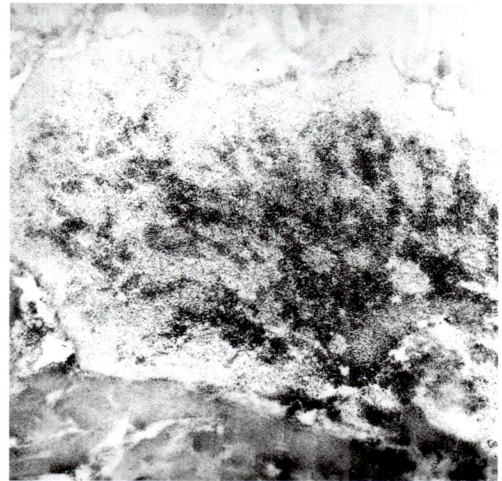

Fig. 4. DNase I in the cornified cell. Human epidermis (horizontal section). (× 10,000)

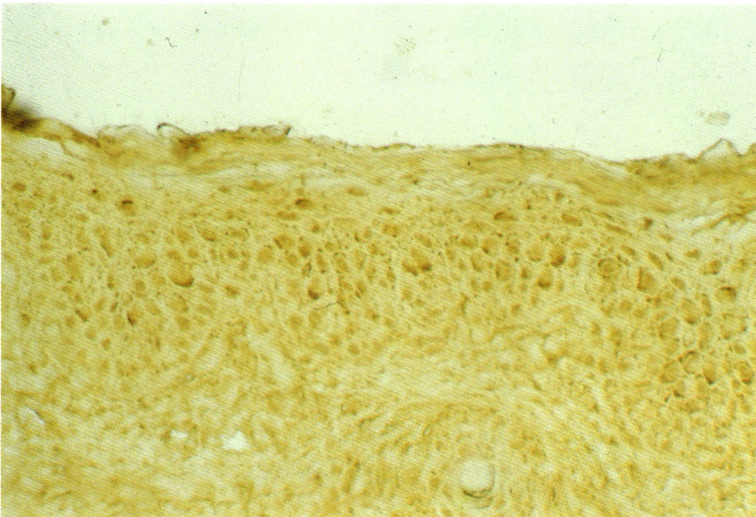

Fig. 5. RNase A. Guinea pig skin. (× 570)

Thy-1 positive d-EC

INTRODUCTION

Thy-1 antigen is a cell surface glycoprotein of restricted tissue distribution which has been studied as the differentiation antigen for T lymphocyte maturation in mice[121]. Recent investigations have revealed that Thy-1 antigen is also expressed on neuronal cells, fibroblasts, mammary myoepithelial cells and haematopoietic cells other than T lymphocytes[122,123]. Although the expression of low amounts of Thy-1 antigen on mouse epidermal cells (EC) had been suggested in 1972 by Scheid et al., based on cytotoxicity studies[124], immunofluorescent studies of EC against Thy-1 antigen were not performed until the discovery of Thy-1 positive dendritic epidermal cells (Thy-1[+]d-EC) in 1983. These cells were identified by two groups as the third dendritic EC population with quite different characteristics from either Langerhans cells (LC) or melanocytes in mice[123,125].

Thy-1[+]d-EC were defined as primarily dendritic but lacked desmosomes, melanosomes, tyrosinase activity, Merkel cell granules and Birbeck granules and they expressed a large amount of Thy-1 antigen but not any Ia antigen on their cell surface[123,125]. In 1984, subsequent investigations demonstrated that Thy-1[+]d-EC were derived from bone marrow precursors as were LC[126,127]. Furthermore, it was shown that Thy-1[+]d-EC were strongly positive whereas LC were negative against anti-acialo GM$_1$ antibody which reacted with natural killer (NK) cells, suppressor cells and foetal thymocytes in mice[128]. At present Thy-1[+]d-EC have only been demonstrated in mouse epidermis and the search for the human analogue of murine Thy-1[+]d-EC has not been successful[129].

IMMUNOFLUORESCENCE STUDIES OF Thy-1[+]d-EC

Thy-1[+]d-EC in epidermal sheets. Acetone-fixed, C57B1/6 mouse ear and tail epidermal sheets, obtained by EDTA separation procedures, were reacted with appropriate dilution of monoclonal anti-Thy 1.2 antibody (New England Nuclear) overnight at 4°C, and then reacted with fluorescein isothiocyanate-(FITC) conjugated goat anti-mouse IgM (Cappel) for two hours at 37°C to visualize Thy-1[+]d-EC, which express a large amount of Thy-1 antigen on their cell surface (1). It has been reported that Thy-1[+]d-EC exhibit a dendritic shape and are distributed evenly over the entire ear epidermal sheet specimen. Also, a small amount of Thy-1 antigen is noticeable on keratinocytes in a 'honeycomb pattern'[128]. In contrast to ear epidermis, Thy-1[+]d-EC are only partially distributed in the 'interscale' region and none are found in the 'scale' region in tail epidermis (3).

Thus density and surface distribution of Thy-1[+]d-EC depend upon the mouse strain and body region. C57B1/6 mice exhibit the highest density of Thy-1[+]d-EC followed by C3H/He, AKR/J, BALB/c and C3H/He nu/nu[125]. Ear and trunk epidermis contain densely and evenly distributed Thy-1[+]d-EC whereas only small numbers of Thy-1[+]d-EC are partially distributed in the 'interscale' region in tail epidermis similar to the distribution of LC in tail epidermis.

Thy-1[+]d-EC in single cell suspensions of EC. Single cell suspensions of C57B1/6 mouse ear epidermis, obtained by standard trypsinization procedures, were stained on ice for one hour for each step using the same reagents as for the sheets (2). Thy-1[+]d-EC show very bright intensity of fluorescence. The frequency of strongly Thy-1 positive EC which depends upon the mouse strain and body region investigated has been reported to range from 0.7 to 2.7% for all EC[125]. One can also note extremely faint membrane fluorescence on approximately 4.1–17.3%[122], or 20–30%[125] of EC suspensions but Thy-1[+]d-EC are easily identifiable by their intense fluorescence[122,125].

Double immunofluorescent studies for Thy-1[+]d-EC using anti-IA and anti-acialo GM$_1$ antibodies. Trunk epidermal sheets of [C57B1/6 × C3H/He]F$_1$ mice were first incubated with mouse anti-Ia^k (ATH anti-ATL)antibody (Cederlane) overnight at 4°C and then with FITC-conjugated goat anti-mouse IgG (Cappel) for two hours at 37°C; or were first incubated with rabbit anti-acialo GM$_1$ antibody (Wako) overnight at 4°C and then with FITC-conjugated goat anti-rabbit IgG (Cappel). These FITC-stained epidermal sheets were again reacted with monoclonal anti-Thy 1.2 antibody overnight at 4°C and were finally reacted with tetramethylrhodamine isothiocyanate-(TRITC) labelled goat anti-mouse IgM (Cappel) for two hours at 37°C (4 and 5).

The Thy-1 and Ia markers never overlap[128]; that is, Thy-1[+]d-EC are different dendritic EC to LC. Thy-1[+]d-EC are strongly positive against acialo Gm$_1$ antibody and these markers clearly overlap.

IMMUNOLOGICAL SIGNIFICANCE OF Thy-1[+]d-EC

Morphological and phenotypical results indicate that in murine epidermis two different types of bone marrow-derived dendritic epidermal cells exist. These are Ia$_+$ and Thy-1$^-$ Langerhans cells and the recently discovered Ia$^-$ and Thy-1[+]d-EC. A large number of immunodermatological studies have revealed that LC plays an important role as antigen presenting cells in many cutaneous immunological events. Although the investigation for LC is quite advanced, the precise function of Thy-1[+]d-EC has not yet been made clear.

At one time Thy-1[+]d-EC had been considered as resident NK cells in murine epidermis because Thy-1[+]d-EC possessed a large amount of cell surface acialo GM$_1$, which was thought to be a fairly specific surface marker for NK cells. However, no investigation has revealed NK cell activity of Thy-1[+]d-EC until recently[128]. So far it has been suggested that Thy-1[+]d-EC play a role in murine cutaneous immunological responses as distinctive leucocytes, perhaps related to NK cells[128].

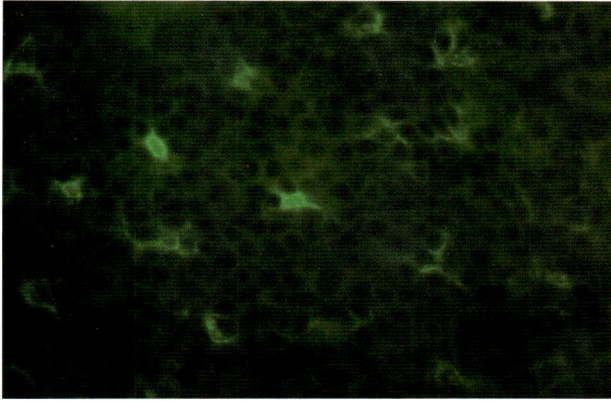

Fig. 1. Thy-1⁺d-EC in ear epidermal sheets (C57B1/6).
Thy-1⁺d-EC are highly dendritic and have many cell surface Thy-1 antigens (× 400). Note few Thy-1 antigen on keratinocytes in a 'honeycomb pattern.'

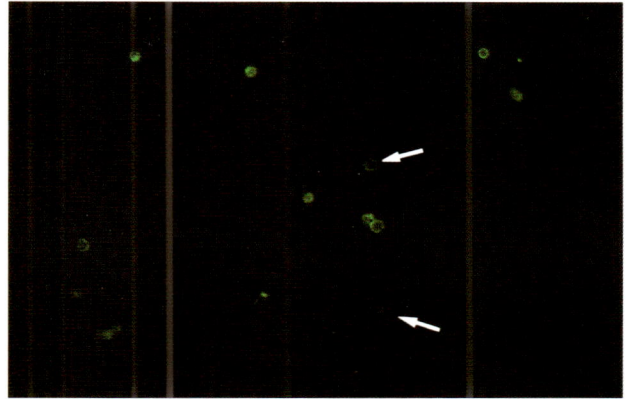

Fig. 2. Thy-1⁺d-EC in single cell EC suspension (C57B1/6, ear).
Thy-1 antigens are strongly positive on the entire cell surface of Thy-1⁺d-EC (× 200). Note extremely dull positive Thy-1 antigens on the cell surface of some keratinocytes (arrow).

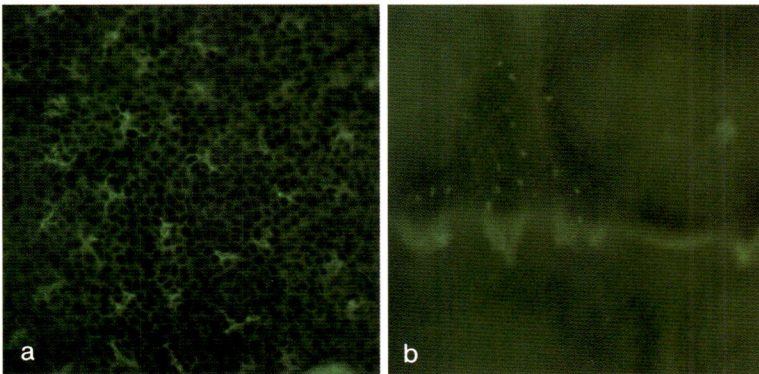

Fig. 3. The density and surface distribution of Thy-1⁺d-EC in ear *versus* tail epidermal sheets (C57B1/6).
Thy-1⁺d-EC are evenly distributed on the ear epidermal sheets overall (a. × 200), whereas only a small number of Thy-1⁺d-EC are partially distributed in the 'interscale' region of the tail epidermal sheets (b. × 100).

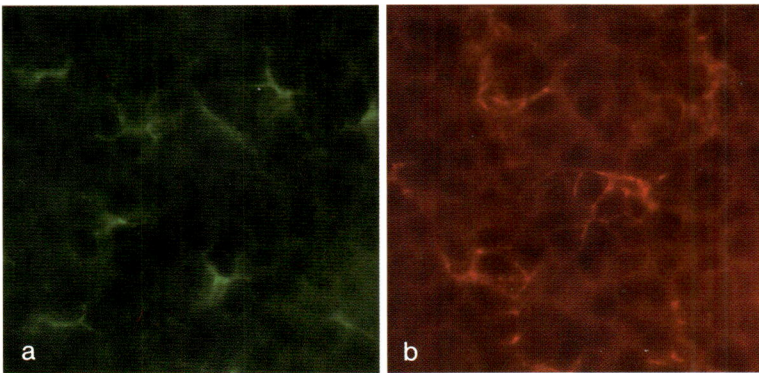

Fig. 4. Double immunofluorescent studies of Thy-1⁺d-EC using anti-Ia and anti-Thy-1 antibodies (B6C3F₁).
A particular field was photographed using FITC (a) and TRITC (b) filter setting. Ia antigens stained with FITC (a) and Thy-1 antigens stained with TRITC (b) are found on different cells (× 400). Thy-1⁺d-EC are a different type of dendritic epidermal cells from Ia⁺ Langerhans cells.

Fig. 5. Double immunofluorescent studies for Thy-1⁺d-EC using anti-acialo GM₁ and anti-Thy-1 antibodies (B6C3F₁).
Acialo GM₁ antigens stained with FITC (a) and Thy-1 antigens stained with TRITC (b) are found on the same cells (× 400). Thy-1⁺d-EC are highly positive against anti-acialo GM₁ antibodies.

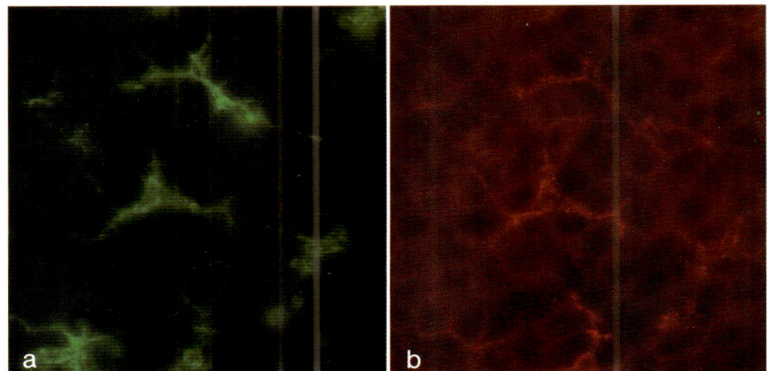

Langerhans cells

INTRODUCTION

Langerhans cells (LC) were first described by Paul Langerhans in 1868 as dendritic cells in the suprabasal regions of the epidermis which stained with gold chloride[130]. These cells were first considered as neural cells because of their affinity with gold chloride, and later were considered to be of melanocyte origin[131]. In 1961, Birbeck described the unique LC granules, which are now referred to as Birbeck granules or Langerhans cell granules. These granules are similar to those found in cells in Histiocytosis X. These findings suggested that LC were of mesenchymal origin. In 1977,

Stingl *et al.* found that LC possess an FcIgG receptor, a C3 receptor and also express Ia antigen. Since then, much progress has been made and it has been shown that LC can act as stimulator cells in a mixed leucocyte reaction, antigen-presenting cells, and accessory cells in the induction of cytotoxic T lymphocytes. The role of LC has also been investigated *in vivo*, particularly in contact hypersensitivity and in skin graft rejection[132,133]. LC have been shown to be detectable by ATPase, alkaline phosphatase, and non-specific esterase staining. Recently it was shown that LC can be detected using OKT-6, S-100, and T-200 antibodies[134,135].

DERMATOLOGICAL SIGNIFICANCE

LC are regarded as antigen-presenting cells in the skin. These cells play an important role in immune reactions in the skin as described above.

TECHNICAL POINTS

For the epidermal cell suspension, trypsin and DNase have been widely recommended. The conditions for trypsin and DNase vary from species to species[136].

For some antibodies, deparaffinized specimens can be used.

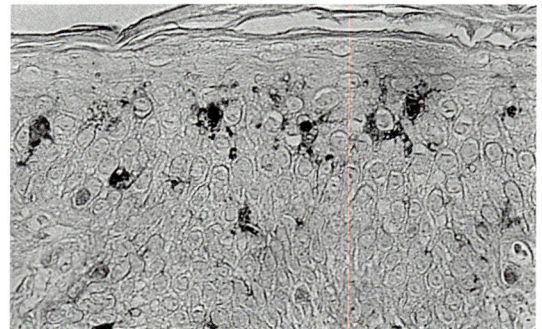

Fig. 1. Human LC stained with OKT-6 antibody as dendritic cells in the epidermis (peroxidase anti-peroxidase method, × 400).

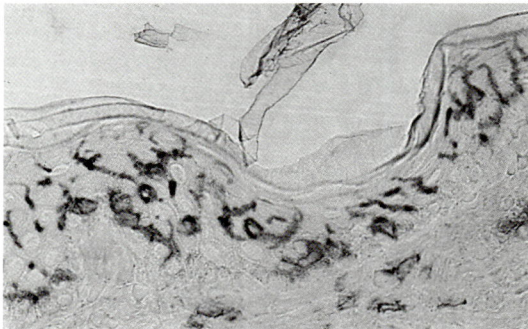

Fig. 2. Human LC stained with S-100 antibody (PAP method, × 400).

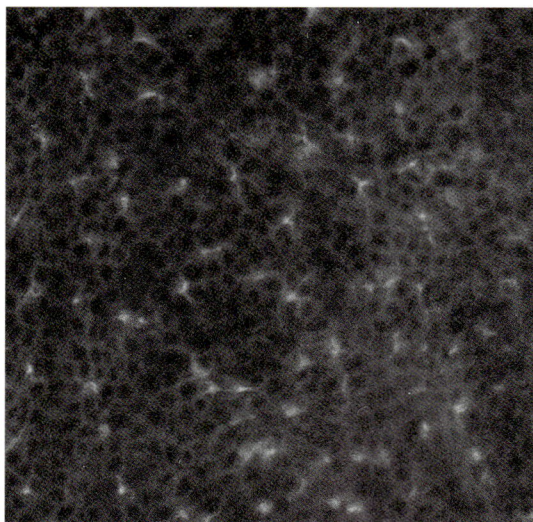

Fig. 3. C3H/He mouse epidermis separated from dermis with EDTA. LC stained with A.TH anti-A.TL antibody followed by FITC-conjugated goat anti-mouse IgG (× 200).

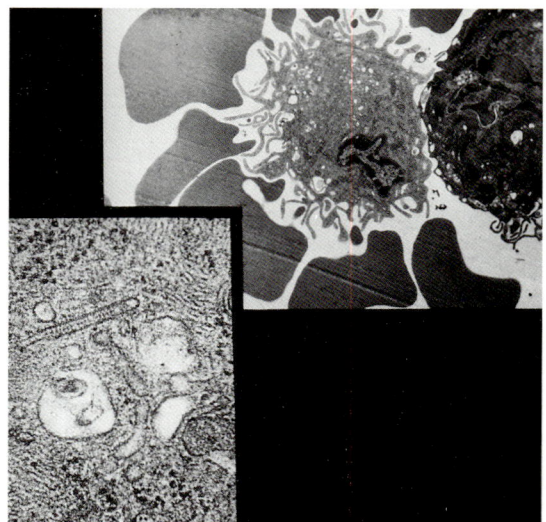

Fig. 4. Electron microscopy of Fc-IgG rosette forming LC (× 3,000). Insert indicates Birbeck granule in LC (× 38,000).

Melanocytes

4.1 Tyrosinase in melanocytes

ORIGIN AND CHARACTER

Tyrosinase, the enzyme responsible for the formation of melanin pigment, is the only enzyme known as the marker for melanocyte. Hearing et al.[137] purified four forms of tyrosinase from mouse melanoma, designated as T_1, T_2, T_3 and T_4 in order of decreasing electrophoretic mobility. According to their report, T_4 was the melanosome-bound form of the enzyme and T_3 represented the *de novo* form of the enzyme; T_3 was thought to be converted to T_1 *in vivo* by the addition of sialic acids and neutral sugars and converted to T_4 by forming a complex with melanosomal membrane constituents. We reported that two forms of the enzyme, T_1 and T_2, separated from the soluble fraction of mouse melanoma are not precursors but are degraded enzymes of T_4 from melanosomes[138]. T_4 is known to be inactivated during melanin formation *in vivo* and *in vitro*[139]. Thus, enzyme activity cannot usually be detected in a mature melanosome.

We have recently produced three monoclonal antibodies, termed TMH-1, TMH-2 and TMH-3[140]. These monoclonal antibodies specifically bind to mouse T_4-tyrosinase. These monoclonal antibodies cross-react with human tyrosinase, as determined by immunofluorescence staining[141], and can now be utilized for immunohistological diagnosis and also for experimental research of human skin diseases[142].

FINDINGS

Since the reactivity of TMH-1, TMH-2 and TMH-3 is specific for tyrosinase, all cells containing tyrosinase, such as normal melanocytes, pigmented nevus cells and melanoma cells, can be immunofluorescence-stained using these antibodies, as shown in figure 1. Unpigmented melanocytes present in amelanotic melanoma or in albino skin are not stained with these antibodies.

DERMATOLOGICAL SIGNIFICANCE

We can affirm that a cell immunohistologically stained with TMH-1, TMH-2 or TMH-3 is either a melanocyte or a melanoma cell, since these antibodies can specifically bind to tyrosinase. But it is not possible to conclude that all of the melanocytes or melanoma cells reacted with these antibodies because unpigmented melanocytes and amelanotic melanoma cells having no tyrosinase cannot be immunohistologically stained by these antibodies. Most of the melanin deposited in the tissue is an aggregation of many melanin granules which are secreted from the melanocytes as mature melanosomes containing little or no native tyrosinase protein.

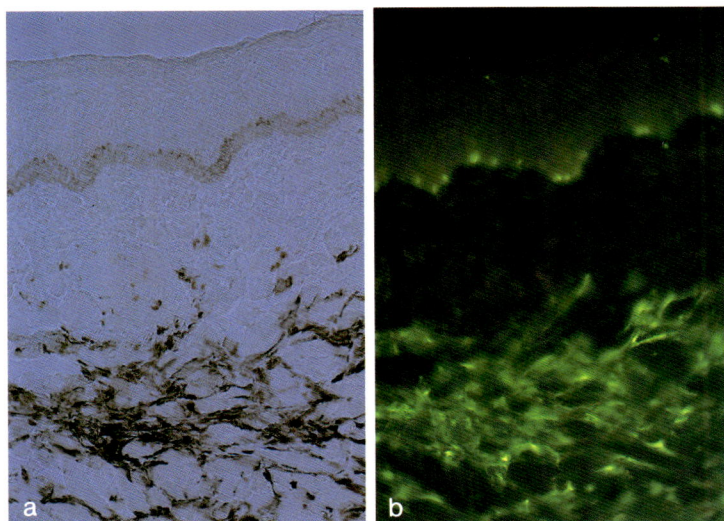

Fig. 1. Blue nevus.
(a) without staining ($\times$ 65). Hyperpigmentation in the basal layer of the epidermis and coarse melanin granule deposits in the dermis. (b) immunofluorescence staining by the monoclonal antibody to tyrosinase ($\times$ 65). Fluorescent areas do not always consist of melanin deposits.

That is the reason why melanin granules deposited in tissues such as nevus and melanoma often show no reactivity to antibodies to tyrosinase.

TECHNICAL POINTS

Paraffin-embedded tissue cannot be used for immunohistological staining. Melanocytes cannot be stained immunohistologically by any of the three antibodies in the sections obtained from paraffin-embedded tissue. This is probably due to the deformation of tyrosinase epitopes during the paraffin embedding process.

4.2 Cell membrane and organelle (melanosome) in melanocytes and melanoma cells

INTRODUCTION
Melanocytes produce a secretory granule, melanosome. Melanosome is a membrane delimited organelle with a structural unit consisting of tyrosinase and matrix protein[143]. In the malignant melanocyte, the composition and structure of the melanosome become markedly deranged. The morphological derangement of melanosome derives largely from abnormally structured matrix proteins, other than tyrosinase[144, 145]. In certain forms of pigmentary disorders, the derangement in structure and composition of melanosome is unique and may often be diagnostic[146–8]. We have recently developed, with the use of hybridoma technology and mouse myeloma cells, four monoclonal antibodies (MoAbs) against the melanosome of human malignant melanoma. The melanosome was isolated from fresh autopsy materials, dissociated by detergents, and partially purified by DE 52 column chromatography (0.25 M KC1). The MoAbs developed were designated MoAb HMSA-1, HMSA-2, HMSA-3 and HMSA-4. HMSA is an abbreviation of human-melanosome associated-antigen[149–53].

FINDINGS
MoAb HMSA-1 and HMSA-2 belong to IgG_1 k subclass while MoAb HMSA-3 and HMSA-4 are of IgM k subclass. The four MoAbs identify the cytoplasmic antigen on the neoplastic melanocyte, but not on the normal melanocyte by the ABC (avidin-biotin complex) method. The epitopes recognized are localized in the cytoplasm, but vary depending on the cell type. By SDS-PAGE analysis, the size of HMSA-1 and HMSA-2 have been found to be different. By immunoelectron microscopy and ELISA (enzyme-linked immunosorbent assay), HMSA-1 is localized in the melanosome, ribosome and endoplasmic reticulum. HMSA-1 and HMSA-2 appear to be the melanosomal matrix protein and precursor forms.

DIAGNOSTIC SIGNIFICANCE
MoAbs HMSA-1 and HMSA-2 react with cells of malignant melanoma and melanocytic nevi. In melanocytic nevi, MoAb HMSA-1 and HMSA-2 homogeneously react with dermal nevus cells giving positive cytoplasmic staining from the top to the bottom of nevus-cell nests. In contrast, malignant melanoma cells reveal heterogeneous reactivity, i.e., weak and intense reactivities scattered randomly throughout the entire tumour-cell nest. Importantly, MoAb HMSA-1 and HMSA-2 react with epidermal melanocytes of dysplastic melanocytic nevi. MoAb HMSA-1 and HMSA-2 tend to have a much stronger reaction to amelanotic melanoma cells than to melanotic cells.

TECHNICAL POINTS
MoAb HMSA-1 and HMSA-2 react with formalin-fixed and paraffin-embedded sections. For indirect immunoperoxidase staining using the ABC technique, paraffin sections are soaked in a methanol solution containing 0.3% hydrogen peroxide for twenty minutes to eliminate endogenous peroxidase, and treated with 0.1% trypsin containing NaF in phosphate buffered saline (PBS) to remove the antigen protein-masking materials. After twenty minutes' incubation with 2% normal horse serum, sections are treated with the MoAbs (supernatant of cultured fluid) for thirty minutes. After washing the PBS, the sections are made to react with biotinylated horse anti-mouse immunoglobulin. ABC solution (Vector Lab., Inc., Burlingam) is then applied to the sections for sixty minutes. After washing with PBS, the final incubation

is made in 0.025% diaminobenzidine and 0.01% hydrogen peroxide buffered with 0.1 M Tris-HC1, pH 7.2. The sections are counter-stained lightly with Giemsa's stain to differentiate the reaction product from melanin pigments.

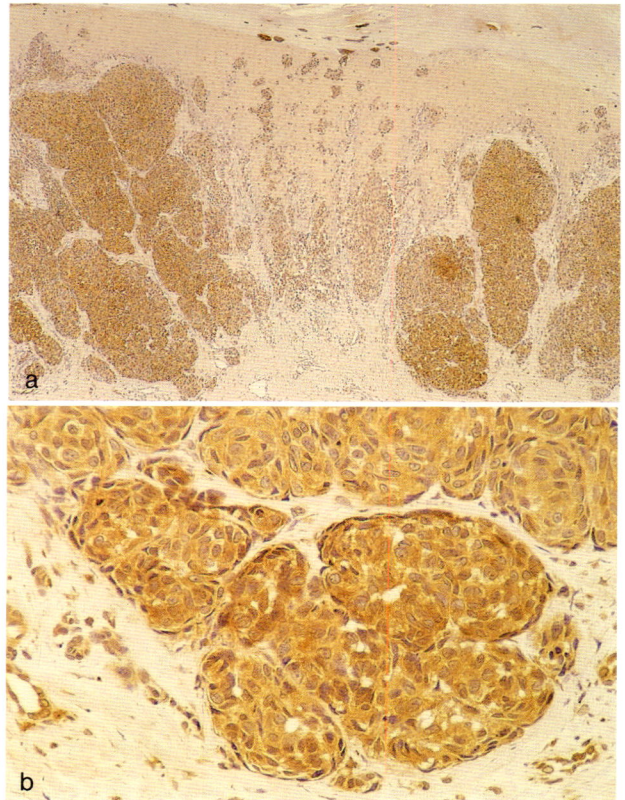

Fig. 1. Subungual malignant melanoma. Amelanotic melanoma with SSM subtype reacted with MoAb HMSA-1 using the ABC technique.
(a) Low-power view showing the positive reactivity to cells in the epidermis and dermis. ($\times$ 40)
(b) High-power view showing the cytoplasmic reactivity. ($\times$ 200)

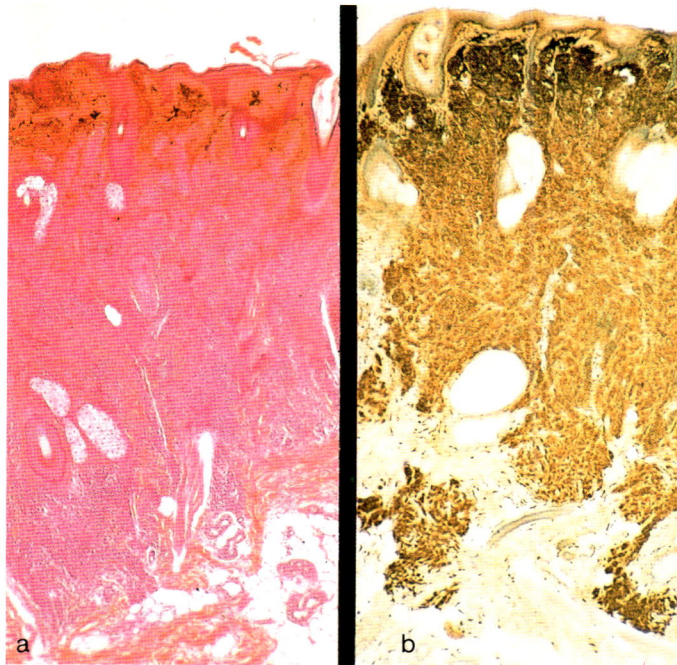

Fig. 2. Pigmented melanocytic nevus.
(a) Control, HE section. (× 40)
(b) Dermal nevus cells reacted but diffusely to MoAb HMSA-2.
ABC technique. (× 40)

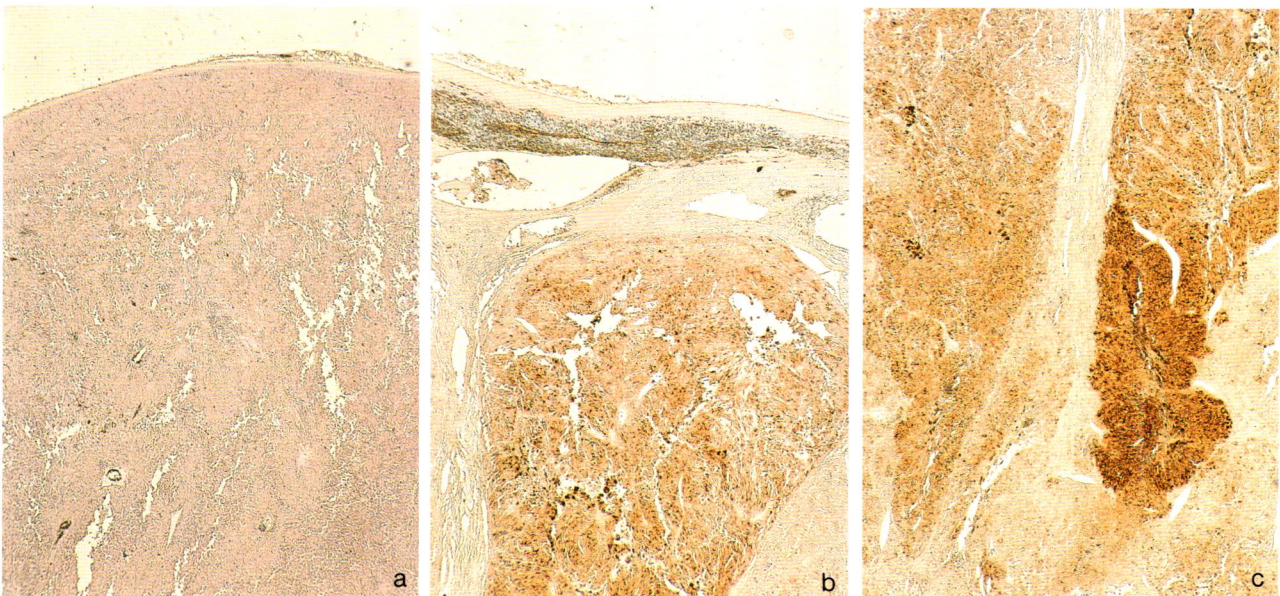

Fig. 3. Amelanotic metastatic melanoma in lymph node.
Reaction with MoAb HMSA-1.
(a) Control specimen. (× 40)
(b) Positive tumour cells below the capsule of the lymph node.
(× 80)

(c) Lymph node centre. Tumour cells are more intensely stained than those below the capsule (Fig. 3-b), and reveal heterogeneous reactivity. (× 80)

Sweat gland cells

ORIGIN AND CHARACTERISTICS

Sweat gland cells originate from embryonal epidermis. Eccrine gland germs begin from the basal layers of the epidermis whereas apocrine gland germs develop from the upper bulge of hair follicles. Because both types of sweat glands develop from embryonal keratinocytes, they share common characteristics with epidermal keratinocytes. However, the cells which differentiate toward secretory portions also show common characteristics with the secretory cells of other internal organs. Myoepithelial cells which lie at the outermost layer of secretory portions are also developed from embryonal epidermis and show epithelial cell characteristics. Additionally, these cells contain myofibrils and share some common characteristics with smooth muscle cells.

It is generally accepted that the sweat glands are classified into two types; i.e., eccrine glands and apocrine glands. However, a recent report has shown that a third type exists, called apoeccrine glands which show intermediate characteristics of both types[154].

Immunohistochemically, carcinoembryonic antigen (CEA) and S-100 protein are commonly used as sweat gland markers[155-8]. Recently monoclonal antibodies EKH5, EKH6[159] smf D-47[160] are reported to react with sweat glands. In addition, antibodies against IgA secretory components (SC)[161], epithelial membrane antigen (EMA)[162], gross cystic disease fluid protein (GCDFP-15)[163] and DBA lectin[164] have also been reported as useful for sweat gland research.

FINDINGS

Normal sweat gland cells. The reactivities of normal sweat gland cells with various antibodies are summarized in Table I. Anti-CEA antibody strongly reacts with secretory cells (1) and positively reacts with the luminal side of ducts to the acrosyringium through dermis (2)[155]. Anti-CEA antibody also reacts with apocrine glands, although the reaction is relatively weak when compared to the reaction with eccrine glands[156]. Anti-S-100 protein antibody reacts with clear cells of the secretory portion of eccrine glands and the myoepithelial cells of eccrine glands, as well as with

apocrine glands[158]. Monoclonal antibody EKH5 reacts with eccrine secretory cells (3) and EKH6 reacts with secretory cells and also partially reacts with coiled ducts[159] (4). Myoepithelial cells are also positively stained with anti-keratin antibody, such as monoclonal antibody EKH4 (specific to 50kd keratin)[165-6] (5). Monoclonal antibody D-47 reacts with eccrine secretory cells[160], GCDFP-15 with appropriate secretory cells[163], EMA with secretory cells of both types of sweat glands[162].

Abnormal sweat gland cells. The reactivities of appendageal tumour cells with these markers has been well investigated. CEA is demonstrated in most benign and malignant sweat gland tumours which form luminal structures along the inner aspect of the lumen. In contrast, S-100 protein is positive in tumours which are rich in myoepithelial components, such as mixed tumour. It is also positive in tumours which are closely related to the secretory portion, such as eccrine spiradenoma, papillary adenoma or hidro-cystoma (7). Monoclonal antibodies EKH5 and EKH6 react predominantly with eccrine derived tumours; not only with luminal structures but also solid tumour masses[167].

In general, one must be careful when assessing the results of immunohistochemical staining because tumour cells may show altered marker profiles compared to the original normal cells. The origin of extramammary Paget cells is still debated because they show the following eccrine and apocrine marker profiles: CEA(+), S-100 protein(−), EKH5(+), EKH6(+), D-47(−), GCDFP-15(+) and DBA lectin(−).

SIGNIFICANCE IN DERMATOPATHOLOGY

Studies of origin or differentiation of appendageal tumour cells rapidly progressed after the introduction of immuno-histochemical techniques. Anti-CEA is useful to differentiate sweat gland-related tumours from other appendageal tumours and anti-S-100 is useful to classify sweat gland tumours into their subclasses. To study the origin and/or direction of differentiation of appendageal tumours, however, a single marker is insufficient. Multiple markers should be used or other techniques such as electron microscopy or histo-chemistry should be combined.

TECHNICAL POINTS

Most markers can be used on both frozen sections and paraffin-embedded sections. However, anti-S-100 protein is not suitable for fresh frozen sections and anti-D-47 cannot be used on paraffin-embedded sections. Both EKH5 and EKH6 can be used on alcohol-fixed paraffin-embedded sections but the best results are achieved on fresh frozen sections. Several types of anti-CEA and anti-S-100 staining kits are commercially available and in most cases, good results can be obtained using paraffin-embedded sections.

TABLE I   REACTIVITIES OF SWEAT GLANDS WITH VARIOUS ANTIBODIES

	CEA	S-100	EKH5	EKH6	keratin (EKH4)	D-47	SC	EMA	GCDFP-15
ECCRINE SWEAT GLAND									
Secretory portion	+	+	+	+	−	+	+	+	−
Myoepithelial cell	−	+	−	−	+	−	−	−	−
Dermal duct	+	−	−	+/−	+	−	−	−	−
Acrosyringium	+	−	−	−	+	−	−	−	−
APOCRINE SWEAT GLAND									
Secretory portion	+	−	±	±	−	−	−	+	+
Myoepithelial cell	−	+	−	±	+	−	−	−	−
Dermal duct	+	−	−	−	+	−	−	−	+

+   Positive   ±   Weak reaction   +/− Partially positive   −   Negative

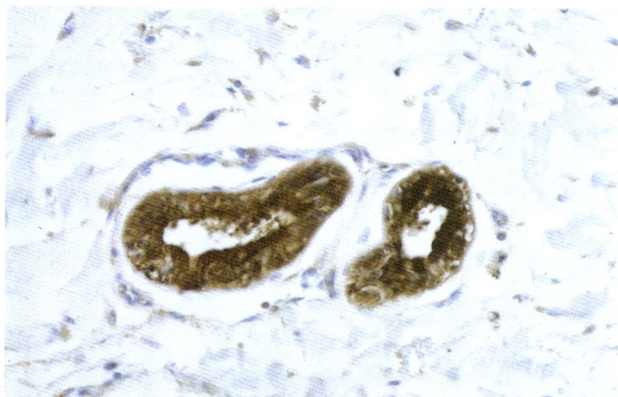

Fig. 1. Secretory portion of eccrine gland. Secretory cells show positive staining. (CEA-PAP staining) (× 230).

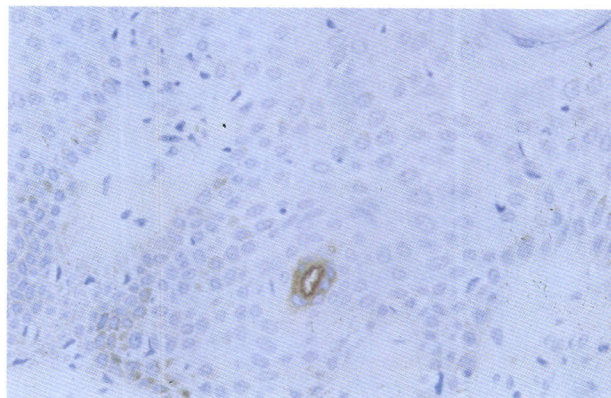

Fig. 2. Acrosyringium. Inner surface of luminal structure is positively stained. (CEA-PAP staining) (× 115).

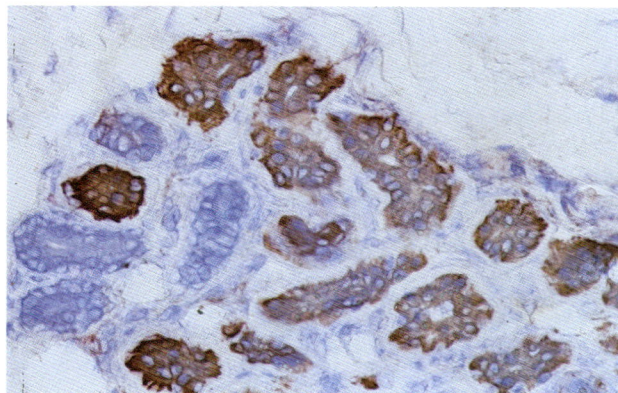

Fig. 3. Secretory portion of eccrine gland. Secretory cells are selectively stained. (EKH5-ABC staining) (× 115).

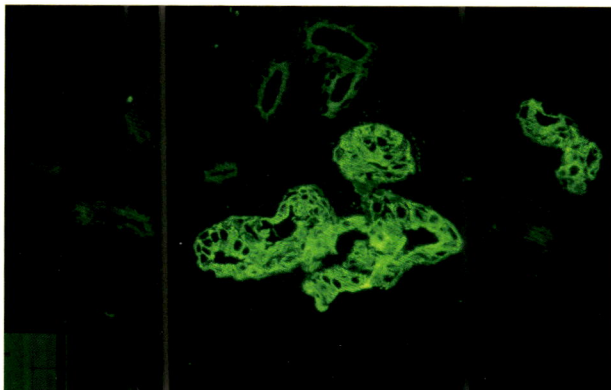

Fig. 4. Secretory cells and some coiled ducts show positive staining. (EKH6-indirect immunofluorescence staining) (× 180).

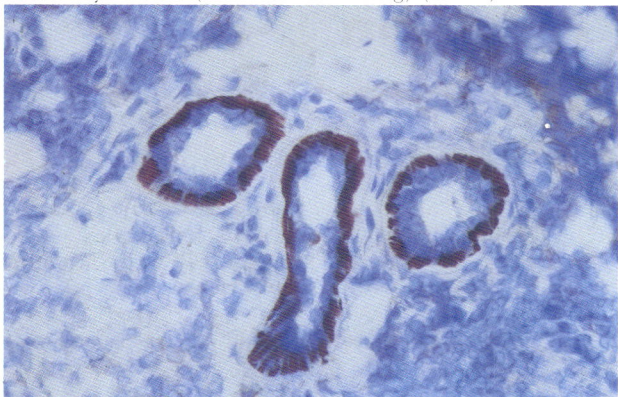

Fig. 5. Secretory portion of eccrine gland. Myoepithelial cells are positively stained. (EKH4-ABC staining) (× 230).

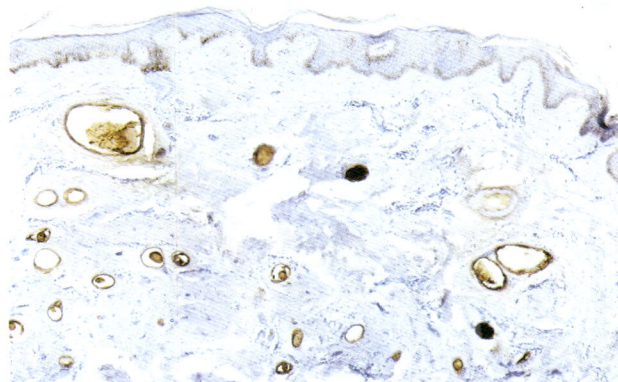

Fig. 6. Syringoma. Syringoma cells show positive staining. (CEA-PAP staining) (× 45).

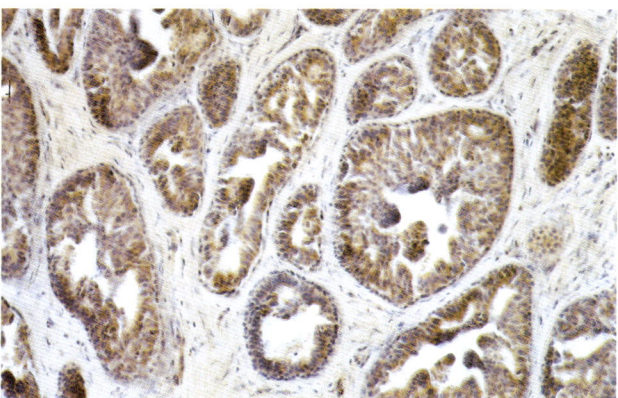

Fig. 7. Eccrine papillary adenoma. Tumour cells are positively stained. (S-100 protein-PAP staining) (× 50).

Pilosebaceous cells

DEVELOPMENT AND CHARACTERISTICS OF PILOSEBACEOUS CELLS

Pilosebaceous cells and sweat gland cells are derived from epidermal keratinocytes in the early embryonic stage in humans[168]. Therefore, the basic characteristics should be similar in these cells although these cells and organs are entirely different in their morphology and function. This is probably why there is no available unique monoclonal antibody which specifically recognizes a certain cell or organ. Great efforts have been made to obtain such a unique monoclonal antibody. At present, there are a few monoclonal antibodies (EKH5[169–171] and HKN6[172]) which react fairly specifically to eccrine glands and the inner root sheath of hair follicles. Since the morphological and biological differences are so great in these epidermal appendages, it is expected that truly specific monoclonal antibodies will be developed in the future.

Some questions, however, will remain as to whether truly specific monoclonal antibodies are obtainable or not in the case of tumours, benign or malignant, because benign epidermal appendage tumours are often pluripotent[173]. This means that cells within a tumour have some characteristics of different types of tumours. This idea is supported by the fact that two or more histologically different tumour cells are often observed in a tumour. We have demonstrated this phenomenon using the human trichilemmoma cell line in tissue cultures *in vitro*. Initially the cell line (K-TL-1) differentiated towards hair follicles in three-dimensional structures[174, 175], but eventually the cell line cells differentiated towards eccrine gland-producing domes and ducts[171]. This *in vitro* phenomenon was also observed in nude mice *in vivo*.

As regards malignant tumours, monoclonal antibodies to specific tumours are not easily available because these cells are ill-differentiated. Monoclonal antibodies which react to a certain normal cell or organ may not react to malignant, transformed cells.

Above all, it is very difficult to obtain a monoclonal antibody to certain epidermal appendage tumours; but there is always the possibility that it may be obtained by chance.

FINDINGS FROM A MONOCLONAL ANTIBODY AGAINST PILOSEBACEOUS CELLS

Normal pilosebaceous cells and sweat gland cells. We have developed a monoclonal antibody which is specific for normal pilosebaceous cells. This antibody was obtained by immunizing mice with whole cells of an *in vitro* established human malignant trichilemmoma cell line (IK-TL-2). The antibody (3D6-2) reacted to the cytoplasm of pilosebaceous cells (**1a**), but only weakly reacted to a portion of the eccrine gland, the submembranous area of the transitional part (**1b**).

Hair follicle and eccrine gland tumours. Immunohistochemical techniques are very useful for diagnosis in tumours of pilosebaceous apparatus; it is possible to determine whether the tumour is pilosebaceous-related or not. Research in this area must continue; the differentiation of malignant tumours from benign ones using a monoclonal antibody is just one of the many promising possibilities.

In this chapter, we show the usefulness of the monoclonal antibody 3D6-2, in the differentiation of hair-follicular tumours and eccrine gland tumours. This antibody strongly reacted to malignant trichilemmoma (**2a**). The reaction was distributed evenly in the cytoplasm of all tumour cells. The resultant products using the PAP method were coarse and granular (**2b**). In contrast, an eccrine benign tumour (eccrine poroepithelioma) did not react to this monoclonal antibody, with the exception of a few outermost tumour mass layers. The reaction products were observed along the cell membrane, not in the cytoplasm (**3a**). Moreover, this monoclonal antibody did not react at all to malignant eccrine tumour (**3b**).

These results showed that this monoclonal antibody differentiates pilosebaceous tumours from eccrine tumours and similarly, malignant eccrine tumours from benign eccrine tumours.

DERMATOLOGICAL SIGNIFICANCE

As mentioned above, differentiation of various skin tumours will be made easily and more accurately when suitable monoclonal antibodies are available. It may be difficult, however, and may well be impossible, to obtain various monoclonal antibodies which uniquely react to certain specific organs or tumours.

TECHNICAL POINTS

No special techniques are required to perform immunohistochemical studies. However, it is desirable to obtain monoclonal antibodies which react not only to frozen sections but also to paraffin-embedded specimens to study past cases. Once such monoclonal antibodies are available, great advances in tumour diagnosis are anticipated.

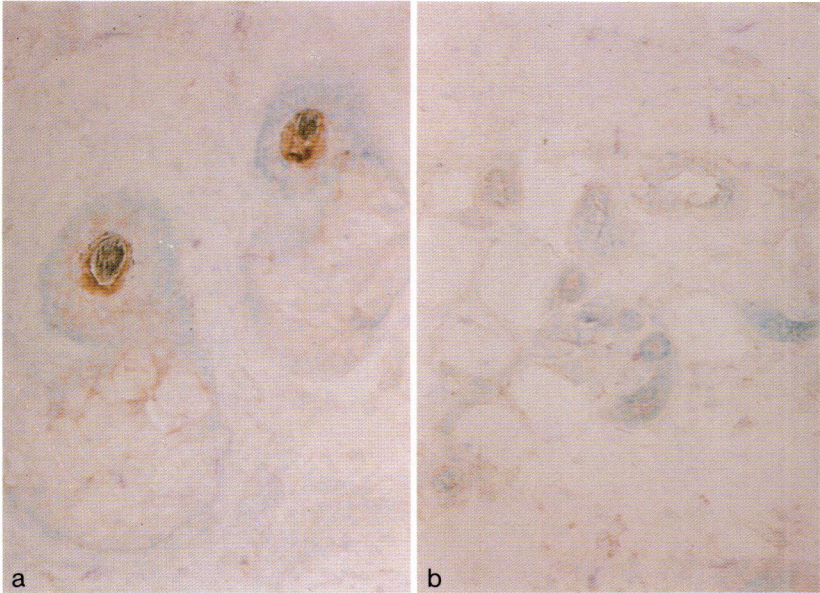

Fig. 1a. Normal human hair follicles and sebaceous glands. Hair follicles and sebaceous cells stained positively. (× 50)

Fig. 1b. Normal human eccrine glands. Cells in transitional area faintly stained along cell membrane. (× 50)

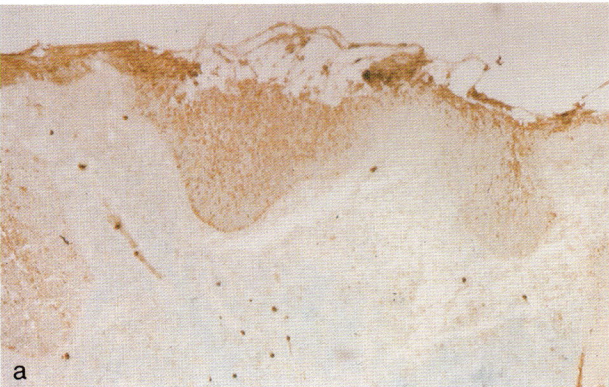

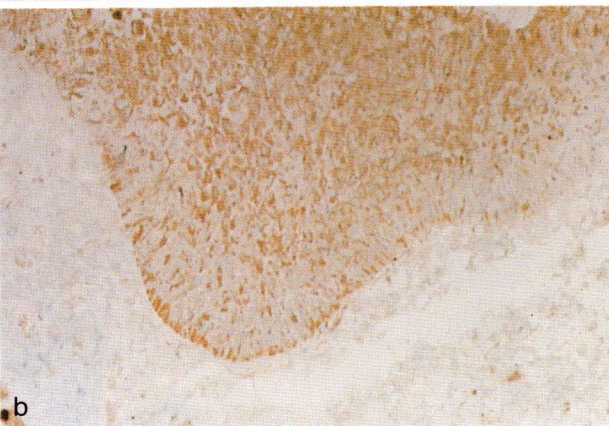

Fig. 2a. Malignant trichilemmoma. All cells stained. (× 20)

Fig. 2b. Enlargement of Fig. 2a. Coarse granular reaction products diffusely present in the cytoplasm. (× 50)

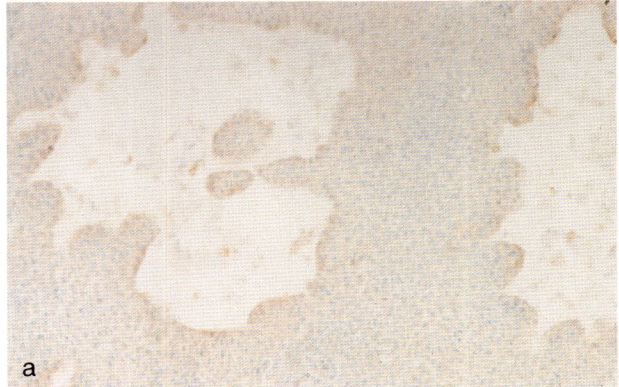

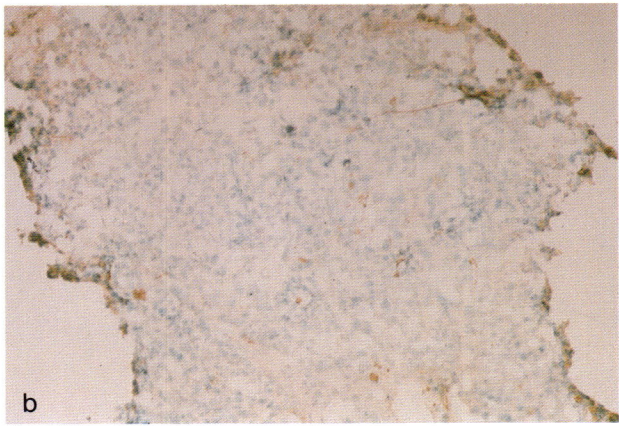

Fig. 3a. Eccrine poroepithelioma. Weak positive reaction is observed in the cells of the outermost layers. The staining product is located along cell membrane. (× 50)

Fig. 3b. Eccrine carcinoma. No reaction observed at all. (× 50)

Fibroblasts

Cytoskeleton

INTRODUCTION

A variety of higher vertebrate cells contain cytoskeleton composed of three major fibrous proteins, microtubules, microfilaments and intermediate filaments. These proteins have been shown to form filamentous meshwork structured to dominate various functions such as: the determination of cellular shape, adhesion, cell locomotion, intracellular movement of organelles and mitosis. These proteins act individually or by interaction with other proteins. In 1974, Lazarides was the first to report arrays of microfilaments by immunofluorescence microscopy, using an antibody to actin in cultured fibroblasts[177]. After that, immunofluorescence techniques have been used in addition to electron microscopy for the observation of cytoskeletal arrangements.

FINDINGS

Cell motility and mechanical support are the chief functions of actin filaments. Actin filaments are observed by immunofluorescence in ruffles and stress fibres (**1a**) and are seen in close association with the plasma membrane and fibronectin (**1b**)[178].

Microtubules form a tubular fibrous structure. One of the important functions of microtubules is the leading role in mitosis. In interphase, microtubules are present as a cytoplasmic microtubular complex oriented along the long axis of the fibroblast. During mitosis, microtubules undergo a cycle of disassembly and re-emerge into the mitotic spindle (**2**)[179].

Intermediate filaments are divided biochemically and immunologically into five different types. Vimentin filaments are those of the fibroblast. These form a reticular arrangement in the cytoplasm. Reorganization of intermediate filaments is also reported during the cell cycle and when treated by cytostatic drugs such as colchicine and cytochalasins[180].

DERMATOLOGICAL SIGNIFICANCE

The observation of the behaviour and reorganization of the cytoskeleton is useful for studying cellular functions and the transmembrane interaction between cells and extracellular matrix for wound healing or for several skin diseases caused by metabolic or secretory disorders.

TECHNICAL POINTS

After fixation with cold methanol, specimens are treated with 0.5% Triton X-100, which eliminates unnecessary cell membrane and cytoplasm, and are stained with specific antibodies to each protein-forming cytoskeletons. Recently, fluorescent phalloidin or the antibodies to tropomyosin, heavy meromyosin or α-actinin have been widely used to visualize actin filaments[181].

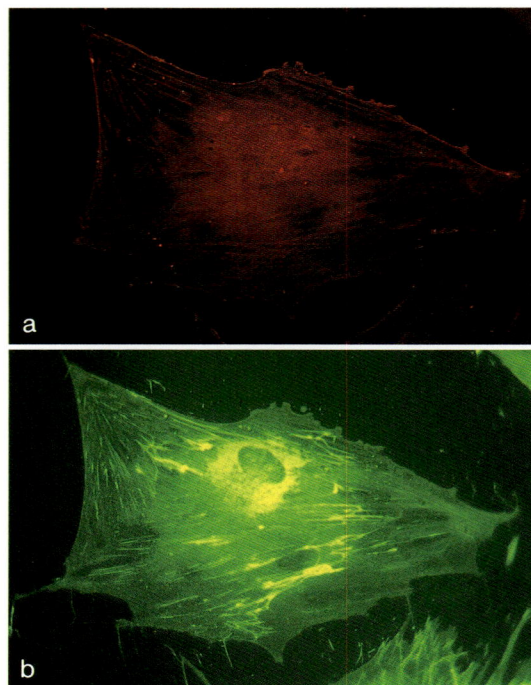

Fig. 1. Double-labelled immunofluorescence staining of cultured human fibroblasts with rhodamine-conjugated anti-actine (a) and FITC-labelled anti-fibronectin (b). Many stress fibres correspond to fibronectin fibrils.

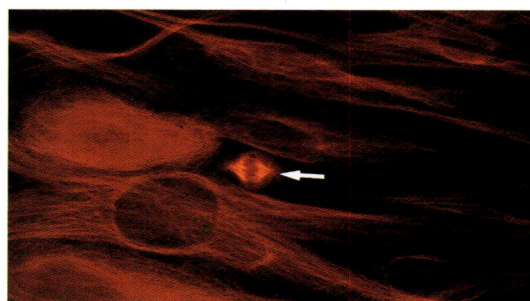

Fig. 2. Microtubules stained with anti-tubulin display fibrous arrays and mitotic spindle in the bipolar fibroblasts.

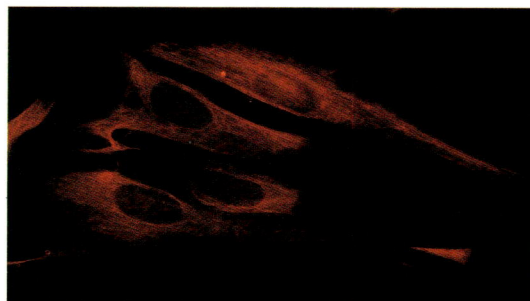

Fig. 3. Vimentin intermediate filaments stained with anti-vimentin spread fine meshworks.

INTRODUCTION

Fibroblasts synthesize and secrete various collagens, fibronectin, and proteoglycans, which have a close relationship to the biological functions of the extracellular matrix. Recent studies have shown that fibroblasts have membrane receptors for the third complement component (C3)[182] and synthesize all three subcomponents (Clq, Clr and Cls) of the first complement component (C1)[183, 184]. Consequently, it is suggested that fibroblasts participate closely and quite directly in immunological phenomena in connective tissue disorders.

FINDINGS

C3 receptor. Normal fibroblasts adhere to sensitized sheep red cells coated with C3, and form so-called 'C3-rosettes' (**1a**). The adherence, in the higher magnification of scanning microscopy, has been found to be carried out by fine cytoplasmic processes of fibroblasts, or C3 receptors[185] (**1b**).

Synthesis and secretion of subcomponents of C1. Normal fibroblasts synthesize and secrete all sub-components (Clq, Clr and Cls) of C1. The Clq molecule secreted by fibroblasts has a higher molecular weight than that in serum[184].

DERMATOLOGICAL SIGNIFICANCE

The biological significance of the presence of C3 receptors on the fibroblast membrane is so far unknown. These C3 receptors, however, possibly play a very important part in localizing harmful agents, such as immune complexes. If so, C3 receptors on fibroblasts also participate in the initial stages of causing immune complex diseases.

The synthesis of Clq in skin has been reported to be enhanced by physical stimuli[183].

TECHNICAL POINTS

C3-rosette formation by cultured fibroblasts can be observed easily but only in early cultures. Synthesis of Clq can be best observed immunohistologically in mildly fixed fibroblasts.

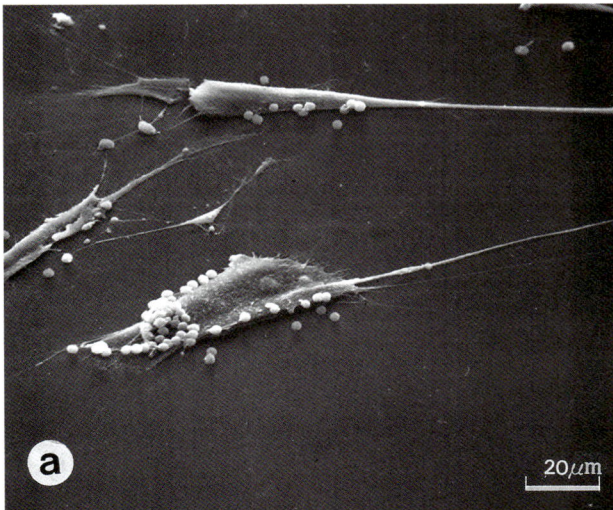

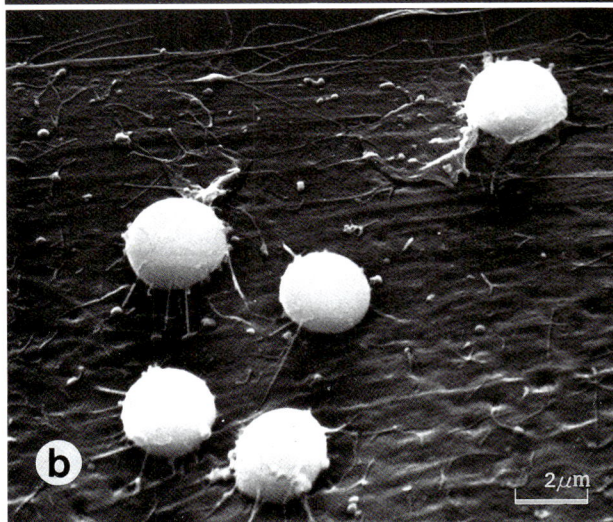

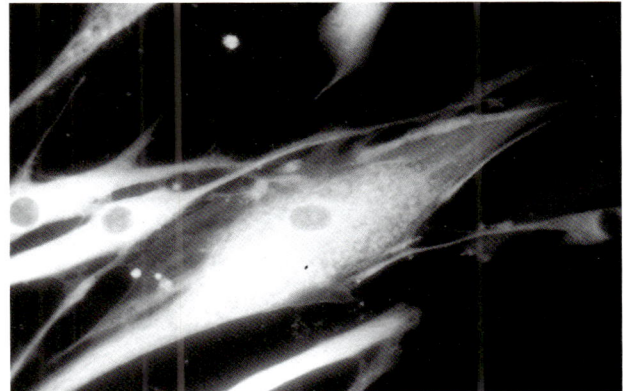

Fig. 2. Location of Clq in cultured human fibroblasts. The cells were treated with fluorescein-labelled antibody to human Clq.

Fig. 1. Scanning electron micrograph of C3-rosette. (This phenomenon may be related to viral infection.)
a. Rosette formation by cultured human fibroblasts and sensitized sheep red cells coated with C3.
b. Binding sites between these cells.

45

Vascular endothelial cells

INTRODUCTION

Vascular endothelial cells (ECs) originate from peripheral flat cells of blood islands that appear in the latter half of the third week of gestation as grouped mesenchymal cells which are derived from mesoderm. These primitive ECs form primitive blood vessels and then anastomose to form blood vessel networks. They connect to a heart germ that appears in the fourth week of gestation. After that, each vessel gradually matures and differentiates into an artery or vein.

Blood vessels serve many important functions for the preservation of tissue life, such as transportation and distribution of nutrition and hormones, gas exchange, exclusion of waste matter, blood coagulation and fibrinolysis. Furthermore, blood vessels have organ-specific characteristics. These functions are always performed through or on ECs. For these reasons, vascular ECs are considered as multifunctional cells with the various properties listed in Table I.

FINDINGS

Vascular ECs grow in a monolayer and have a cobblestone-like appearance (**1a**). For identification of ECs, antibodies against Factor VIII-related antigens (FVIIIRg) are widely used[186]. The staining pattern of FVIIIRg is granular in the cytoplasm or ECs (**1b**). Although localization of FVIIIRg occurs not only in ECs but also in megakaryocytes and platelets, it is possible to detect tissue blood vessels using this antibody (**2**)[187]. Immature ECs also have FVIIIRg, but in smaller amounts than in normal matured ECs. On the other hand, malignant ECs lose the capacity for vascular formation and do not express FVIIIRg (**3a**).

Ulex europaeus agglutinin I (UEA I) lectin is well known[188] as another useful marker for vascular ECs. UEA I binds specifically to alpha-L-Fucose residues on ECs. These fucose residues are factors of antigen determination for the ABO blood group. The staining is not affected by the blood group type of the tissue donor. Thus malignant ECs can be identified (**3b**).

It is highly important to distinguish blood vessels from lymphatics by using these markers. Lymphatic ECs are partially stained by using both anti-FVIIIRg and UEA I. The staining pattern for lymphatic ECs is different to that of vascular ECs which stain uniformly[189].

Fibrinolysis is one of the important functions of vascular ECs. Following the report of Todd[190], ECs have become recognized as synthetic cells of plasminogen activators. Immunohistocytologically, plasminogen activators are observed in vascular ECs[191], and also in lymphatic ECs (**4**).

In normal tissue, complement components do not bind to ECs, but after treatment with a detergent, complement binding sites appear on ECs (**5**)[192], although these are not EC-specific. Binding of complement components except Clq is inhibited by the action of EDTA and EGTA. Depositions of Clq and C4 are not observed when C4-deficient serum is used as the complement source. Taken together, it is possible that complement is activated on ECs independent of immunoglobulins and immunocomplexes[192]. This complement-binding activity is still preserved in malignant ECs (**6**).

DERMATOLOGICAL SIGNIFICANCE

Microvascular vessels in skin have been investigated by various methods[193]. ECs composing microvascular vessels have angiogenetic activity to promote granulation and tumour growth. On the other hand, their injury brings about tissue damage. Their existence is relevant to the appearance of many skin diseases; it is valuable, therefore, to identify vascular ECs, to discuss their differentiation or malignancy, and to examine immunohistocytologically several functions and activities of ECs. Recently, methods of culturing micro-

TABLE I   PROPERTIES OF VASCULAR ENDOTHELIAL CELLS

1 MORPHOLOGY	Monolayer
	Cobblestone-like appearance
	Weibel-Palade body
	Pinocytic vesicle
	Basement membrane
2 PRODUCTS	Factor VIII-related antigen
	von Willebrand factor
	ABO blood group antigen
	HLA-DR antigen
	Angiotensin covering enzyme
	Alkaline phosphatase
	Xanthine oxidase
	Fibrinolysis activators and inhibitors
	Collagenase
	Fibronectin
	Collagen (type I, III, IV, V)
	Prostacyclin (PGE_1 & E_2, PGI_2)
	Thrombospondin
3 RECEPTORS OR BINDING ACTIVITIES	Insulin
	Oestrogen
	Histamine
	Low density lipoprotein
	Ulex europaeus agglutinin I lectin
	Complement components (Clq, C4, C3)

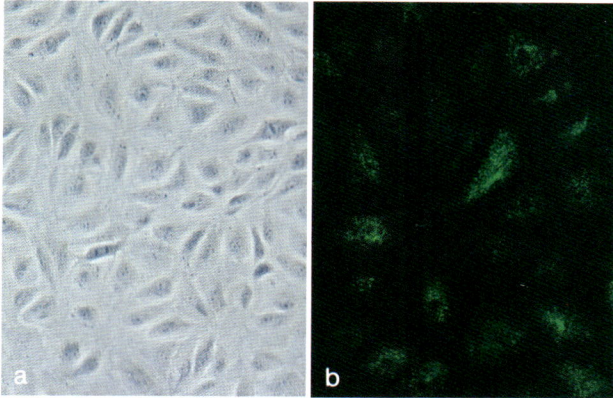

Fig. 1a. Cultured human microvascular ECs from adult skin.
(× 400) **1b.** Factor VIII-related antigen or cultured
microvascular ECs. (× 320, immunofluorescence method)

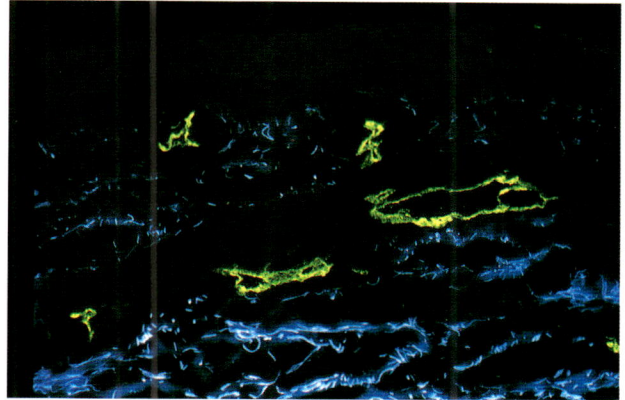

Fig. 2. Factor VIII-related antigen in normal skin. (× 160,
immunofluorescence method)

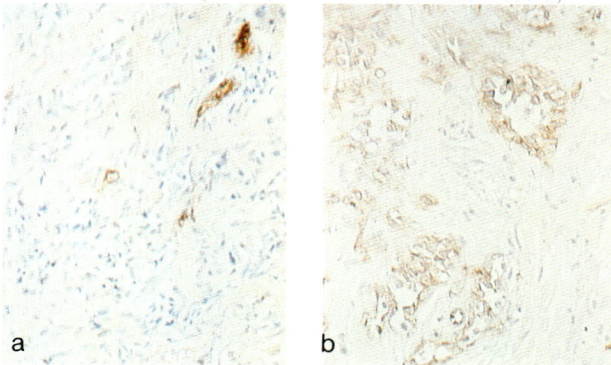

Fig. 3a. Factor VIII-related antigen in malignant
haemangioendothelioma. (× 200, PAP method)

Fig. 3b. UEA 1 binding sites in malignant
haemangioendothelioma. (× 200, PAP method by Dr. Yuhsuke
Suzuki, Kitasato University)

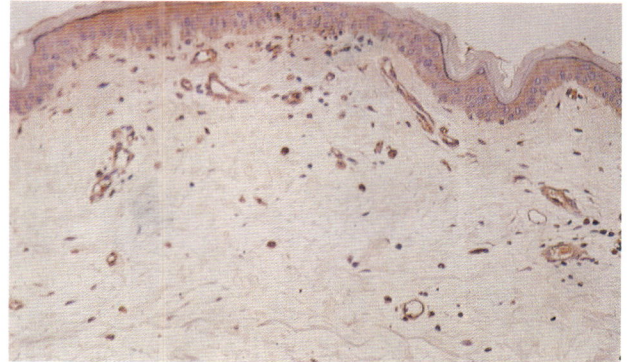

Fig. 4. Localization of tissue plasminogen activator in normal
skin. (× 200, ABC method)

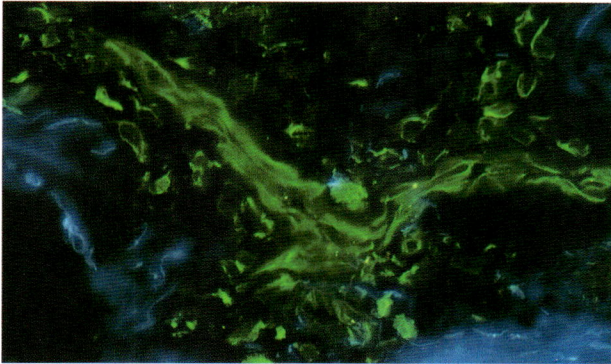

Fig. 5. Clq binding sites in vascular ECs at subpapillary plexus.
(× 600, immunofluorescence method)

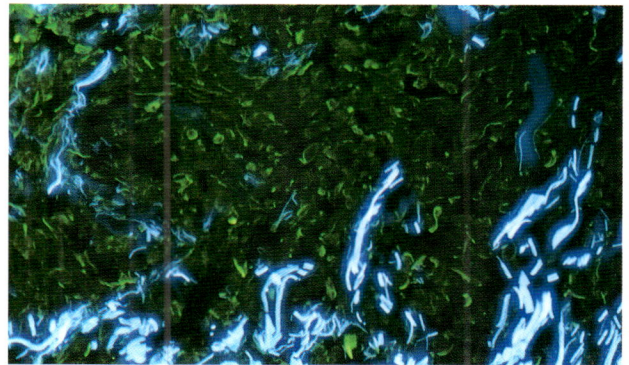

Fig. 6. Clq binding sites in malignant hemangio-endothelioma.
(× 600, immunofluorescence method)

vascular ECs from skin have been established[194]. Specific
markers to investigate specific functions and properties of
cutaneous microvascular ECs are anticipated in the future.

TECHNICAL POINTS

To preserve antigenicity, fresh frozen tissue sections should
be used as the substrate for immunofluorescent methods.
Paraffin sections are good for detecting the localization of
FVIIIRg and UEA I binding sites using enzyme-labelled

antibody methods (PAP method and ABC method). In order
to observe complement component binding, it is necessary
to pre-treat the fresh frozen sections with NP-40 detergent
for expression of binding sites, following fixation with
paraformaldehyde[192]. Antibodies against plasminogen activators and angiotensin converting enzyme are now available
for the demonstration of vascular ECs[191, 195].

47

Nerve cells

INTRODUCTION

In the peripheral nerve system, sensory and autonomic nerves are innervated to maintain a constant state. Sensory nerves possess free nerve endings and, in a few areas, characteristic end-organs which are called Meissner's corpuscles and Pacinian corpuscles. Autonomic nerves, driven by the sympathetic nervous system, supply the blood vessels, arrector pili muscles and sweat glands. Nerve fibres are composed of myelinated or unmyelinated axons covered with Schwann cells, and surrounded by an endoneurium. The cutaneous innervation has been demonstrated by light microscopy using methylene blue and silver staining[196]. Recently, histochemical techniques have been used for cutaneous specimens to demonstrate acetylcholinesterase[197], which is thought to be a marker for cholinergic nerves, and to demonstrate formaldehyde-induced histo-fluorescence in adrenergic nerves[198].

S-100 protein[199], which is soluble in 100% ammonium sulphate at neutral pH, has been demonstrated immunohistochemically in glia of the central nervous system, in glial cells of the peripheral ganglia and in Schwann cells of the cutaneous nerves[200]. Neuron-specific enolase (NSE) is the most acidic isoenzyme of enolase, and was originally described as 14-3-2 protein[201]. NSE is present in the neurons of the central and peripheral nervous systems and the neuroendocrine (APUD) system[202]. Immunohistochemical staining of S-100 protein and NSE is performed for the demonstration of the peripheral nervous system and for the differentiation of neural tissue tumours.

FINDINGS

Normal skin[203, 204]. Since Schwann cells possess a significant amount of S-100 protein, nerve fibres are strongly positive for S-100 protein and can easily be differentiated from connective tissue (**1**). In a transverse section of rat sciatic nerve the perikaryon of Schwann cells surrounding the myelinated axons shows a strong positive reaction (**2**). Axons and the myelin sheath are devoid of S-100 protein. As regards NSE, axons are positive, and the myelin sheath and Schwann cells are negative (**3**). S-100 protein and NSE-positive nerve fibres are differentiated from muscles on the arrector pili muscles. The network of fine nerve fibres which surround the eccrine glands are recognized with NSE (**4**). Meissner's corpuscles and Pacinian corpuscles of the digits are S-100 protein and NSE positive. Lamellar cells of Meissner's corpuscles, which originate from Schwann cells, are S-100 protein positive. The axon enters the Meissner's corpuscle from the bottom side and the spirals of axons are clearly stained with NSE (**5**). The lamellar cells of Pacinian corpuscles are devoid of NSE and S-100 protein. Inner core cells of Pacinian corpuscles, which originate from Schwann cells, are S-100 protein positive and NSE negative (**6**). NSE-positive reaction products are present only on axons which are within the centre of inner core cells.

Tissue pathology[205, 206]. Since denervation of the peripheral nerve causes the degeneration of nerve fibres, nerve axons, including the Meissner and Pacinian corpuscles, are devoid of NSE. However, S-100 protein remains on the Schwann cells, the lamellar cells of Meissner's corpuscles and the inner core cells of the Pacinian corpuscles.

S-100 protein and NSE are present on Schwann cells

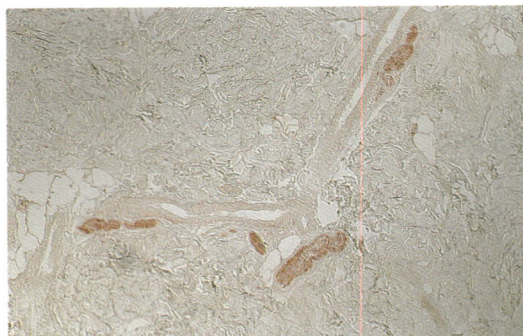

Fig. 1. S-100 protein staining of nerve fibres in the dermis. (× 50)

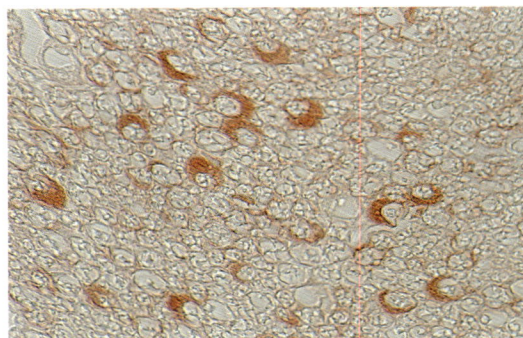

Fig. 2. Transverse section of rat sciatic nerve (S-100 protein). (× 400)

and axons of the peripheral nerves, respectively. S-100 protein and NSE staining are useful markers for the differential diagnosis of neural tissue tumours. Tumour cells of Schwannoma are strongly positive for S-100 protein and negative or weakly positive for NSE (**7**). The spindle cells of neurofibroma are S-100 protein positive, and NSE-positive axons are also present in the tumour nest (**8**). In the case of neuroma, the large nerve bundles and Meissner corpuscle-like structures are both S-100 protein and NSE positive (**9**).

TECHNICAL POINTS

Antibodies against S-100 protein and NSE are commercially available. For immunohistochemical staining, formalin-fixed specimens should be used with the PAP or ABC method.

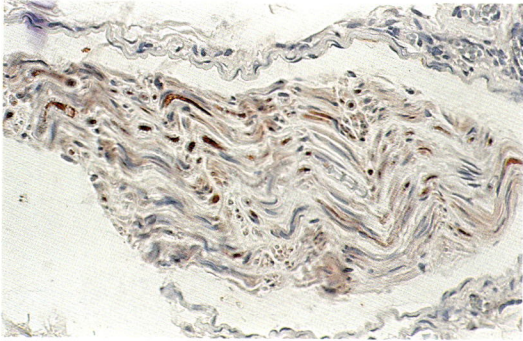

Fig. 3. NSE staining of nerve fibres. Myelin sheath is devoid of NSE. (× 400)

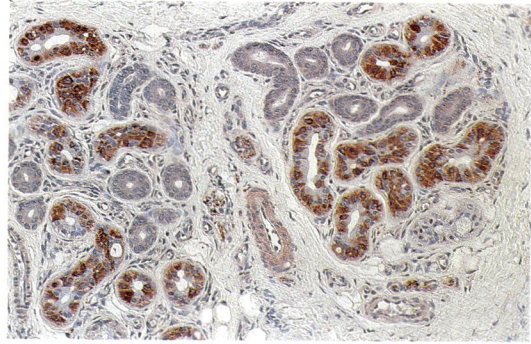

Fig. 4. NSE-positive nerve fibres are surrounded on the sweat glands. Secretory portions of the eccrine glands are also NSE positive. (× 50)

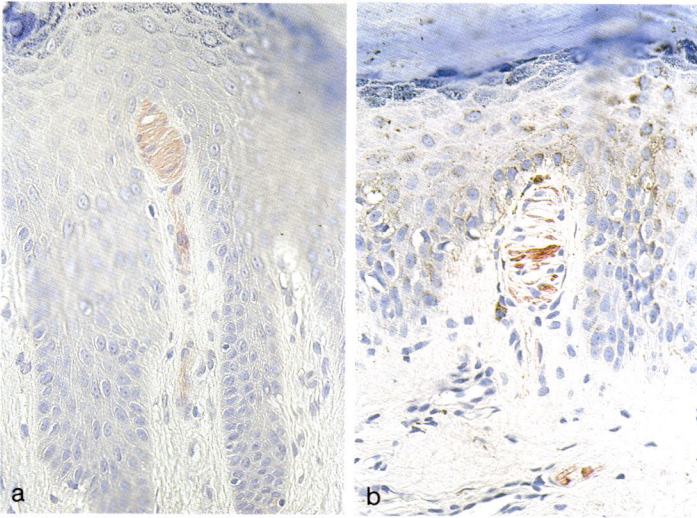

Fig. 5. Meissner's corpuscle. (× 400)
a. S-100 protein is positive in the lamellar cells.
b. NSE is present in an axon.

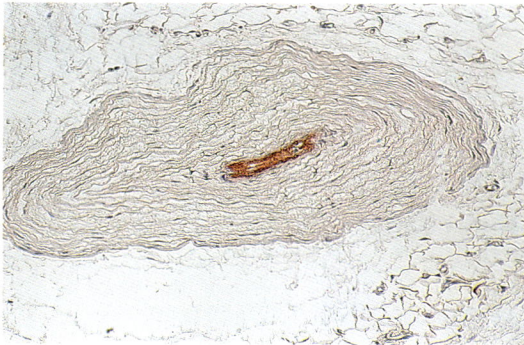

Fig. 6. Inner core cells of Pacinian corpuscle are S-100 protein positive. (× 50)

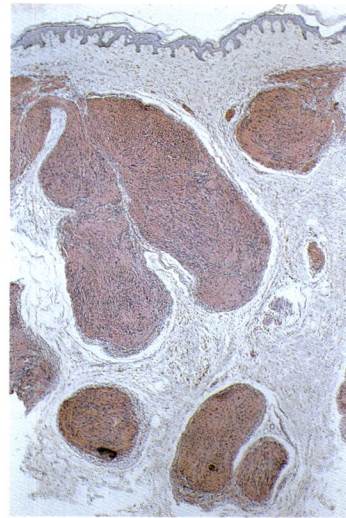

Fig. 7. Schwannoma. (S-100 protein) (× 25)

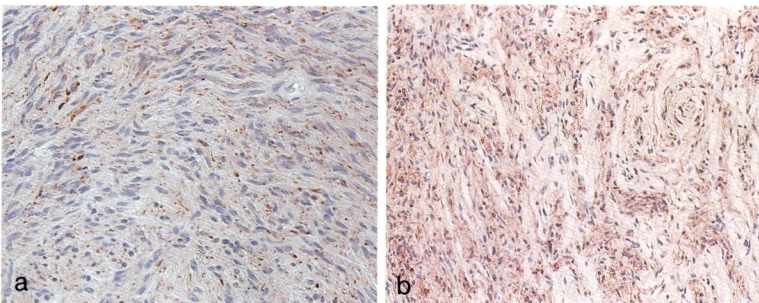

Fig. 8. Neurofibroma. (× 200)
a. S-100 protein.
b. NSE.

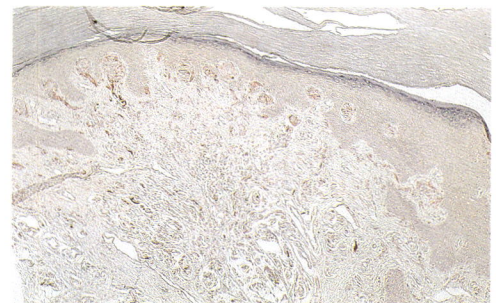

Fig. 9. Neuroma. (NSE) (× 50)

Subsets of infiltrated lymphocytes in the skin

INTRODUCTION

Lymphocytes, which are the principal immunologically competent cells, consist mainly of T and B cells and some T and B cell subsets. Previously, E-receptors, Fc receptors, C3 receptors, surface immunoglobulin and hetero-antisera have been used to analyze the functional subsets of lymphocytes.

Monoclonal antibodies (MoAb), which are generated by hybridoma technology, recognize differentiation antigens on the surface of distinct T cells, B cells, or other immunologically competent cells. The utilization of MoAb with immunohistochemical techniques is useful for identifying the distribution of lymphocyte subsets in the skin, and possibly for probing the interaction of lymphocyte subsets with other cells, such as cancer cells or other immunologically competent cells (e.g., Langerhans cells, monocytes, natural killer cells).

Because there is a wide variety of dermatoses with an immune system disturbance involved in the pathogenesis, it is important to investigate the subsets of infiltrated lymphocytes in the skin. The specificities of the representative MoAb are shown in Table I.

FINDINGS

The results regarding the predominance of T cell subsets reported to date are summarized in Table II and our data are shown in figures 1–8.

DERMATOLOGICAL SIGNIFICANCE

It is considered that an immune system disturbance is of importance to the pathogenesis of a wide variety of dermatoses. Therefore, detailed immunohistochemical studies of lymphocyte subsets will facilitate the analysis of that pathogenesis.

TECHNICAL POINTS

Immunoperoxidase methods using MoAb are commonly employed for tissue analysis of lymphocyte subsets. Fresh-frozen cryostat sections and acetone fixation are used almost exclusively. Recently it has been reported that some MoAb label cell surface antigens by the use of a modified processing technique with formaldehyde-fixed paraffin-embedded sections[219].

TABLE I   MONOCLONAL ANTIBODIES USED IN CHARACTERIZING LYMPHOCYTE SUBSETS

MONOCLONAL ANTIBODIES	SPECIFICITY
OKT 3[a], LEU-1[b]	Peripheral blood T cells, Thymocytes
OKT 4[a], Leu-3a[b]	Helper/inducer T-subset
OKT 8[a], Leu-2a[b]	Cytotoxic/suppressor T-subset
OKT 6[a]	Common thymocytes, Langerhans cells
OKT 11[a]	E-rosetting lymphocytes, Thymocytes
OKI a1[a], HLA-DR[b]	B cells, monocytes, macrophages, Langerhans cells, activated T cells
OKB 7[a], B1[c]	B cells, B cell lymphomas
HNK1 (Leu-7)[b], Leu-11[b]	K and NK cells

[a]OrthoDiagnostic System Inc.
[b]Becton-Dickinson, Monoclonal Center Inc.
[c]Coulter Electronics

TABLE II   PREDOMINANCE OF T CELL SUBSETS IN VARIOUS DERMATOSES[207–218]

helper/inducer T cell predominant	DLE, lichen planus, psoriasis vulgaris, erythema multiforme, atopic dermatitis, contact dermatitis, PPD reaction, mycosis fungoides, Sézary syndrome, granuloma annulare, alopecia areata, adult T cell leukaemia, tuberculoid leprosy (within the granuloma), sarcoidosis (within the granuloma), basal cell carcinoma
suppressor/cytotoxic T cell predominant	SLE, graft-versus-host disease, tuberculoid leprosy (periphery of the granuloma), sarcoidosis (periphery of the granuloma), squamous cell carcinoma

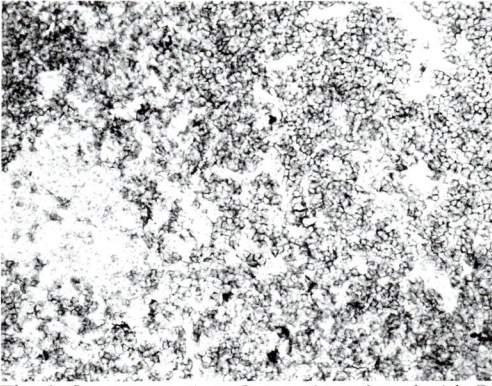

Fig. 1. Cryostat section of a tonsil incubated with OKT 3. Many positively stained cells are observed in the paracortical and interfollicular areas. (× 200)

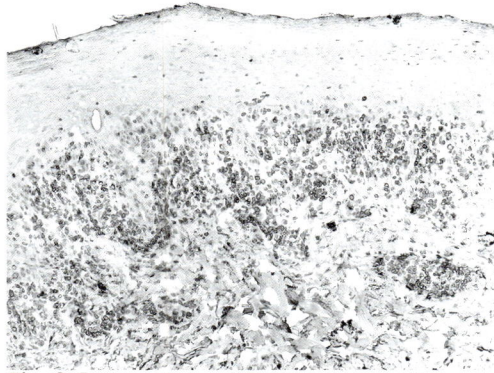

Fig. 2. Lichen planus. OKT 4-positive cells in upper dermis. (× 100)

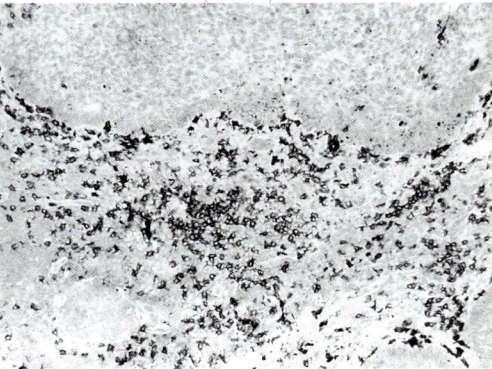

Fig. 3. Basal cell carcinoma (BCC). Many OKT 4-positive cells surround BCC. (× 100)[218]

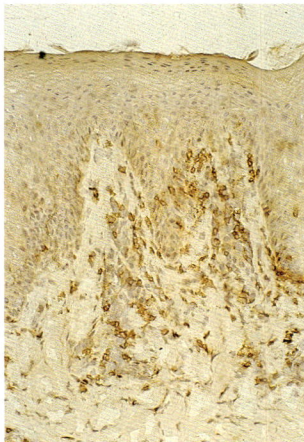

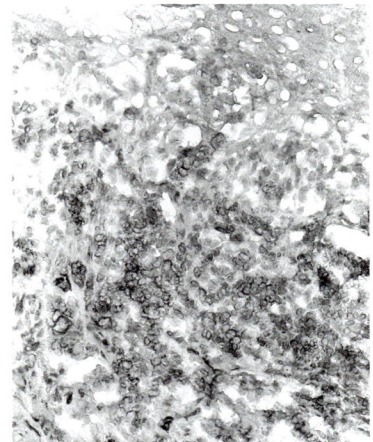

Fig. 4. Systemic lupus erythematosus. OKT 8-positive cells infiltrated the dermis and epidermis. (× 100)

Fig. 5. Discoid lupus erythematosus. OKT 4-positive cells in the dermis. (× 200)

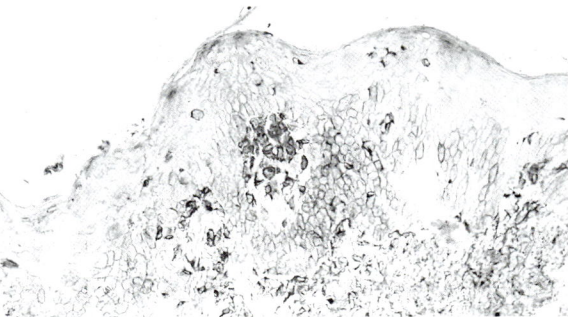

Fig. 6. Mycosis fungoides. HLA-DR antigen demonstrated on the surface of keratinocytes. (× 100)

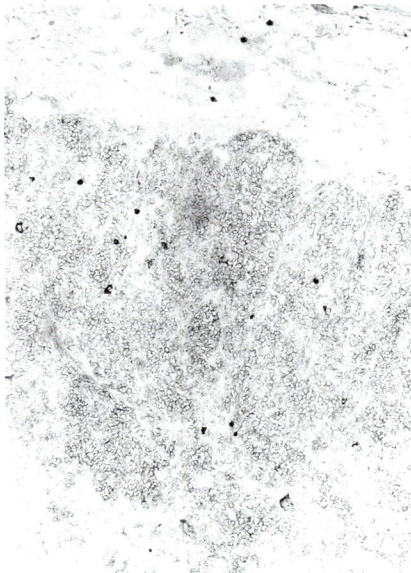

Fig. 7. Adult T cell leukaemia. Most of the atypical infiltrates reacted with OKT 4. (× 100)

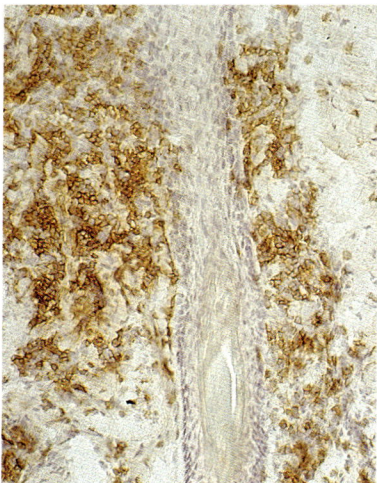

Fig. 8. Alopecia areata. Many OKT 4-positive cells surround the hair follicle. (× 200)

Synopsis

At the outset

Ground substance (Interstitium) is an extracellular matrix constituting the intercellular space of the connective tissue developed from the mesenchyme. This substance is distributed in all tissues and organs of the body, functioning not only as a mechanical supporting tissue for the suitable physiological manifestation of individual locomotive organs and tissues, but also as a medium through which water, ions, all nutrients and metabolic products pass in transit between the blood and the cells of the body.

Recent advances in the research of extracellular matrix have shown the existence of tissue-specific and structurally different collagen molecules in the body (10 types so far) as major fibrous components of the ground substance. Furthermore, among structural glycoproteins, the presence of cell-adhesive components, which are also tissue-specific and function as a scaffolding between the cells and surrounding tissue constituents, has been described. These findings strongly suggest that the ground substance plays an important role *in vivo* in regulating functions of the cells as their microenvironment[220], and may further provide us with an invaluable clue in studies on the pathophysiology of matrix-related diseases, together with accumulating information on the cell responses (expressions of matrix components) to individual humoral factors such as cytokines and growth factors. Thus, the resulting information will make it possible in future for us to diagnose pathogenic or normalizing factor(s) for the cell environments concerned through the analysis of the respective lesions.

Constituting components

COLLAGEN

Collagen is a family of fibrous proteins with common structural features that provide an extracellular framework for all multicellular animals, and accounts for some one-third of total body protein. A collagen molecule is composed of three polypeptide chains (known as α-chains) forming a characteristic triple helical structure.

Each constituent α-chain, which is composed of the approximately 1,000 residues for the helical region of fibrous collagen, can be expressed by $(Gly-X-Y)_{333}$, where glycine occupies every third residue, and X and Y are residues other than glycine. In mammals, the X positions are often occupied by prolyl residues and the Y positions by hydroxyprolyl or alanyl residues. Amino acid residues occupying the remaining X and Y positions depend on the tissue source of collagen and aminal species, such as collagen fibres in the skin and cartilage, which reflect tissue-specific properties.

Biosynthesis[220, 221]. Collagen is synthesized on the ribosome of the producing cell as pre-pro α-chain, which contains a short hydrophobic prepeptide at the extreme amino terminus and two non-collagenous polypeptide extensions at both amino terminal and carboxy terminal ends of the triple helical region composed of (Gly-X-Y)n. During the biosynthetic process within the cell, each pro α-chain is subject to the following 6 different modifications before helix formation: (i) hydroxylation of proline (mainly at 4th position, and much less at 3rd position), (ii) hydroxylation of lysine, (iii) addition of galactose to the OH group of certain hydroxylysines (-Hyl-Gal), (iv) likewise, addition of glucose to certain galactosyl residues of Hyl-Gal formed (-Hyl-Gal-Glc), and then procollagen thus formed is secreted extracellularly in the form of packing into a secretory granule. (v) procollagen is further processed with proteolytic cleavage of the extension peptides from the amino terminal end (by procollagen N-protease) and the C-terminal end (by procollagen C-protease) to form a collagen molecule which proceeds to fibril formation.

During this process, (vi) the ε-amino group of certain registered Lys and/or Hyl residues of collagen molecule is subjected to oxidative deamination by the action of lysyloxidase present in the matrix, being converted to aldehyde group, which preferentially takes part in cross-links formation, and thus the fibres become matured. The number of cross-links in collagen fibres in tissues increases with age. In summary, a collagen molecule is completed by translation of pre-pro α mRNA on the ribosome into pre-pro α-chain followed by several steps of modification. The levels of the enzymes involved in these processes differ from tissue to tissue, thus modifying collagen molecules for appropriate organization of tissues and organs to maintain tissue-specific, well-balanced physiological functions. In other words, once any defect occurs at some of these modification steps, a serious metabolic disease may result (e.g. Ehlers–Danlos syndrome). To clarify defect(s) in collagen metabolic disorders, immunohistochemical analysis and immunoassays of diseased tissues and cells using antibodies to individual collagens and related modification enzymes, as well as studies on collagen-type distribution, and quantitative and qualitative analyses of abnormal component(s) in the lesion, are recommended.

Polymorphism. At least ten genetically distinct types of collagen have been described by now, and more distinct types will be reported in future (**1**). Based on the cell types producing collagens, tissue distributions and functions of the collagens, these collagen types can be classified into (i) fibrillar collagen (type I, type II and type III), (ii) basement membrane collagen (type IV)[222, 223], and (iii) pericellular collagen (type V)[224].

Collagen types VI–X, which were recently described[225–9], distribute in tissues as minor constituents. Although only limited information is available with these collagens, the existence of type IX collagen[228], containing chondroitin sulphate in the cartilage and selective localization of type X collagen[229] in hypertrophic and calcifying hypertrophic cartilage reveals type specific functions of these collagens in the individual tissues.

(i) Fibrillar collagens: Type I, type II and type III collagens

Type I collagen   (the major component of tendon, sclera and
                     bone: ubiquitously distributes in skin and
                     many other tissues)
Type II collagen   (hyaline and elastic cartilage, vitreous body)
Type III collagen   (vascular system, immature tissues,
                     reticular fibres; widely distributed along
                     with type I collagen)

300 nm

Collagen fibres   FLS fibres (fibrous long spacing)   SLS fibres (segment long spacing)

Type IV collagen   (basement membrane of individual
                     tissues)[3, 4]

Monomer NC-1   Network structure: (1) 7-S collagen region
                                                                      (2) NC-1 (noncollagenous) region

H_2N-   400 nm $-COOH$

Tetramer

7S

60 nm

Type V collagen   (distributes in the cell surface and matrix of
                     placenta, muscle, skin, cartilage etc.)[5]

100 nm

Type VI collagen   (placenta, uterus, skin etc.)[6]

Monomer   Monomer

Dimer   Dimer

Tetramer   Tetramer

                                       75 nm
                                       30 nm

Filament
                   100 nm   75 nm   42 nm

                                       Filamentous structure of intima (type VI) collagen

Type VII collagen   (anchoring fibrils associated with
                     subepithelial basement membrane)[7]

                                       Pepsin   Long-chain collagen   Pepsin

                                                        Pepsin

                                       S   S
                                       S   P1   P2   S
                   100 nm   450 nm

Type IX collagen   (cartilage, embryonic avian cornea)[9]

HMW   LMW   HMW   LMW

                                                                    S-S
                                                                    S-S
                 100 nm
                                                  Pepsin   Bound with CS or DS

Type X collagen   (limited localization in hypertrophic and
                     calcifying hypertrophic cartilage)
150 nm

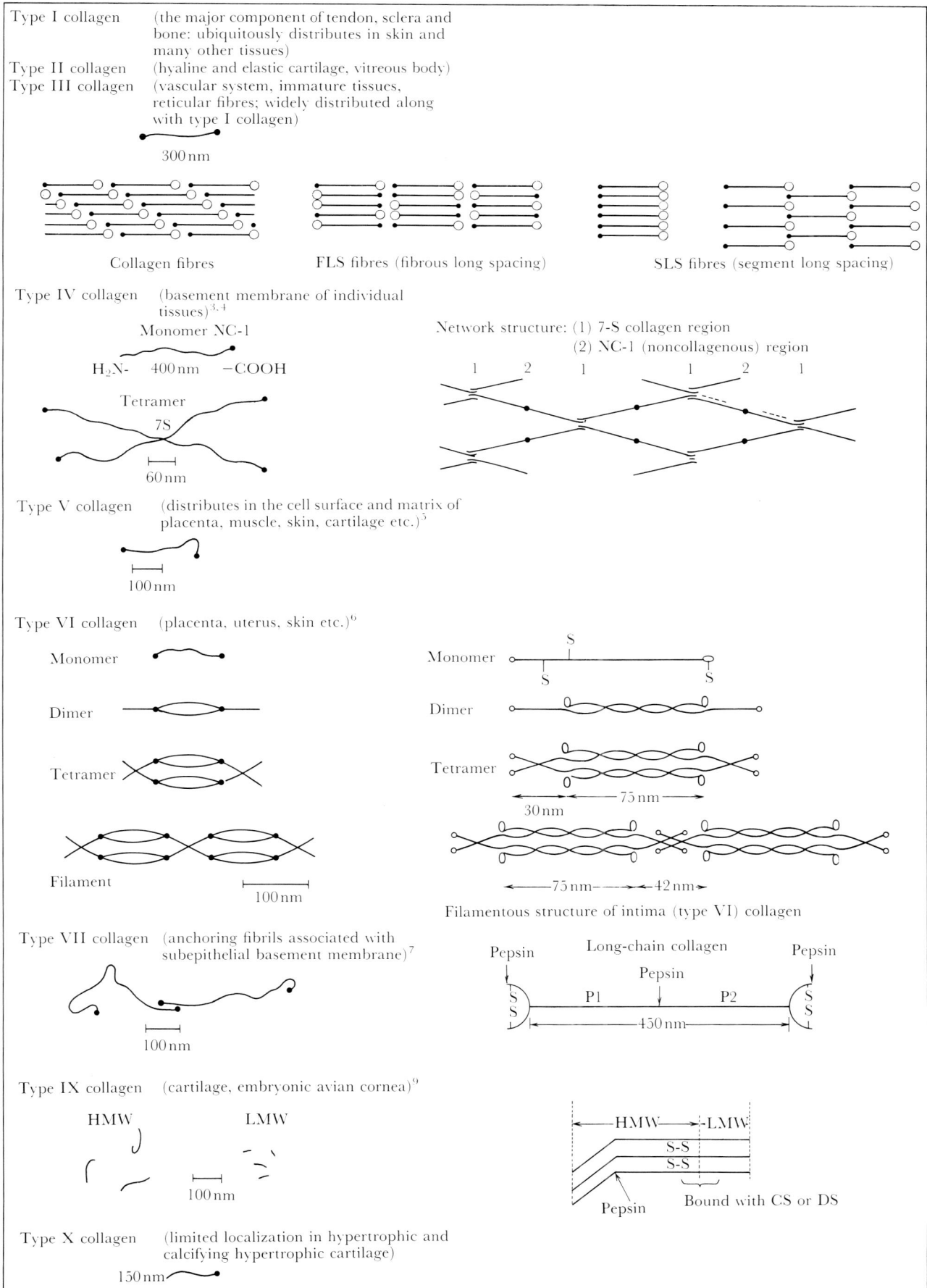

Fig. 1. Schematic diagrams of the molecular structure of various
types of collagen (type I to type X, except type VIII collagen),
as observed under electron microscopy (CS: chondroitin
sulphate; DS: dermatan sulphate).

53

distribute in tissues as fibrous forms with the same characteristic 64–67 nm periodicity, which is generated by the packing of the collagen molecules in a precise axial register of a unique quarter-stagger with overlap. This axial stagger has been precisely defined at 234±1 residues for type I collagen.

Type I collagen, [$\alpha 1(I)_2 \alpha 2(I)$], accounts for about 90% of total collagen in the body and is the major collagenous component of skin, tendon, sclera, bone, and cornea. This collagen appears to be not identical from tissue to tissue, suggesting type I collagen species are closely related products of a family of type I collagen genes[230]. Type II collagen, [$\alpha 1(II)_3$], is also reported to be a family of closely related molecules which are composed of structurally different α chains[231]. Type III collagen, [$\alpha 1(III)_3$], is widely distributed together with type I collagen in a variety of tissues including blood vessel walls. This type of collagen was first described to be foetal type collagen, because of its relatively dense distribution in foetal tissues. However, this can be explained by the increased accumulation of type I collagen in the tissues with age. Type III collagen was thought to be the main component of reticular fibres, since it forms fibrils of smaller diameter. However, reticular fibres also contain type I collagen.

(ii) Pericellular collagens[227-31]: Type V collagen [$\alpha 1(V)_2 \alpha 2(V)$] is distributed surrounding alveolar epithelium of the lung, as well as fibroblasts. This type of collagen can be isolated from placenta, cornea, skin, and blood vessels. A high content of type V collagen is observed in the media of atherosclerotic aorta.

ELASTIN[232]

Elastin fibres are composed of two distinct protein components, i.e. an amorphous elastin core having no distinct periodicity and a sheath of microfibrillar structures 10–13 nm in diameter which distributes in the surrounding region of the amorphous protein core. Elastin fibres constitute 2–5% of the dry weight of dermis, and are the most prominent components of the aorta (30–60%) and ligament nuchae (70–80%), and widely distributed in many other tissues. Elastin fibres can be easily identified by their characteristic tinctorial properties (e.g. with acid-orcein stain), and play a role in maintaining elasticity of the tissues. Amorphous elastin core, which is the predominant component of elastin fibres, contains glycine, alanine, proline and valine, which account for 80% of all the constituting amino acids, but lacks tryptophan, cysteine and methionine. The nature of the elastin core is very hydrophobic, as represented by a characteristic repeating structure of (Pro-Gly-Val-Gly-Val)$_n$. The fibrous elastin core is a polymer of tropoelastin (molecular weight: 72,000) synthesized by elastin-producing cells. When tropoelastin molecules associate to form a fibre, they do so in a way that a limited number of the 38 lysyl residues per molecule aligns at juxtaposition, and is subjected to oxidative deamination by lysyl oxidase of the ε-amino group of these registered lysyl residues, to form cross-links called desmosine and isodesmosine.

The resultant elastin fibres, therefore, are composed of β-spiral regions mainly responsible for elastomeric properties and of α-helical cross-linking regions responsible for fibrous structures to bind constituting tropoelastin molecules together. There is no evidence for the presence of elastin polymorphism so far.

PROTEOGLYCANS

Proteoglycans are complex macromolecules consisting of a core protein of varying size to which mucopolysaccharide (glycosaminoglycan, GAG) chains are covalently linked. In contrast to collagen, proteoglycans constitute only 0.1–3% of the dry weight of the tissues. However, the constituting polysaccharide chains, that is GAG (mostly composed of hexosamine and hexuronic acid), hold a large quantity of bound water, and the sulphate and carboxyl groups on the repeating disaccharide units of most of the GAG chains other than hyaluronic acid (HA) and chondroitin chains result in a high concentration of anionic charges. Thus, the proteoglycans are polyanions, which play a role in holding corresponding amounts of cations, occupy essentially all the interstitial space in the matrix, and serve as a barrier to prevent the escape of water and ions from the tissues.

HA and proteodermatan sulphate (PGDS) are the predominant GAG constituents in the skin[233]. Proteochondroitin 4-sulphate (PGCS) is also present in premature skins at foetal to juvenile stages. Relative ratios of DS content/HA content in the skin increases with age. PGDS consisting of a core glycoprotein (molecular weight: 56,000) linked with 1–4 chains of DS is distributed about the collagen fibrils[234], almost exclusively at the d band in the gap zone and seems to function to promote collagen fibrillogenesis. The ratio of DS content/collagen content is constant through the dermis[233]. The content of HA in papillary layer is higher than that in reticular layer. HA has a promoting function for cell proliferation. Proteoheparan sulphate (PGHS), which is derived from cell membrane and basement membrane, is also present in the skin. The GAG chains are known to show little antigenicity because of their repeating structure of disaccharide units. Therefore, it is recommended to use antibodies rather than individual core proteins of proteoglycans for their immunohistochemical localizations. However, it should be noted that a PGCS, carrying a structurally and antigenically related core protein to that of skin PGDS, has recently been isolated from articular cartilage[235].

CELL ADHESIVE SUBSTANCE

Cell adhesive substance is a group of glycoproteins found in connective tissue, which seems to be involved in the adhesion of fibroblasts and other cell types to their natural substrata in the tissues, and is composed of multi-domains to bind to cell membrane, collagen, proteoglycan and fibrin. The presence of tissue-specific cell adhesive substances such as fibronectin (fibroblasts)[236], chondronectin (chondrocytes)[237], laminin (epithelial cells)[238] has been described so far. These substances seem to be involved in the regulation of cell activities such as the proliferation, differentiation and locomotion of cells. Fibronectin (**2**) is not confined to the cell surface and tissues but occurs also in the blood plasma. Laminin (**3**) has a molecular weight of about 800,000 and, by rotary shadowing, has a flexible cross-like shape consisting of one long (75 nm) and three short (35 nm) arms. Laminin is composed of three subunits: the larger (the long arm of the cross) has a molecular weight of 400,000; the smaller subunits (the short arms) have molecular weights of 200,000 and are involved in the formation of the basement membrane as its constituent. Laminin binds to the epithelial cell at its cross-like region, to type IV collagen at its short arm terminal regions, and to PGHS at its long arm terminus[238]. Pathophysiological significance of laminin in the metastasis of carcinoma cells has recently been described, by the findings that the tumour cells, once bound to laminin, are stimulated to produce collagenase which degrades basement membrane (type IV) collagen.

Basement membrane

Basement membrane components include type IV collagen, laminin, PGHS and entactin (a glycoprotein containing sulphate group with a molecular weight of 158,000)[239]. Type IV collagen is synthesized by epithelial cells and cells resting on the basement membrane as a procollagen ([$\text{pro}\alpha 1(IV)_2 \, \text{pro}\alpha 2(IV)$]) which is secreted extracellularly and incorporated into basement membrane without cleavage of N-terminal and C-terminal propeptide extensions. Most of

Lys residues in both proα1(IV) and proα2(IV) chains are hydroxylated to form Hyl residues, as much as 90% of which are subjected to two step glycosylations to form Glc-Gal-Hyl. All these characteristic features of type IV collagen result in the prevention of the assembly of this particular collagen into the cross-banded fibres, but in the formation of a mesh-like membranous structure as shown in figure 4, where the C-terminal propeptide extensions of two collagen molecules bind together and the N-terminal propeptide extensions of four collagen molecules overlay together by forming S-S linkages. In this way, the mesh-like structure of type IV collagen, predominantly located in the lamina densa, may play a role in regulating the permeability of proteins and other macromolecules over a certain size. Electron microscopic observations show that both negatively charged PGHS and laminin are predominantly distributed in the outer layers (lamina rara) of basement membrane, in which laminin functions as a scaffolding of basal cells through its binding to the cell surface receptors. In summary, the basement membrane functions as a molecular sieve through the mesh-like structure of the constituting type IV collagen, and as an electrostatic regulator for the permeability of the constituents in blood and body fluids by the negatively charged groups of PGHS. Little is known about the physiological function of entactin at present.

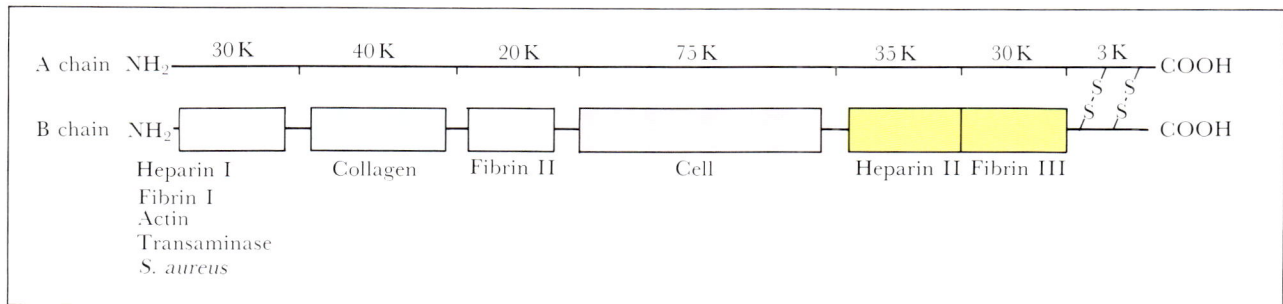

Fig. 2. A schematic diagram of fibronectin structure[236].
A chain, molecular weight 235 K, and B chain, molecular weight 230 K, are linked together at C-terminal region forming S-S bond. The molecule is composed of seven different multi-functional regions including the C-terminal S-S linkage region.

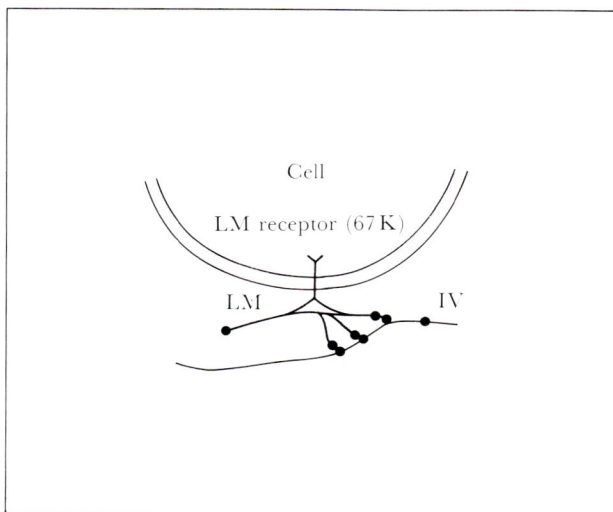

Fig. 3. A schematic diagram showing the mode of binding of laminin molecule with cell and type IV collagen[236,238].
Laminin molecule (LM) consisting of three short chains and one long chain binds with its receptor (molecular weight 67,000) on the cell membrane through the crossing region and with type IV collagen at the end region of individual short chains. While the end region of long chain has a high affinity with heparan sulphate proteoglycan (HSPG).

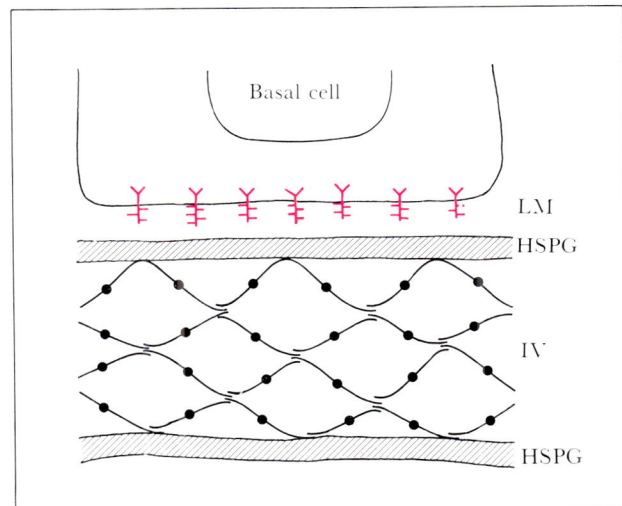

Fig. 4. A schematic diagram showing the structure of basement membrane[222,223,236].
Laminin (LM) receptor is located on the surface layer of the basal cell membrane; Laminin binds with its receptor and heparan sulphate proteoglycan (HSPG) as shown in Fig. 3. In addition, laminin distributes in lamina rara layer (showing diagonal line) as a main component which shows high affinity with mesh-like structures of type IV collagen (IV) and HSPG, while type IV collagen distributes in lamina densa forming mesh-like structure.

Laminin

CHARACTERIZATION

Basement membranes are extracellular structures containing both collagenous (type IV collagen) and noncollagenous glycoprotein (laminin, fibronectin, entactin, proteoglycan). Laminin, a noncollagenous basement membrane protein, plays a role in epithelial adhesion to type IV collagen, and is normally present in the dermo-epidermal junction, but not in the epidermis. Laminin may also have a role in cell differentiation and tissue morphogenesis.

In 1979, Timple et al. isolated laminin from Englebreth-Holm-Swarm sarcoma, a mouse tumour which produces basement membrane components[240]. Meanwhile, Chung et al. isolated laminin (GP-2) from cultured parietal endoderm cells[241]. Recently Sakashita et al. isolated laminin from mouse scrotal carcinoma cells (PFHR-9)[242], and Wewer et al. isolated laminin from yolk sac tumour of rat[243].

Foidart et al. reported that epithelial and endothelial cells in culture synthesize laminin and that laminin is localized to the lamina lucida of human epidermal basement membrane and mouse oesophagus endothelial basement membrane. (Immunoelectron microscopy study)[244].

Two distinct subunit chains had originally been found by SDS polyacrylamide gel electrophoresis under reducing conditions: 200–220 Kd subunit (A chain) and 400–440 Kd subunit (B chain)[245].

The whole laminin molecule when seen by rotary shadowing has an asymmetric cross-like configuration consisting of three identical short (35 nm) arms (220 Kd subunit) and one long (75 nm) arm (400 Kd subunit), linked by disulphide bonds at the centre of the cross[246].

FINDINGS

Normal skin. In immunohistological studies using purified antibody against laminin, laminin was localized with a continuous linear pattern in the dermo-epidermal junction, capillary (**1a**), and surrounding the hair follicles (**1b**), eccrine gland (**1c**) and peripheral nerves.

Abnormal skin. In nevus cell nevus, laminin is demonstrated as a continuous linear pattern around each cell (**2**). In the so-called mixed tumour cell, laminin is demonstrated in the basement membrane and around epithelial cells (**3**)[247]. In basal cell carcinoma, laminin is demonstrated as a continuous linear pattern between tumour nest and stroma (**4**), and in one type of basal cell carcinoma, laminin is seen within tumour nests (**5**)[248, 249]. In squamous cell carcinoma, laminin is demonstrated with linear patterns between tumour nests and stroma, and is also seen at the tumour invasive site.

Hashimoto et al. observed the location of laminin in bladder carcinoma and suggested that laminin is produced by carcinoma cells during the proliferation process and might assist the invasion and metastasis of carcinoma cells[250].

DERMATOLOGICAL SIGNIFICANCE

Functionally, laminin preferentially binds to cells, type IV collagen and proteoglycan. Laminin is a constituent of the basement membrane, and thus may play an important role in tumour proliferation, invasion and metastasis.

TECHNICAL POINTS

In immunofluorescent staining, frozen sections without fixation are the best, but for permanent storage, cold acetone fixation is suggested. It is also possible to use paraffin sections with the PAP and ABC methods.

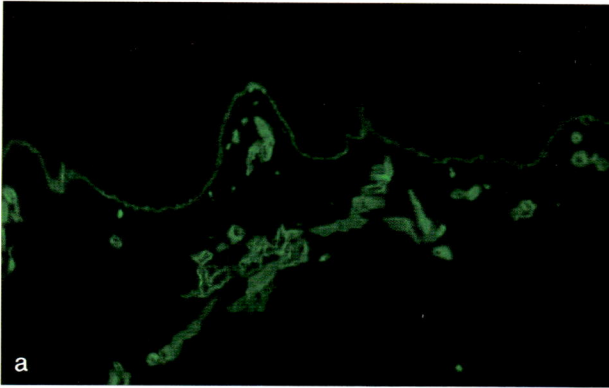

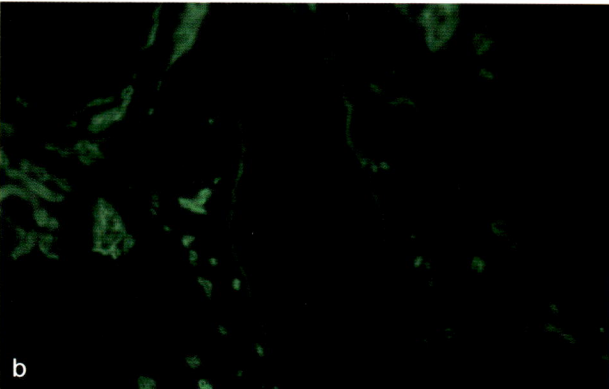

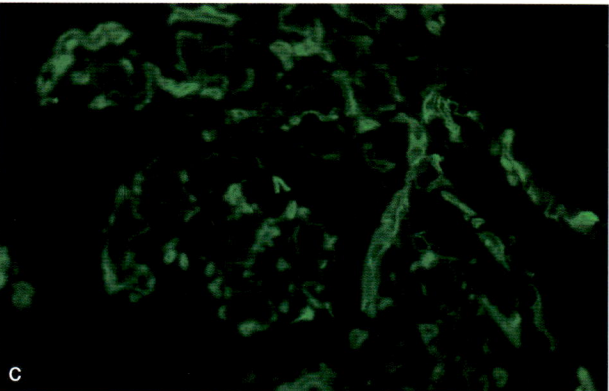

Fig. 1. Normal human skin.
(a) Anti-laminin antibody reveals intense linear fluorescence at the dermo-epidermal junction and in blood vessel walls (× 200), and (b) in hair follicles (× 500), and (c) in eccrine glands.(× 500)

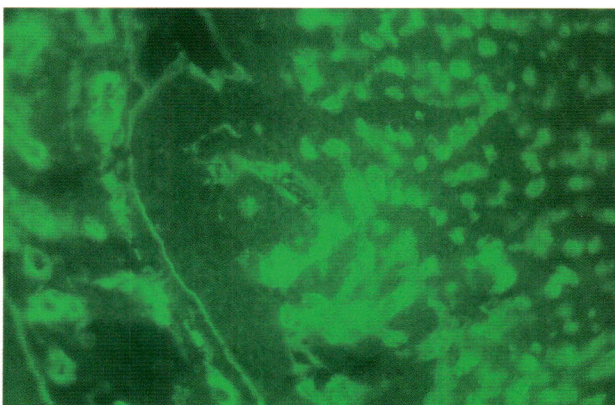

Fig. 5. Basal cell carcinoma.
Annular, granular, spongy fluorescence pattern within the tumour nests. (× 400)

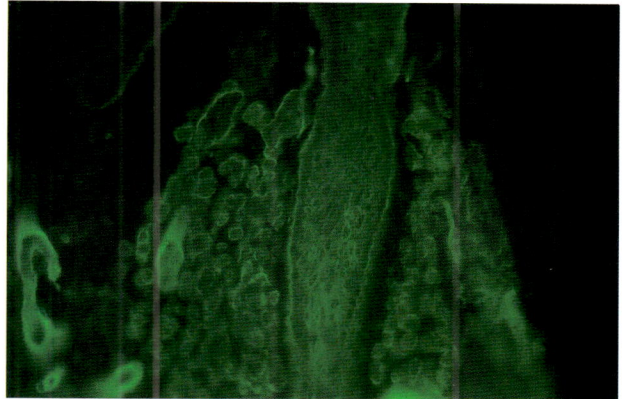

Fig. 2. Nevus cell nevus.
Anti-laminin antibody reveals intense linear fluorescence surrounding each tumour cell and tumour nest. (× 400)

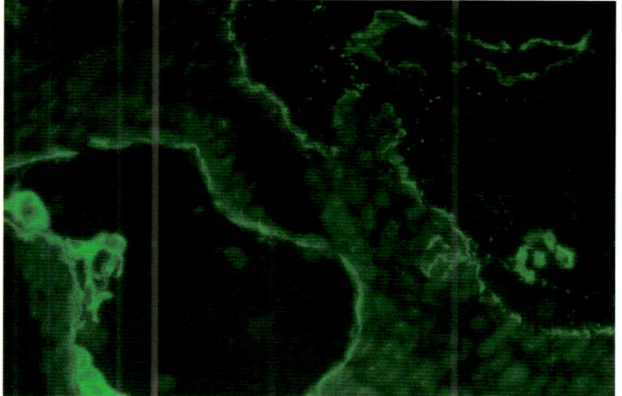

Fig. 3. Mixed tumour.
Anti-laminin antibody reveals intense linear fluorescence at the zone of basement membrane surrounding tumour and stroma. (× 400)

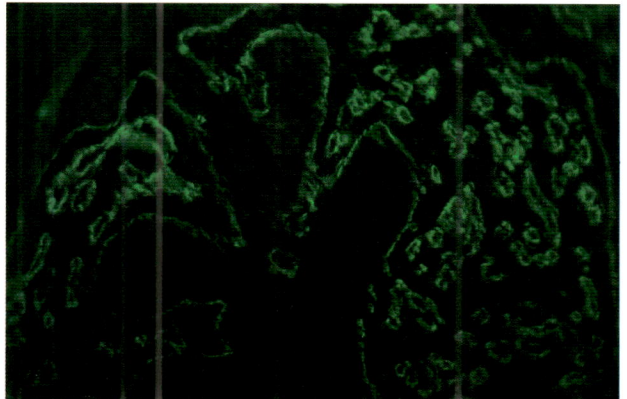

Fig. 4. Basal cell carcinoma.
Anti-laminin antibody reveals a discrete boundary of fluorescence surrounding all tumour nests. (× 200)

Fibronectin

INTRODUCTION

Fibronectin (FN), a high molecular weight glycoprotein of about 440,000 dalton, is synthesized and secreted by fibroblastic cells, endothelial cells, macrophages and other mesenchymal cells. FN is widely distributed in connective tissues, basement membrane and plasma. It is well known that FN has a special affinity to collagen, fibrin, heparin, hyaluronic acid, Clq and others.

FN plays an important role in multibiological activities, including cell to cell adhesion, cell to substrate adhesion, migration and differentiation of cells, maintenance of cellular structure, wound healing, blood coagulation and opsonic function[251]. There are two types of FN: cellular FN and plasma FN, which are immunologically similar but not identical[252]. Some biological activities and molecular structures vary between the two FN.

Using antihuman FN antibody, it is now possible to study the quantity and localization of FN in plasma and connective tissue. The localization of FN in skin diseases has been previously reported by Stenman et al.[253], Fyrand[254], Fleischmajor, et al.[255]. In the near future, investigation of the mechanism and physiological significance of FN may contribute to the treatment of various skin diseases. In this chapter, localization of FN in various dermatoses using an immunofluorescence technique is described.

FINDINGS

Normal human skin. It seems that FN is co-distributed with collagen, fibrin, hyaluronic acid and other three-dimensional structures in the skin. Immunologically, FN can be found linearly along the dermo-epidermal junction, and reticulated in the papillary dermis, vascular walls of papillary dermis (**1a**), and perifollicular spaces (**1b**), and intercalated between arrector pili muscle cells (**1c**) and along eccrine sweat glands (**1d**).

On the contrary, the cornified layer, epidermis and deep dermis did not show any specific FN immunofluorescence. FN was formed in the extracellular matrix secreted by cultured human fibroblasts (**2**). Recently human keratinocytes have been shown to synthesize, secrete and deposit FN in the pericellular matrix in vitro[257].

Various dermatoses. It has been suggested that there are both cellular and plasma FNs in inflammatory cutaneous changes. The intra-epidermal deposition of FN was found in eczematous changes including contact dermatitis and angiodermatitis. FN increased remarkably in the spongiosis and around perivesicular areas in contact dermatitis (**3**). The intercellular deposition of FN in the epidermis was demonstrated in pemphigus vulgaris, which is associated with the location of immunoglobulin and complement.

FN was observed in the thickened basement membrane zone of systemic lupus erythematosus and at the bottom of the bulla of bullous pemphigoid (**4**). It is suggested that these findings are due to the affinity between FN and Clq. In progressive systemic scleroderma tissue and morphoea tissue, FN was only faintly observed in the dermo-epidermal junction and papillary dermis. FN was sometimes found as a cytoplasmic distribution in the granular layer and in Munro's microabscess as a cytoplasmic distribution of psoriasis vulgaris (**5**). FN was also located on the crust and epidermis above the elongated papilla. These findings suggest that deposition of plasma FN is caused by inflammatory or exudative reactions within the lesion. FN is also easily detectable in perivascular walls of papillary dermis in angiodermatitis.

FN can be abundantly found as a linear, netformed or curling arrangement in the whole dermis of granulation tissues which develop immediately following injury, such as hypertrophic scar and keloid tissues (**6**). FN decreased gradually in the deep dermis of mature scar tissue and was found to resemble the localization of FN in normal skin[258]. In dermatofibroma, FN is also distributed conspicuously in the dermis (**7**).

FN may be localized along the newly synthesized immature collagen fibres from proliferative fibroblastic cells. There are no obvious inflammatory or exudative reactions in dermatofibroma, therefore the increased amount of FN may indicate mainly the increase in production of cellular FN from fibroblastic cells.

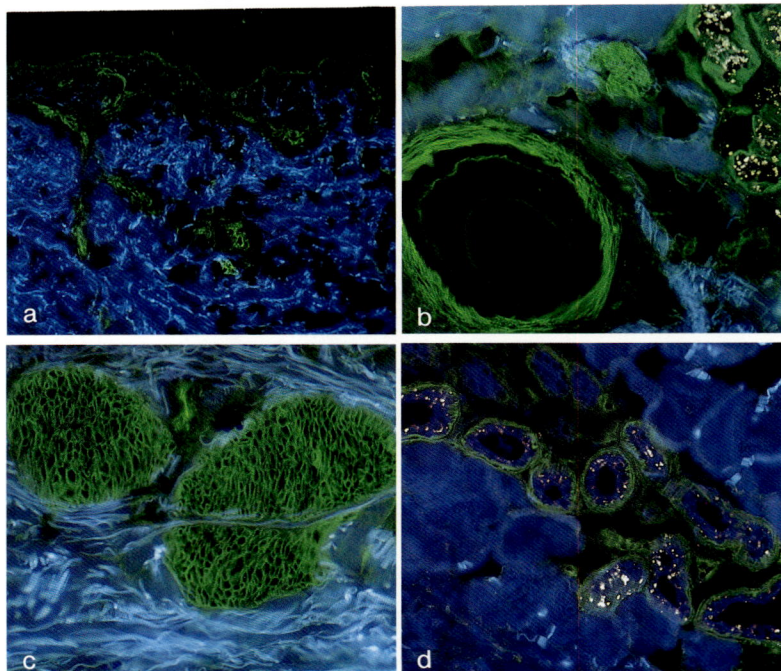

Fig. 1a. Normal human skin. FN on the dermo-epidermal junction in the papillary dermis, and on the vascular walls. (The indirect IF stain, × 100)

Fig. 1b. FN on the perifollicular spaces. (× 400)

Fig. 1c. FN on the cell membrane of arrector pili muscles. (× 400)

Fig. 1d. FN on the perieccrine sweat glands. (× 400)

Dermatological significance. The kinetics and pathological significance of FN in the skin lesion are still unknown. Further studies of plasma and cellular FN may clarify more pathophysiological functions in dermatological conditions. FN may play important roles not only in wound healing, but also in chemotaxis, inflammation and immune response against tumours.

Technical points. Using an immunofluorescent technique, the unfixed frozen sections gave the best results with clear localization. Postfixation of frozen sections did not give good results, with the exception of cold acetone fixation. In addition, fixation in 10% formaldehyde solution and 95% alcohol resulted in nonspecific staining and unclear localization of FN.

The biopsy specimens and frozen sections should be thoroughly washed in PBS before fixation to wash out the nonspecific deposits of plasma protein which contain plasma FN. The direct immunofluorescence method shows more specific distribution of FN than the indirect method. It is important to be aware of the cross-reaction between hetero-geneous IgG fractions, when the indirect method is used for tissue. Monoclonal anti-FN antibody and the enzyme-labelled antibody method using paraffin-embedded sections are also useful for FN studies.

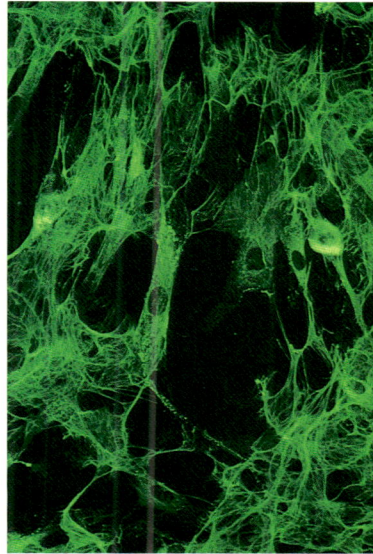

Fig. 2. FN is detectable in the pericellular matrix and cytoplasma of cultured human fibroblasts. (× 600)

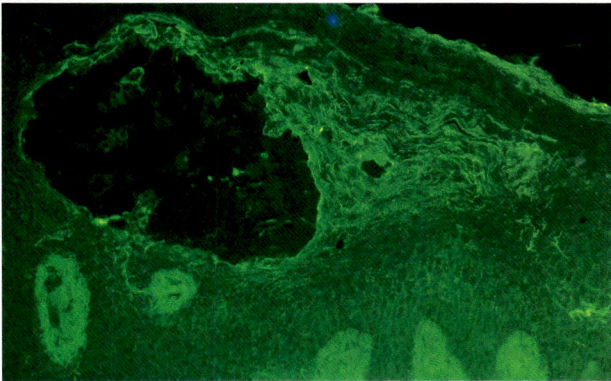

Fig. 3. Intra-epidermal deposition of FN in contact dermatitis, particularly in the spongiosis and perivesicular area. (× 200)

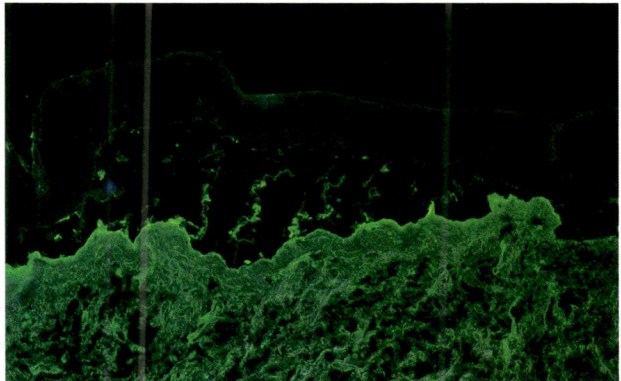

Fig. 4. Prominent deposits of FN in the bottom of the bulla of bullous pemphigoid. (× 200)

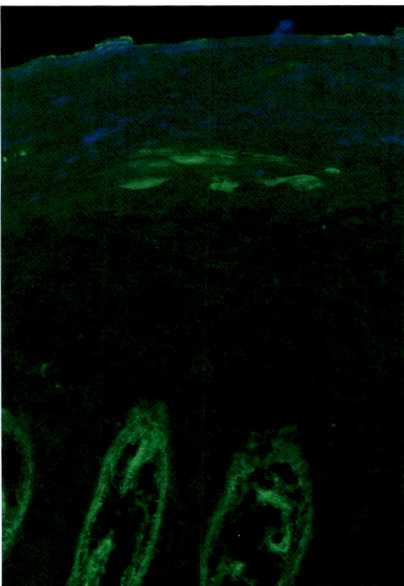

Fig. 5. In psoriasis vulgaris, FN is found in the intra-epidermal spaces as cytoplasmic distribution. (× 400)

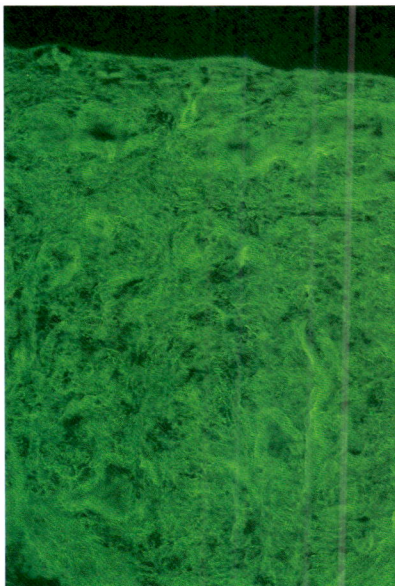

Fig. 6. FN is detected in the whole dermis of hypertrophic scar tissue. (× 200)

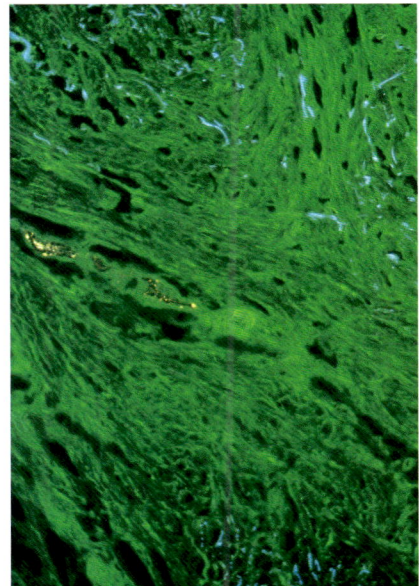

Fig. 7. FN, in a curling arrangement, is abundant in the dermis of dermatofibroma. (× 200)

Type I, III, V collagens

INTRODUCTION

To identify collagen-producing cells, Ooshima carried out an immunohistological study on the localization of the specific antiserum to prolyl hydroxylase[259]. The presence of this enzyme, which is involved in collagen biosynthesis, indicates a high possibility that the cell produces collagen. The study revealed positivity for this enzyme in vascular and uterine smooth muscle cells, vascular endothelial cells, chondrocytes, hepatocytes, and alveolar epithelial cells in addition to fibroblasts, suggesting that various cells (both mesenchymal and epithelial) produce collagen. As in the synthesis of other proteins, collagen synthesis starts in the ribosome in the form of preprocollagen. Preprocollagen is modified in the cell and accumulates in the rough endoplasmic reticulum as procollagen, which is then secreted from the cell via the Golgi apparatus. Procollagen (collagen molecules) and aggregates form mature collagen fibres[260]. Type I collagen (I), $[\alpha1(I)]_2 \alpha2$ molecules, consisting of two $\alpha1(I)$ chains and one 2 chain, are distributed in various organs such as the dermis, tendons, bones, arterial wall, liver, lungs, kidneys, and intervertebral disc. The trimer, $[\alpha1(I)]_3$, has been detected in various kinds of cell cultures, dermis, and tendons. Type III collagen (III) forms molecules in the form of $[\alpha1(I)]_3$ and is present along with type I in the dermis, arterial walls, liver, lungs and kidneys, but is found only in minute amounts in bones and tendons. Type V collagen (V) forms molecules in various combinations of $\alpha2(V)$ chain (A chain), $\alpha1(V)$ chain (B chain), and $\alpha3(V)$ chain (C chain), and has been found in the dermis, lungs, cornea, nerves, tendons, aorta, bones and cartilage. The distribution pattern of these collagens in the skin has been investigated immunohistologically. Using different antibodies to each collagen type, Meigel et al.[261] reported (1977) that type I is present throughout the full thickness of the dermis, but type III is only found in the papillary layer of the dermis. In 1978, Epstein et al.[262] suggested by biochemical analysis that the quantitative proportion between types I and III in the dermis is nearly uniform throughout the entire dermis. Because of these discrepancies, we studied the localization of types I and III using polyclonal antibodies to both collagen and a monoclonal antibody to type III. Konomi et al.[263] studied the distribution pattern of type V in 1984 using antibodies to A, B and C chains, and showed that collagen is normally present in the interstitial tissue but not in the basement membrane. Other studies suggested, however, that collagen is present only in the basement membrane in some pathological (tumoural) conditions of the skin[264, 265]. To clarify this point further, we also examined the localization of type V using antibodies to A and B chains.

FINDINGS

All our evaluations of the distribution patterns of types I, III and V using polyclonal antibodies and those of type III using monoclonal antibody yielded similar results. The epidermis and subepidermal basement membrane were negative, and the entire thickness of the dermis was positive for the collagens (1–3). The degree of positivity was relatively even throughout the dermis, but tended to be greater in the papillary layer (4). The positivity was also notable around the adnexa of the skin, being observed as bands surrounding the external limits of the basement membrane of the eccrine and apocrine glands (5). More intense positivity was observed around the basement membrane of the hair follicles, diffusely in the upper portion, and in bands in the lower portion (6). Perivascular areas were moderately positive for types I and III, but were positive for type V. These findings were obtained from the examination of skin samples at 36 sites in 16 subjects ranging in age from 2 to 85 years. These samples are considered to apply to a wide spectra of ages and skin sites.

DERMATOLOGICAL SIGNIFICANCE

The conventional view that type I is present in the entire thickness of the dermis and type III is present only in the papillary layer was refuted by our results, obtained using monoclonal antibodies, that both types I and III are distributed in the same pattern throughout the dermis. Consequently, the idea that reticulin fibres are composed primarily of type III[266], which is based on the similarity in the distribution patterns of the two materials, is not valid, at least in skin. Since Type V was also distributed in a pattern similar to types I and III, the manner of mixing, arrangement and special relationship of the three collagens as well as morphological differences between them emerge as new problems to be clarified by immunoelectron microscopic investigation. Localization of the C chain of type V is as yet unknown, and monoclonal antibody studies are considered necessary to approach this problem.

TECHNICAL POINTS

Although the best antigen preservation was performed on the unfixed frozen section, we used cold acetone fixing for a more clear and distinct demonstration of the positive reaction. To avoid a non-specific fluorescence of the epidermis, liver powder absorption should be done repeatedly and the antigen-antibody reaction time should also be carefully checked.

(This study was conducted jointly with Kazuyoshi Fukai, Hiromi Kobayashi and Miyako Chanoki of the Department of Dermatology, Osaka City University Medical School, and Yasuteru Muragaki of the First Department of Pathology, Wakayama Medical College.)

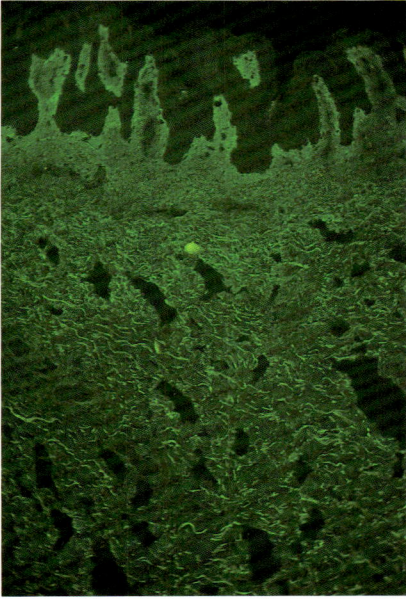

Fig. 1. Staining pattern with polyclonal anti-type I collagen antibody. Whole dermis stained positively. (× 60)

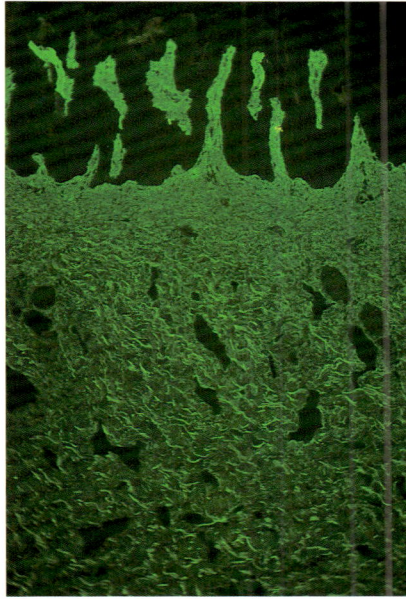

Fig. 2. Staining pattern with monoclonal anti-type III collagen antibody. Whole dermis stained positively. (× 60)

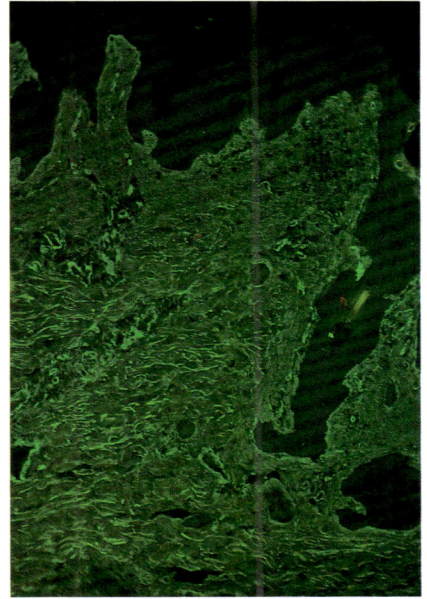

Fig. 3. Staining pattern with polyclonal anti-type V collagen antibody. Whole dermis stained positively. (× 60)

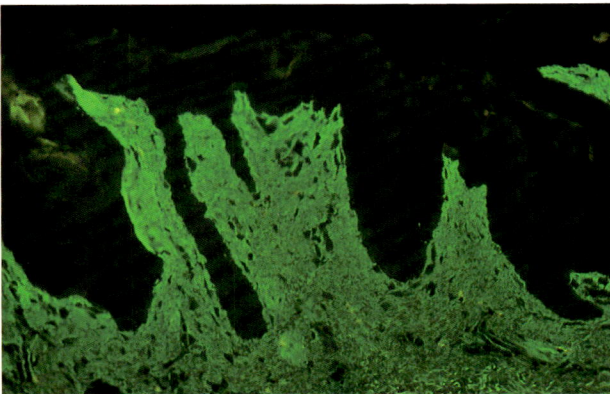

Fig. 4. Enlargement of the papillary dermis stained with monoclonal anti-type III collagen antibody. Stronger fluorescence is shown in this area. (× 120)

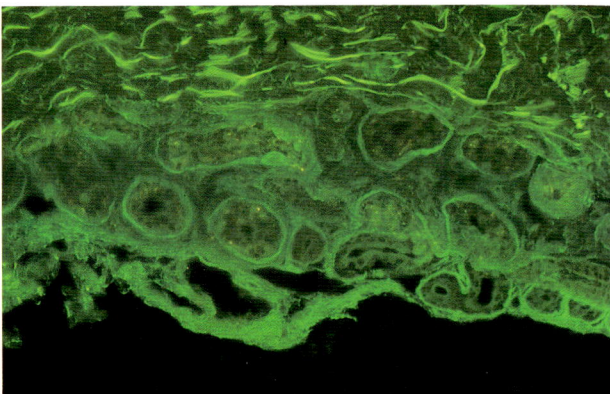

Fig. 6. Staining pattern of a hair follicle with polyclonal anti-type I collagen antibody. Upper part is diffusely positive and lower part shows band-like staining around the basement membrane zone. (× 60)

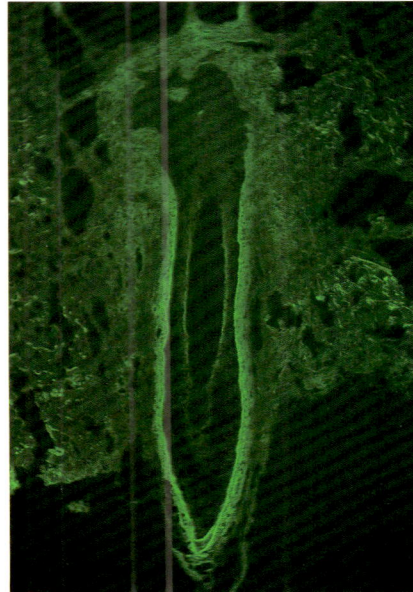

Fig. 5. Staining pattern of eccrine sweat glands with polyclonal anti-type V collagen antibody. Positive fluorescence is shown around the basement membrane zone. (× 120)

Type IV collagen

INTRODUCTION

Type IV collagen is known as a component of basement membrane collagen and is called membrane collagen.

The characteristics of type IV collagen are as follows: (1) Type IV collagen molecules consist of 3-hydroxyprolines and hydroxylysines. Almost all hydroxylysines have disaccharides (galactose or glucose); (2) type IV collagen exists in tissues as procollagen (propeptides are present in both the NH_2-terminal and the COOH-terminal extensions in the triple-helical segment of chains) and are not present in fibrillar array[267].

The metabolism of type IV collagen is not very well known. Type IV collagen is not digested by tissue collagenase[268] but by bacterial collagenase and elastase[269]. Uitto *et al.*[270] have reported that human leucocyte collagenase digests type IV collagen.

FORM

By light microscopy, the basement membrane is not clearly defined. It is thought to be a zone which includes the dermal side of plasma membrane of basal cells and upper dermis. Type IV collagen forms complexes with other non-collagenous glycoproteins, such as laminin, entactin, fibronectin and glycosaminoglycans. By immunohistochemical examination, type IV collagen has been found in vascular, glomerular, lens capsule and parietal yolk sac basement membrane. By immunoelectron microscopy, the main structure of basement membrane zone of the human skin was determined as lamina densa, which is thought to be type IV collagen[271].

FUNCTION

Basement membrane (type IV) collagen has the following functions:

1. Filtration. In ultrastructural studies of the glomerular basement membrane, the basement membrane ultrafilter has a limited diameter of about 10 nm and a molecular weight of about 40,000 dalton.
2. Type IV collagen plays an important role in the division, growth, rebirth and maintenance of cells.

ABNORMAL CONDITION

In abnormal conditions, the structure of type IV collagen varies. The main changes are destruction, thickness and stratification of the basement membrane.

TECHNICAL POINTS

Soluble type IV collagen is sometimes contaminated with laminin. Thus immunoelectron microscopy must be performed with pure antibodies to type IV collagen.

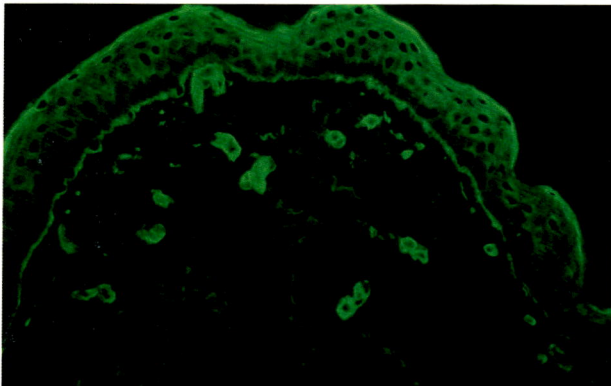

1

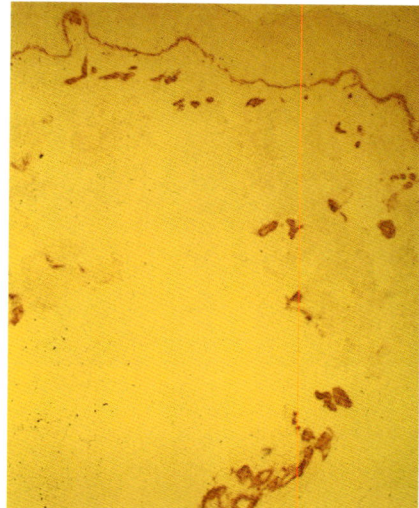

2

Bullous pemphigoid antigen

INTRODUCTION

Bullous pemphigoid (BP) antigen is a normal component of the basement membrane zone of the epidermis, and is known to be synthesized by epidermal basal cells. It is a high molecular weight protein with disulphide linked chains with an approximate molecular weight of 220–240 Kd[272,273]. This antigen can be identified immunologically by the circulating autoantibody of a BP patient, and defined as the substance reactive to the autoantibody of the BP patient.

FINDINGS

The skin of vertebrates reacts with BP autoantibodies producing the typical linear staining of the basement membrane zone by indirect immunofluorescent technique (1). This antigen is localized in the basement membrane zone of mammalian stratified squamous epithelia, including the mucosa of the oral cavity and upper oesophagus. It has been reported that the basement membrane zone of epithelia of the gallbladder, bladder, urethra, trachea and bronchi contain antigens which react with BP antibodies[274]. Immunoelectron microscopic studies have demonstrated that BP antigen is localized in the lamina lucida and is closely associated with the plasma membrane of basal cells[275].

DERMATOLOGICAL SIGNIFICANCE

At the epidermal-dermal junction of re-epithelializing wounds, BP antigen can be detected by immunofluorescence microscopy under the migrating epidermis as soon as epidermal cells make contact with the wound surface, whereas laminin and type IV collagen cannot be detected as early as BP antigen in this interaction[276]. In epidermal cell suspension obtained by trypsinization of guinea pig epidermis, about 50% of the cells adhere to type IV collagen-coated glass coverslips. These selectively attached cells were small round cells which revealed positive immunofluorescence with BP sera, while the unattached cells showed negative immunofluorescence[277].

Therefore BP antigen seems to play an important role in cell migration and basal cell-substrate adhesion.

BP antigen can be synthesized by cultured epidermal keratinocytes and has a coarsely granular perinuclear pattern within the cells (2). When the Ca^{2+} concentration of the medium is lowered to less than 0.1 mM, epidermal keratinocytes lose desmosomal connections, do not stratify, and thus proliferate rapidly. BP antigen can be detected in more than 90% of the cells of these cultures[278]. This staining pattern is similar to that observed in Pam cells[273] and SV40-transformed keratinocytes[279]. When the Ca^{2+} concentration of the medium is changed to 1.2 mM, the synthesis of BP antigen decreases. In this environment, cell-to-cell contact and desmosome formation occur, and cells are stratified. Cornification takes place on the top of stratified cells and DNA synthesis is diminished. Thus BP antigen is the marker for rapidly proliferating epidermal cells which possess basal cell characteristics.

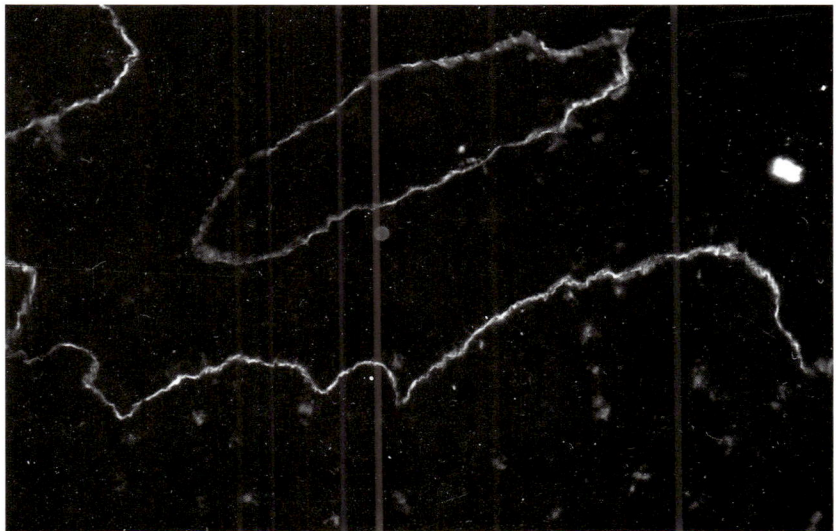

Fig. 1. Indirect immunofluorescence staining of BP antigen of the guinea pig jaw skin. (× 225)

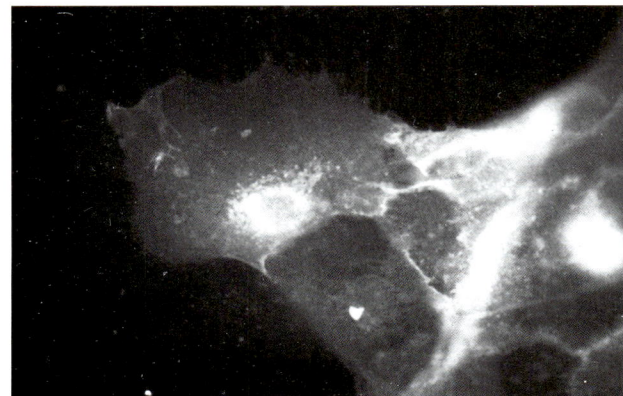

TECHNICAL POINTS

For immunofluorescence, an unfixed frozen section is the best. When fixation is necessary, cold acetone fixation is recommended.

Fig. 2. Indirect immunofluorescence staining of BP antigen of human keratinocytes in culture. BP antigen is seen as fine granules in the perinuclear zone. (× 900)

Glycosaminoglycan

INTRODUCTION

Glycosaminoglycan (GAG) in the skin is produced mainly by fibroblasts and is located between the collagen fibrils and the matrix of dermal connective tissue in the epidermo-dermal junction and the epidermis. In adult skin, GAG is 1–5% of the dry weight of the skin, 60–70% of which is hyaluronic acid (HA) and 15–20% is dermatan sulphate.

Ishikawa and Maeda have reported that the filamentous HA and granular GAG-protein complex (proteoglycan:PG) is present in the matrix around the collagen fibrils and that the HA chain is connected to the collagen fibrils[280, 281], as observed by electron microscopy (1).

Anti-GAG and anti-PG antibodies have been made and utilized by many researchers. We prepared an antibody toward bovine nasal cartilage PG according to the method of Wieslander and Heinegård[282]. The reactivity of human PG with the antiserum against bovine cartilage PG was examined using human skin[283].

FINDINGS

Normal skin. Using an immunofluorescent technique, specific fluorescence was seen in the subepidermal zone, the blood vessel walls and faintly between the collagen fibres. By immunoelectron microscopy, horseradish peroxidase-positive granules, compatible with PG, were attached to the collagen fibrils and thin filaments in the interfibrillar matrix, thus possibly representing HA[283].

Lesional skin. Clinically uninvolved skin tissue of systemic scleroderma (SS) showed the same characteristics as normal skin tissue (**2a**). Moderately involved skin demonstrated disseminated, fine granular PG deposits surrounding the blood vessels (**2b**). In markedly involved skin tissue, coarse granular PG deposits were seen in a random arrangement between the collagen fibres (**2c**).

In the lesion tissue of circumscribed scleroderma, more intense fluorescence was seen between the collagen fibres (**3**). Keloid tissue showed fine granular PG deposits regularly arranged along the collagen fibres. The lesional skin of *Scleroderma adultorum* (Buschke's disease) demonstrated a thin layer PG deposition along the collagen fibres. However, no fluorescence was visible in the lesional skin of lichen myxoedamatosus. These results and the fact that the skin of lichen myxoedematosus lacks PG around the HA filament are compatible with the electronmicroscopic study of Maeda, Ishikawa and Ohta[284].

DERMATOLOGICAL SIGNIFICANCE

GAG and PG in skin are thought to play important roles not only in normal skin – in the fibre formation of connective tissue and the transportation of materials between the epidermis and dermis – but also in various diseases.

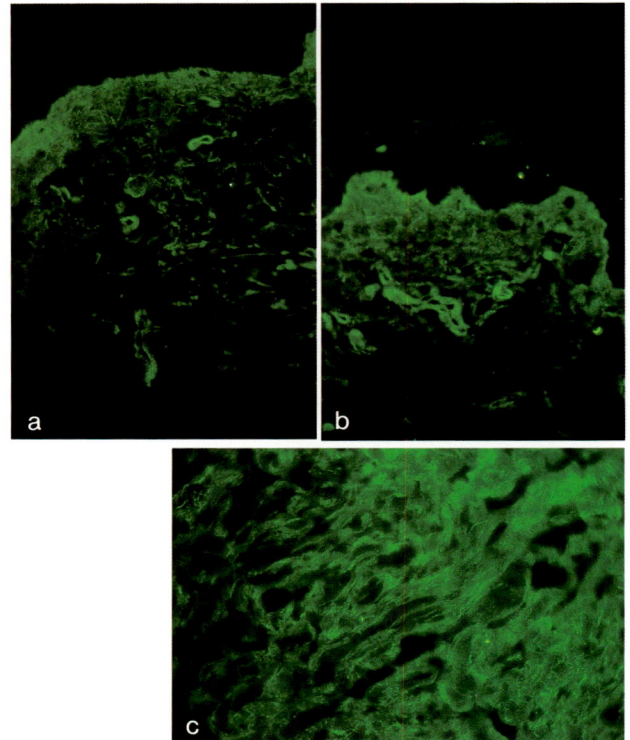

Fig. 2. Systemic scleroderma. (× 350)
a. Clinically uninvolved skin tissues. PG deposits are seen in the subepidermal zone, the blood vessel walls and faintly between the collagen fibres.
b. Moderately involved skin tissue. Disseminated, fine granular PG deposits are seen surrounding the blood vessels.
c. Markedly involved skin tissue. Coarse granular PG deposits are seen in a random arrangement between the collagen fibres.

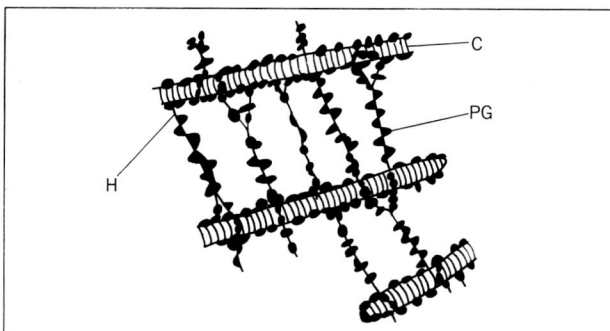

Fig. 1. A schema of the features of the collagen fibrils and PG macromolecules. The short chains of PG are attached surrounding the collagen fibrils (c) and the HA chains (H) are located between the collagen fibrils. (Hidekazu Ishikawa, Hidebumi Maeda: Nishinihon J. Dermatol. **43**: 1024, 1981.)

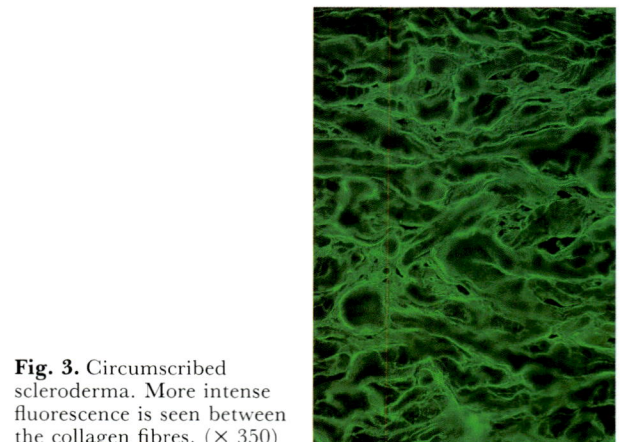

Fig. 3. Circumscribed scleroderma. More intense fluorescence is seen between the collagen fibres. (× 350)

FINDINGS IN VARIOUS DERMATOSES

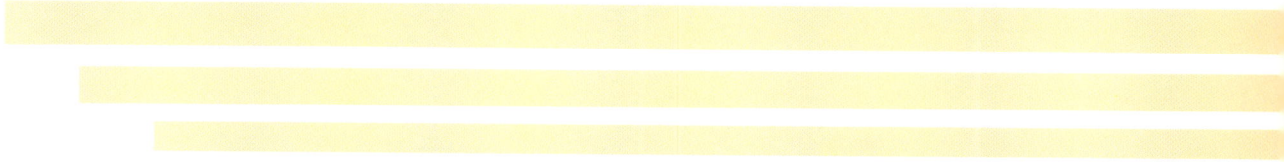

Bullous dermatoses

Pemphigus

INTRODUCTION

Pemphigus is a skin disease which shows acantholytic blister formation in the epidermis. Pemphigus is divided into four major subgroups: pemphigus vulgaris, pemphigus vegetans, pemphigus foliaceus and pemphigus erythematosus. Histologically, the former two groups show acantholysis in the suprabasal area and the latter two groups in the subcorneal area (**1**).

Among various skin disorders, pemphigus was the first discovered to have immunological disturbance, the presence of intercellular autoantibodies in the serum and the deposition of IgG in the intercellular area of the lesional skin[285-7]. Since then, it has been well recognized that these immunological abnormalities are very important for the diagnosis and pathogenesis of pemphigus.

FINDINGS

By direct immunofluorescence the deposition of IgG is observed in the intercellular area of the biopsy specimen from lesional skin (**2a**). Pemphigus vulgaris tends to demonstrate a stronger reaction in lower epidermis, in contrast to the preferential staining in upper viable epidermis in cases of pemphigus foliaceus. Additionally, deposition of complement components, such as C1q, C4, C3, properdin and factor B, is frequently seen in the same area (**2b**)[288].

By indirect immunofluorescence staining, IgG intercellular antibodies are found in the sera of most pemphigus patients (**3a**). These autoantibodies were considered not to have complement binding activity by *in vitro* complement immunofluorescence techniques[289]. However, it has recently been reported that complement binding intercellular antibodies are found in the sera of some patients (**3b**)[290]. By immunoelectron microscopy using peroxidase, reaction products are seen continuously in the intercellular space of lesional skin (**4**).

In cases of pemphigus erythematosus, the skin biopsies taken from a sun-exposed area show deposition of IgG and complement at the dermo-epidermal junction as well as IgG intercellular deposition. This suggests a relationship between this type of pemphigus and systemic lupus erythematosus.

RELEVANCE FOR DIAGNOSIS AND PATHOGENESIS

The immunopathological findings are now considered to be the most important for the differentiation of pemphigus from the diseases with different immunological characteristics (bullous pemphigoid, dermatitis herpetiformis, etc.) and from those with no immunological abnormality (Hailey-Hailey's disease, transient acantholytic dermatosis, etc.). This technique is also useful for the diagnosis of cases with atypical skin lesion, such as herpetiform pemphigus. Furthermore, because it is known that the titres of circulating intercellular antibodies are well correlated with the disease activity and IgG deposition disappears in the remission stage, repeated examinations of these immunological changes are important as indices for treatment.

It has been suggested that intercellular antibodies play an important role in the pathogenesis of pemphigus. However, the real mechanisms of blister formation have not yet been clarified. Recently, it has been recognized that, when normal skin explants are cultured in media with patient serum or IgG purified from it, acantholytic changes in the epidermis occur (**5a**)[291]. It is believed that complement is not necessary for this change. On the other hand, the relevance of complement in the pathogenesis of pemphigus is suggested by several facts: (1) the deposition of complement components in lesional skin, and (2) the reduced level of complement activity in blister fluid. Furthermore, it was reported that, by means of the *in vitro* leucocyte attachment technique, migration and attachment of normal human leucocytes were seen in the epidermis of skin section which had been previously reacted with pemphigus serum. This change was dependent on the presence of complement (**5b**)[292]. This phenomenon may be important for understanding the pathogenesis, because infiltration of eosinophils in the epidermis (eosinophilic spongiosis) is frequently observed in early lesions. Apart from these immunohistological studies, recent biochemical studies have suggested the possibility that blister formation is induced by some proteinases, particularly plasminogen activator, which are produced by keratinocytes following IgG binding[293].

BIOPSY METHODS

For immunofluorescence tests, it is preferable to take the erythematous peribullous margin of early vesicles or bullae. At the same time, it is convenient to excise whole bullae and use the other edge for routine histopathological examinations.

Immediately following the biopsy, the tissue is mounted with OCT compound on a piece of cork and then quick frozen in a hexane bath which has been cooled in an alcohol-CO_2 pellet mixture. The tissue should be sectioned in a cryostat while frozen.

TECHNICAL POINTS

Intercellular antibodies are not detectable in some cases. The reactivity of these antibodies sometimes shows specificity for species and organs. Rabbit skin, guinea pig mucous membrane or monkey skin were used in the past as the substrate for indirect immunofluorescence. However, it appears that normal human skin is the most reliable[294]. As the antibodies are often negative in the early stages, repeated examinations are necessary.

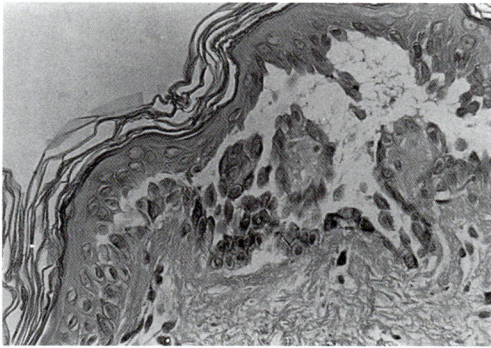

Fig. 1. Histopathology of pemphigus vulgaris. (H & E staining: × 200)

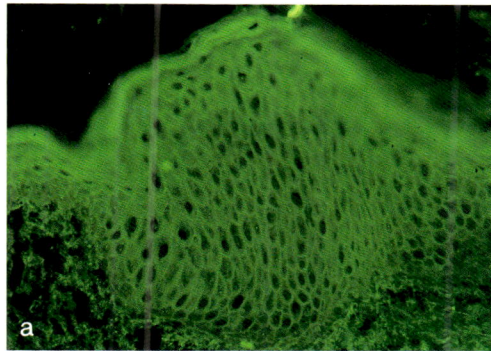

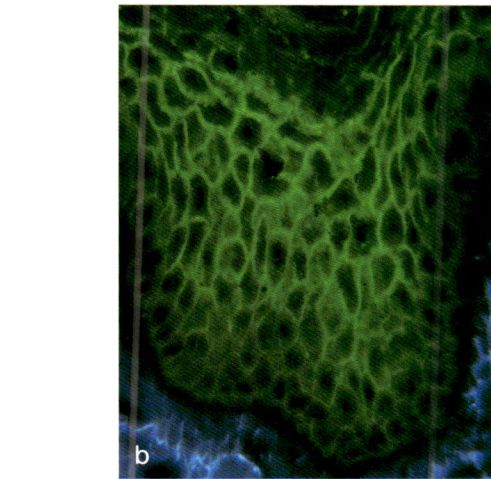

Fig. 2. Direct immunofluorescence staining patterns in the lesional skin of pemphigus vulgaris.
a. IgG deposition. (× 200) b. C3 deposition. (× 200)

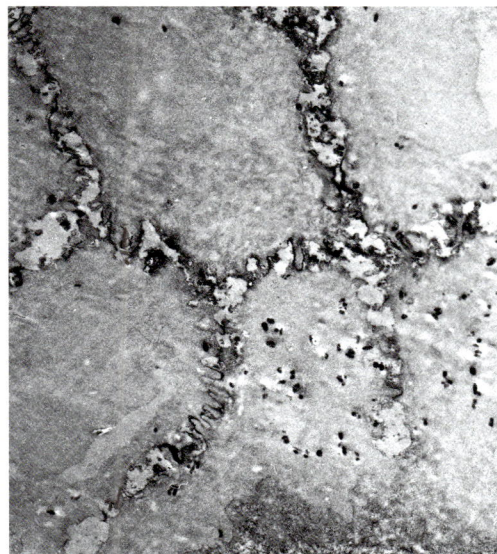

Fig. 3a. Intercellular binding of IgG by indirect immunofluorescence, using human skin as substrate. (× 200)

Fig. 3b. Binding of C4 via intercellular antibodies by complement immunofluorescence staining. (× 400)

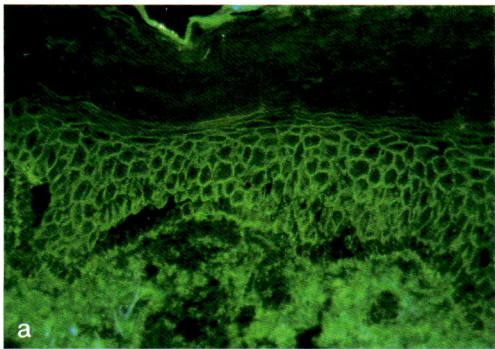

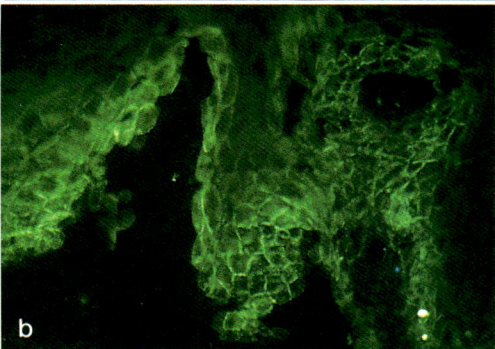

Fig. 4. Immunoelectron microscopy using peroxidase conjugate. Reaction products are seen along the intercellular space.

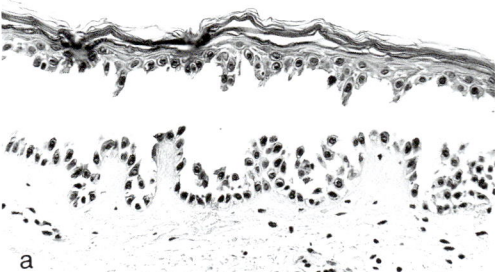

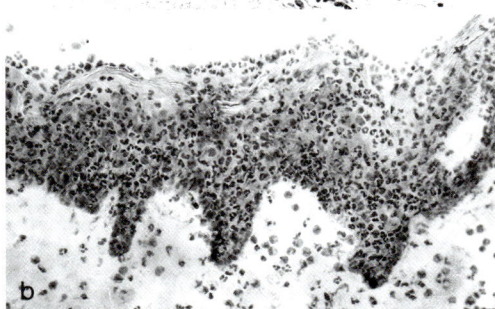

Fig. 5a. Suprabasal acantholysis-like change of normal human skin explants previously cultured in pemphigus serum medium for 48 hours at 37°C.

Fig. 5b. Migration and attachment of normal human leucocytes in epidermis of skin section reacted with intercellular antibodies.

67

Pemphigoid

INTRODUCTION
Pemphigoid is a group of bullous diseases characterized by damage in the cohesion between the basal cells of the epidermis and the dermis[295]. The skin eruptions consist of large tense bullae and pruritic erythematous lesions appearing over the entire body of aged persons. Autoimmune mechanisms are considered to be involved in the pathogenesis of the disease. Bullous pemphigoid is the typical type but other atypical types, such as cicatricial pemphigoid, are included in this group.

IMPORTANT FINDINGS AND THEIR SIGNIFICANCE
Pathological examination. The blisters are formed beneath the epidermis without acantholysis of the epidermal cells. Lymphoid cells, eosinophils and a few neutrophils infiltrate the upper dermis as well as the blister cavity. Eosinophilic cytoid bodies (or ghost cells) due to degenerated basal cells are occasionally seen just beneath the blister roof (**1a**)[296]. Ultrastructurally, the blister formation results from the separation between the plasma membrane of the basal cells and the basal lamina (namely in the lamina lucida). The basal lamina is well preserved on the blister floor, but the hemidesmosomes of the basal cells of the blister roof are remarkably reduced (**1b**).

Direct immunofluorescence test (observation of *in vivo* bound immunoglobulin and complement). *In vivo* bound immunoglobulin and/or complement is found in the lesional and perilesional skin. These are present in a continuously linear pattern along the basement membrane zone of the epidermis (epidermal-dermal junction) in the non-separated skin. In separated skin the deposits are mostly localized, not along the blister floor but along the basilar surface of the blister roof, and occasionally along both (**2**). Among the serum factors, IgG and C3 are the most frequently detected; IgA, IgM and Clq are detected less frequently. IgG and/or C3 depositions are detectable in non-lesional skin, too, in about 60% of the patients.

Indirect immunofluorescence test (detection of circulating anti-BMZ antibodies in patients' sera). Indirect immunofluorescence tests using normal human skin, lip mucosa of the guinea pig or oesophageal mucosa of the monkey as the substrate, and the patients' sera as the first antibody (two-fold dilution method), reveal the presence of autoantibodies in various titres of patients' sera (IgG class) reacting to the basement membrane zone of the substrate. The incidence of positive findings is 60–70% in patients with bullous pemphigoid and 15–20% in those with cicatricial pemphigoid. When sera are applied to substrate frozen sections of normal human skin treated with 1 M sodium chloride solution and partially separated at the epidermal-dermal junction, anti-BMZ antibodies react to the epidermal side of the separated skin, namely beneath the basal layer of the epidermis (**3**)[297].

Immunoelectron microscopy. (a) Localization of *in vitro* bound immunoglobulin and complement: Electron microscopy of immunoperoxidase-stained sections reveals that the reaction products, indicating deposits of immunoglobulin or complement, are in some cases distributed between the basilar surface of basal cells and basal lamina, and in other cases localized on the basilar surface of the basal cells or on the basal lamina. Occasionally, the deposits are seen in the dermis in association with the detached basal lamina (**4, a–c**). The reaction products are generally not seen between the basilar surface of the melanocytes and the basal lamina (**5**)[298], but a weak reaction is rarely seen[299]

(b) *In vitro* binding sites of anti-BMZ antibodies: Electron microscopy of immunoperoxidase-stained sections (anti-human IgG) of normal human skin pieces incubated with patients' sera using an organ culture system[300] shows ultrastructural reaction sites of anti-BMZ antibodies in patients' sera. The reaction products are discretely distributed along the basilar surface of the basal cells. Distribution of tonofibrils indicates that the reaction sites are on the basilar surface of the hemidesmosomes (**6**). Treatment of epidermal sheets or isolated basal cells with saponin enhances the penetration of antibodies into the cytoplasm of the basal cells and allows the anti-BMZ antibodies to react with hemidesmosome-tonofibril complexes[301].

Vertical observation of indirect immunofluorescence test. When the epidermal sheets, detached from the dermis by treatment with 1 M sodium chloride solution, are incubated with patients' sera as the first antibody and next with FITC-conjugated anti-human IgG, reaction sites of anti-BMZ antibodies can be observed upward from the dermal side of the epidermis. Anti-BMZ antibodies react with the dermal surface of the basal cells in a granular pattern (**7**).

TECHNICAL POINTS
In order to histologically or immunohistologically study the border between the bullae and surrounding skin, it is necessary to obtain an entire biopsy specimen of a small, newly-formed blister. After fixation with PLP (periodic acid-lysine paraformaldehyde) solution, the biopsy specimen is cut into two parts, one of which is processed for routine histological examination and the other for immunohistological examination using the immunoperoxidase method for light and electron microscopic observation.

DIAGNOSTIC SIGNIFICANCE AND PATHOGENESIS
The diagnosis of pemphigoid cannot be established without immunohistological studies; a positive finding by direct or indirect immunofluorescence examination is required to differentiate the cases from other various subepidermal bullous diseases. When neither examination is positive, the case cannot be diagnosed as pemphigoid. Furthermore, diagnosis of the clinically atypical cases and the cases that should be differentiated from epidermolysis bullosa acquisita must be established on the basis of salt-treated indirect immunofluorescence test and immunoelectron microscopic study.

Anti-BMZ antibodies in pemphigoid patients' sera are considered to play an important role in the pathogenesis of blister formation. Briefly, the reaction of anti-BMZ antibodies and BP antigen(s)[302] activates the complement system, which induces white blood cells to migrate[303]. Some proteolytic enzymes released from the white blood cells harm the cohesion of the epidermis and the dermis at the lamina lucida[304].

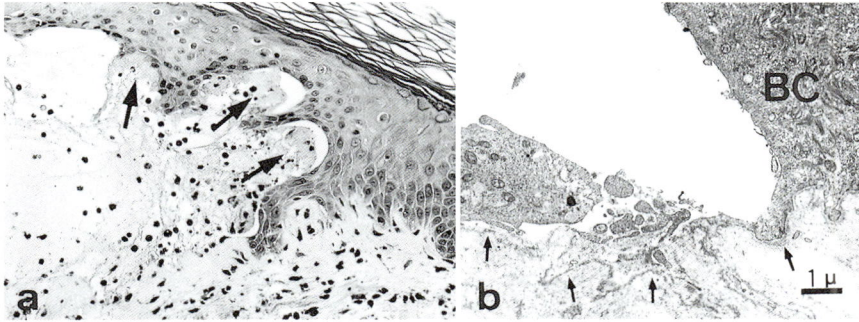

Fig. 1a. Subepidermal blister. Mononuclear cells, eosinophils and neutrophils infiltrate the upper dermis and the blister cavity. Eosinophilic degeneration (arrows) occurs in the epidermal cells of the blister roof.

Fig. 1b. Blister formation results from the separation of the basal cells (BC) and the basal lamina (arrows).

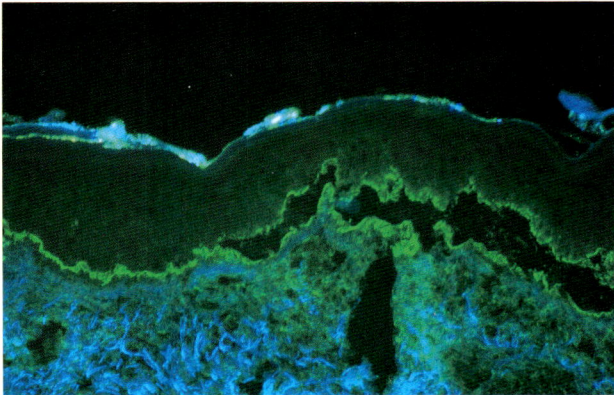

Fig. 2. Direct immunofluorescence test shows IgG deposits along the basement membrane zone, basilar surface of the blister roof and on the blister floor.

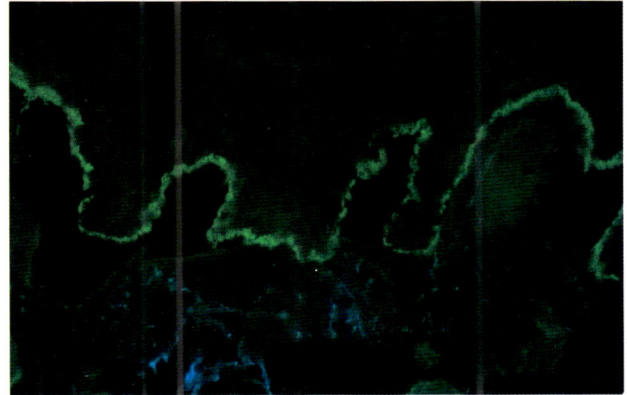

Fig. 3. Indirect immunofluorescence test, using 1 M salt-treated normal human skin, shows the reaction of the anti-BMZ antibodies (IgG) with the epidermal side of the separated skin.

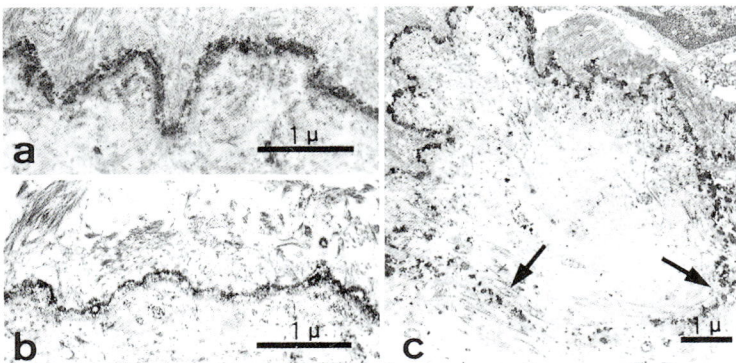

Fig. 4. Immunoelectron micrographs showing the deposition of complement[299].

Fig. 4a. Deposition in the lamina lucida.

Fig. 4b. Deposition along the basilar surface of the basal cells.

Fig. 4c. Deposition in the dermis associated with the detached basal lamina (arrows).

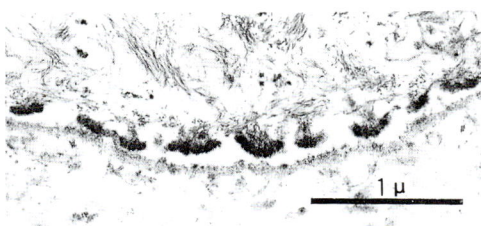

Fig. 5. Immunoelectron micrograph showing the deposition of IgG (arrows). Reaction products are absent beneath the melanocyte (MC).

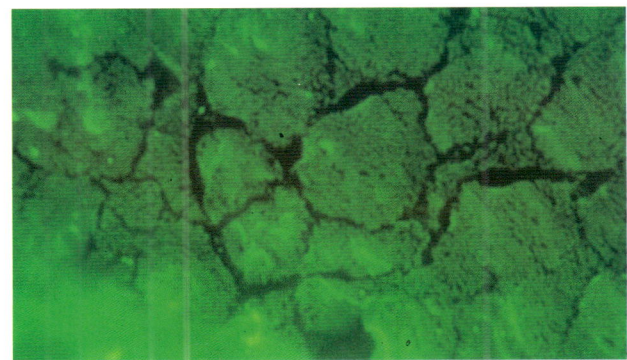

Fig. 6. Anti-BMZ antibodies (IgG) react with the basilar surface of the hemidesmosomes.

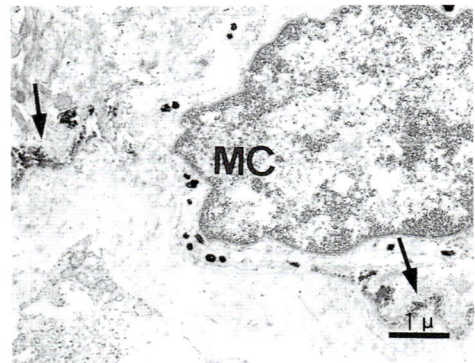

Fig. 7. Vertical observation of an indirect immunofluorescence study, using 1 M salt-separated epidermal sheet as the substrate, reveals a granular fluorescence pattern on the dermal surface of the basal cells.

Herpes gestationis

INTRODUCTION
Herpes gestationis (HG) is a rare pruritic subepidermal bullous dermatosis of pregnancy and the postpartum period. It is thought to be mediated by IgG anti-basement membrane zone antibodies which avidly fix complement. Definitive diagnosis can be made with specific immunopathologic studies.

STUDIES FOR DIAGNOSIS
Histopathology. The histopathology of the early erythematous lesion of HG shows epidermal and papillary dermal oedema with occasional foci of eosinophilic spongiosis. The bullous lesions are subepidermal and contain numerous eosinophils (**1**)[305]. Ultrastructurally, the level of the split is within the lamina lucida and the blister seems to be formed secondarily to basal cell necrosis[306]. The dermal infiltrate consists of mononuclear cells, eosinophils, and occasionally a few neutrophils.

Immunologic features. Direct immunofluorescence examination of the lesional or perilesional skin shows that in all active cases of HG there is C3 deposition in a linear pattern at the basement membrane zone (**2**)[307]. Other components of the classical as well as alternative complement pathway may also be detected. Approximately 30–40% of these patients also demonstrate deposition of IgG. IgA and IgM basement membrane zone deposition have only been rarely noted. Dense deposition of C3 at the basement membrane zone of lesional skin, however, is the diagnostic hallmark in patients with HG[307, 308]. *In vivo*-bound C3 and IgG are localized in the lamina lucida (**3**)[306, 309].

Indirect immunofluorescence studies have demonstrated that only 10–20% of patients with active HG possess anti-basement membrane zone antibodies[307]. Almost all HG sera, however, avidly fix C3 to normal skin basement membrane zone when tested by *in vitro* C3 staining (**4**).

Initially labelled as HG factor, this C3 fixing factor has been shown to be serum IgG autoantibodies which fix complement, but in such small quantities that it escapes detection by routine indirect immunofluorescence staining[310, 311].

Infants born of affected mothers may manifest a transient blistering eruption. C3 deposition in the basement membrane zone has also been noted in the skin of these infants[312, 313], and cord sera has been shown to contain HG factor activity[310, 311]

DIFFERENTIAL DIAGNOSIS
Direct immunofluorescence studies are necessary to distinguish HG from a variety of other pregnancy-related dermatoses, such as erythema multiforme and dermatitis herpetiformis. The unique deposition of C3 along the basement membrane zone in HG is an important differential factor.

The possible relationship between HG and bullous pemphigoid is as yet unresolved, though both have many features in common[314]. The localization of the antibodies to lamina lucida in both diseases and recognition of the same antigens by immunoblotting[315] would suggest that these diseases are quite similar or even identical. However, the role of pregnancy and hormones, the complement-fixing avidity of the anti-basement membrane zone antibodies in HG, and the fact that basal cell necrosis is distinct in HG but uncommon to bullous pemphigoid suggest that these two diseases are different[316].

AETIOLOGY AND PATHOGENESIS
The exact aetiology of HG is unknown. However, HG appears to be an autoimmune disorder which is triggered when women with an immunogenetic susceptibility to high immune responsiveness are exposed to an antigenic factor derived from pregnancy.

Many findings suggest that the disease is generated by the avid complement-fixing IgG anti-basement membrane zone antibodies. It is theorized that interaction of antibodies with antigens located in the lamina lucida of the basement membrane zone activates the complement cascade. The subsequent inflammatory responses produce the clinical features that are recognized as HG.

TECHNICAL POINTS
See A-2 bullous pemphigoid (p. 68).

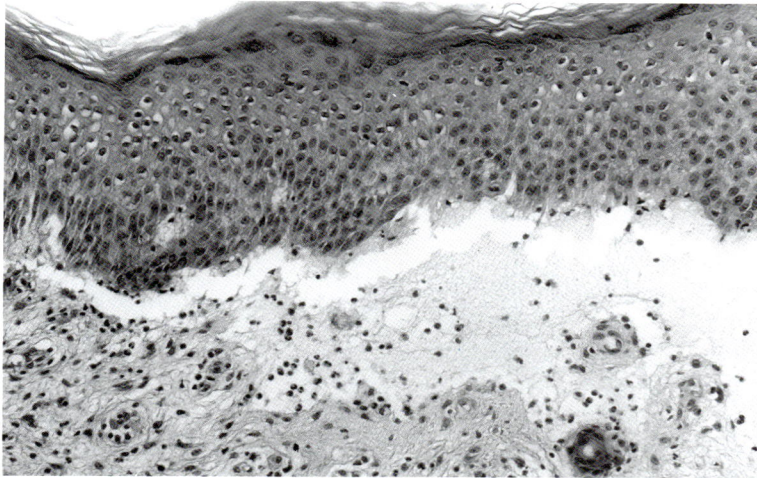

Fig. 1. Subepidermal bulla arising on erythematous skin. The dermis and the cavity of the bulla contain many eosinophils. (× 200)

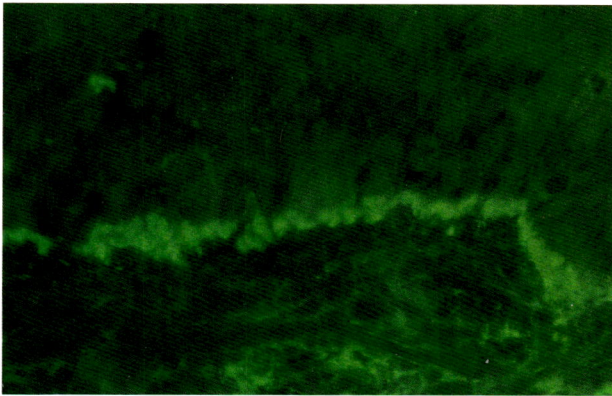

Fig. 2. Linear deposition of C3 along the basement membrane zone[316]. (Lesional nonbullous skin, × 400.)

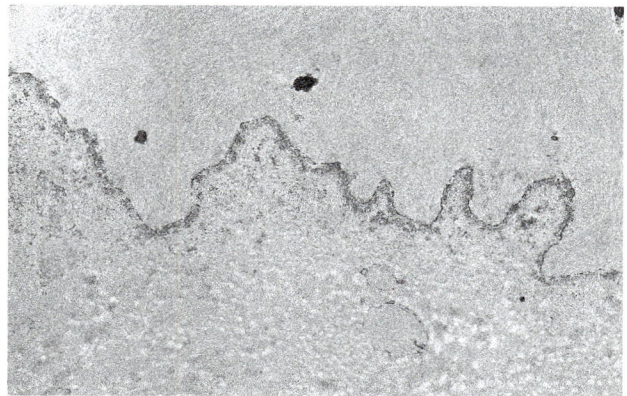

Fig. 3. *In vivo* localization of C3 to lamina lucida of lesional skin[306]. (Courtesy of H. Yaoita, M.D., × 10,200.)

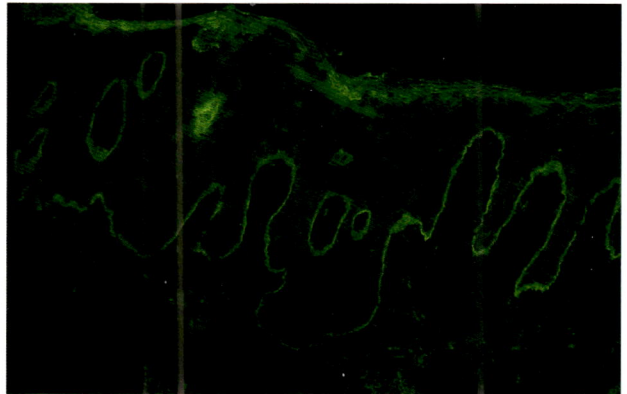

Fig. 4. *In vitro* C3 staining of normal human skin with HG serum. (× 200) Positive basement membrane zone staining is evident.

Epidermolysis bullosa acquisita

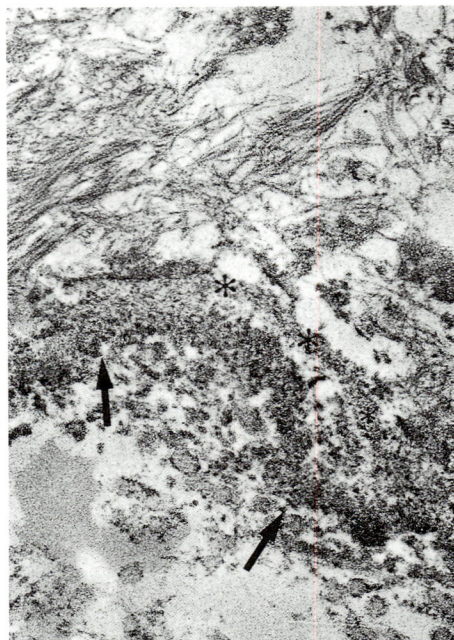

Fig. 1a. Indirect immunoelectron microscopic study.
The deposition of anti-DEJ antibodies from a patient with EBA
(arrow) is noted at the dermal side below the basal lamina (*).

INTRODUCTION

Epidermolysis bullosa acquisita (EBA) was first described in 1904 by Kablitz as a subgroup of epidermolysis[317]. Similar cases had already been reported by Elliot in 1895[318] and Fox in 1897[319]. Originally, this disease was believed to be non-hereditary, late-onset dystrophic epidermolysis. The diagnostic criteria proposed by Roenigk *et al.* in 1971 established EBA as a clinical entity in general[320]. However, since Kushniruk discovered that there is deposition of immunoglobulins and complement along the dermo-epidermal junction (DEJ) in the skin of those patients[321] and then Nieboer *et al.*[322] and Yaoita *et al.*[323] elucidated the characteristic immunoelectron microscopic findings, a different concept (autoimmune mechanism) has been introduced for the pathogenesis of EBA. Furthermore, the identification of EBA antigen by Woodley *et al.* emphasized a physiological role as one of the new BMZ antigens[324].

FINDINGS

Immunofluorescence (IF) and immunoelectron microscopic (IEM) tests are necessary for the diagnosis of EBA. IEM tests are particularly important for the differential diagnosis of bullous pemphigoid (BP) and EBA as mentioned below.

Immunofluorescence test. IgG deposition is noted along the DEJ similar to BP (**3d**). Out of 33 cases reported from 1973 to 1984, IgA deposition was described in 10, IgM in 11 and complement in 25, along with IgG deposits. The deposition of more than two classes of immunoglobulin is found more frequently in EBA than in BP[325]. Circulating anti-DEJ antibodies were demonstrated in 7 out of 33 cases by the indirect IF test.

Immunoelectron microscopic test. The deposition of immunoglobulin is noted at the subbasal lamina area (**1**). This finding is very important for the diagnosis of EBA since it is quite different from BP[326] and cicatricial pemphigoid[327] in which immunoglobulin deposits are seen in the lamina lucida (*see* A-2 pemphigoid).

The distribution of EBA antigen and BP antigen. Direct IF tests carried out on the various organs of an autopsied patient with EBA show linear deposition of IgG and C3 in the skin, tongue, oesophagus and trachea. EBA antigen is also demonstrated in skin, tongue, oesophagus, cornea and bladder of mouse, guinea pig, rabbit and human by indirect IF test. The distribution of EBA antigen is quite similar to that of BP antigen (Table I).

TECHNICAL POINTS

The biopsy for IF study should be taken from an unaffected area or from an area adjacent to the skin lesion. Studies using blistered skin may result in a false-negative test. IEM study is the most valuable for the differential diagnosis of EBA and BP; however, in general it is technically too difficult to perform in a standard clinic. Simple IF procedures have been described which discern the difference between these two diseases without the use of IEM, if circulating anti-DEJ antibodies are detected in the patient's serum[328, 329] (**2**).

DEJ separation method. One can separate artificially the epidermis from the dermis of a normal skin using 1 M NaCl. This skin can then be utilized for indirect IF with the serum in question. EBA antibodies bind to the dermal side of the separated surface, while BP antibodies delineate the epidermal side[328, 329] (**2**).

Ethanol fixation method. BP antigen loses antigenicity after ethanol fixation. When the indirect IF test is performed on ethanol-fixed human skin sections (for thirty minutes at room temperature), BP antibodies no longer bind to the DEJ, whereas EBA antibodies still bind and show bright linear fluorescence (**3**).

Similar results have been obtained in mouse, guinea pig and rabbit skin, and rabbit cornea[329].

TABLE I ORGAN AND SPECIES SPECIFICITY OF EBA AND BP SERA

| | DIRECT IF | INDIRECT IF | | | | INDIRECT IF | | | |
| | PATIENT | MOUSE (a) | | GUINEA PIG | | RABBIT | | HUMAN (c) | |
	EBA	EBA	BP	EBA	BP	EBA	BP	EBA	BP
skin	+	+	+	+	+	+	+	+	+
tongue, oesophagus	+	+	+	+	+	+	+	+	+
stomach, intestine	−	−	−	−	−	−	−	−	−
pancreas	−	ND	ND	ND	ND	ND	ND	−	−
liver, lung	−	−	−	−	−	−	−	−	−
kidney	+(b)	−	−	−	−	−	−	−	−
trachea	weak	ND	ND	ND	ND	+	+	+	+
aorta	−	−	−	−	−	−	−	−	−

ND   not done
(a)   Substrates used
(b)   Granular staining pattern noted in glomeruli, considered to be related to the immune complex
      recognized in this patient
(c)   65 y, female cadaver

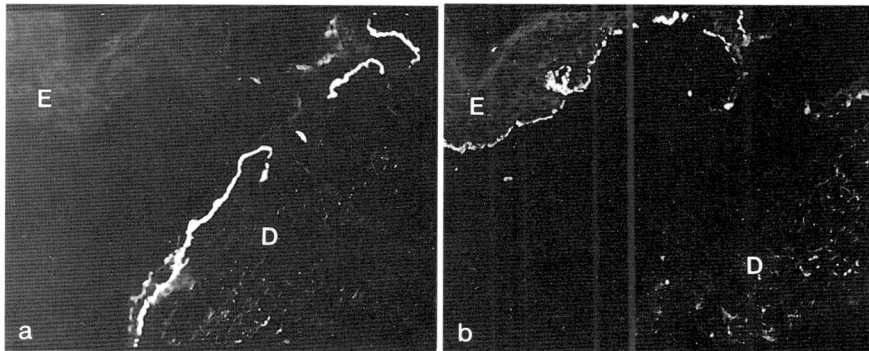

Fig. 2. DEJ separation method.
Indirect IF study performed on normal human skin artificially separated at DEJ with 1 M NaCl. EBA antibodies (a) bind to the dermal side, whereas BP antibodies (b) delineate the epidermal side. E: epidermis, D: dermis.

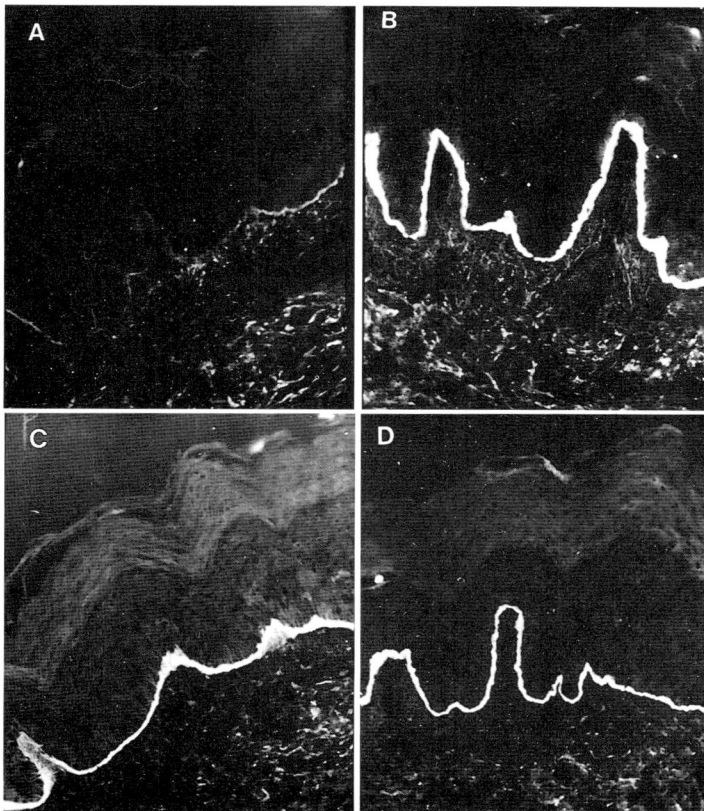

Fig. 3. Ethanol fixation method.
Human skin is used as substrate.
a. substrate: ethanol fixed, antibody: BP antibody
b. substrate: untreated control, antibody: BP antibody
c. substrate: ethanol fixed, antibody: EBA antibody
d. substrate: untreated control, antibody: EBA antibody
The binding of BP antibody decreased markedly when an ethanol-fixed substrate was used (A).

Linear IgA bullous dermatosis

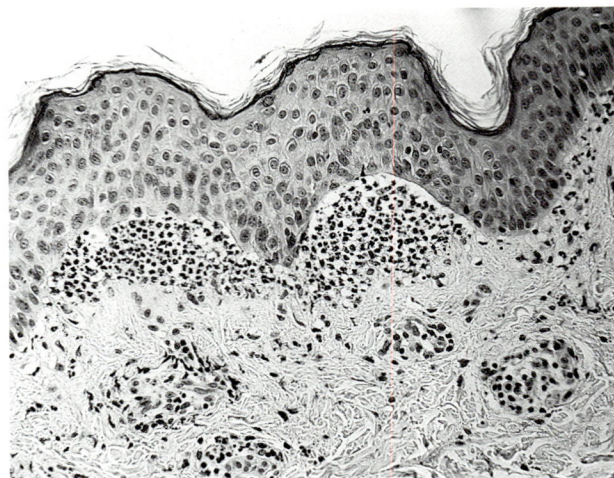

Fig. 1. Histopathological findings.
Characteristic papillary microabscess composed of neutrophils. (H & E, × 100)

INTRODUCTION

Recently a group of bullous dermatoses of unknown aetiology, which are characterized by *in vivo* linear IgA deposition at the dermo-epidermal junction, have been increasingly reported. Some of these cases were described as the subtype dermatitis herpetiformis (DH)[330] and others were included in bullous pemphigoid[331]. Chorzelski *et al.* regarded these dermatoses as a clinical entity, and named them linear IgA bullous dermatosis[332].

FINDINGS

Two clinical subtypes have been reported. One is benign chronic bullous dermatosis of childhood, which is characterized by the outbreak of annular erythema and blisters of various sizes in the perioral, orbital, perineal and other regions in the first decade. Mucous membranes are rarely involved, and itching is not too marked.

The other is adult linear IgA bullous dermatosis, which is more common in females. Polymorphous eruptions composed of erythematous, vesicular and large bullous lesions appear on the trunk and limbs in adults between the ages of 20 and 70. Mucous membrane involvement is frequently recognized. In contradistinction to classical DH, these cases usually lack the characteristic gluten hypersensitivity and correlation to HLA-B8 antigen.

Histopathological findings reveal subepidermal blister formation and neutrophilic papillary micro-abscess in both juvenile and adult types, like those of classical DH (**1**). Direct immunofluorescence studies using patients' skin reveal linear IgA deposition at the dermo-epidermal junction *in vivo* (**2**). The IgA deposition can be observed not only in lesional and perilesional skin but also in normal appearing skin. Circulating IgA class anti-basement membrane auto-antibodies have also been demonstrated in several cases[331,333,334].

The treatment is similar to that of classical dermatitis herpetiformis; sulfapyridine and dapsone are usually effective. However, Chorzelski *et al.* pointed out that sulfones are not as effective in linear IgA bullous dermatosis as in classical DH, and that corticosteroids are necessary in such cases[332].

DIAGNOSTIC SIGNIFICANCE AND PATHOGENESIS

By considering the clinical, histopathological and immuno-pathological findings, the diagnosis can be made. Classical DH and bullous pemphigoid should be considered in the differential diagnosis. The pathogenesis of linear IgA dermatosis is still unknown.

BIOPSY PROCEDURE

Under local anaesthesia, a small blister should be resected together with perilesional skin. This biopsy specimen is cut into two pieces, one of which contains a blister. The specimen is fixed in formaldehyde for light microscopic examination and also in glutaraldehyde for electron microscopy. The other piece is examined by immunopathological methods, and biopsy specimens obtained from normal appearing skin are also examined.

TECHNICAL POINTS

Light microscopic investigation. Frozen sections are cut in a cryostat, and *in vivo* IgA deposition is observed using the direct immunofluorescence method. For beautiful pictures of specific fluorescence, careful repeated rinsing with phosphate buffered saline (PBS) should be performed. For attachment of the frozen sections, albumin-coated glass slides may be employed.

Electron microscopic investigation. For electron microscopic observation of IgA binding sites, the enzyme-labelled antibody method (immunoperoxidase method) should be used. This technique has been described in previous reports[335-7]. For good observation, the following three points are essential: (1) preservation of antigenicity of deposited IgA, (2) preservation of ultrastructural morphology, (3) penetration of specific antibodies. Generally, paraformaldehyde or McLean-Nakane's PLP fixative[335] may be employed for fixation. However, the dermo-epidermal junction, observed mainly in linear IgA bullous dermatosis, usually reveals a well-preserved, fine structure even without fixation. Although glutaraldehyde is a strong fixative, antigenicity may easily be lost with this fixative and thus it should not be employed for immunoelectron microscopy.

Excised skin samples are immersed immediately after biopsy in 0.01 M PBS with 10% glycerol for two hours at 4°C, and then are embedded in OCT for cryostat preparation. Glycerol inhibits ice crystal formation during the freeze and thaw procedure. The frozen sections are stained using the immunoperoxidase method and dehydrated with alcohol, and then embedded in epoxy resin. The embedded materials can be observed by a light microscope, and the reaction product is demonstrated at dermo-epidermal junction with linear continuity (**3**).

Ultrastructural localization of IgA in linear IgA dermatosis is classified into two types: localization in the lamina lucida, and localization in the subbasal lamina region[336]. In some case reports, both patterns of IgA deposition were observed in the same specimen (**4**)[332,337]. Yaoita suggests that these two different IgA deposition patterns are responsible for the varied clinical features of linear IgA dermatosis[336].

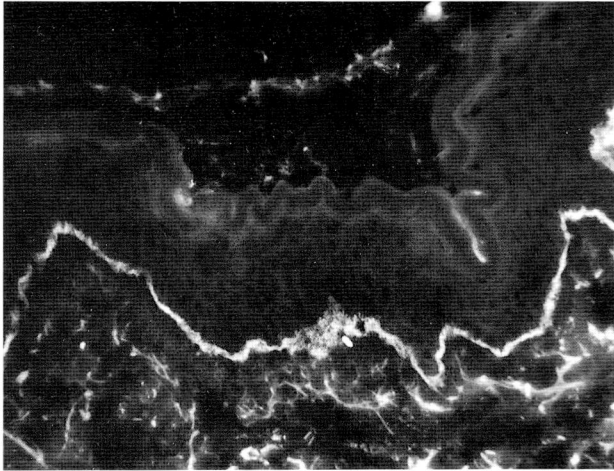

Fig. 2. Direct immunofluorescence.
Linear IgA deposition is observed at the dermo-epidermal junction *in vivo*. (× 100)

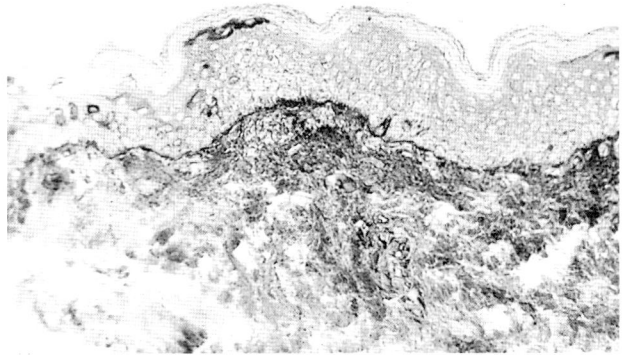

Fig. 3. Light microscope findings with immunoperoxidase staining.
Linear deposition of reaction products at the dermo-epidermal junction. (× 100)

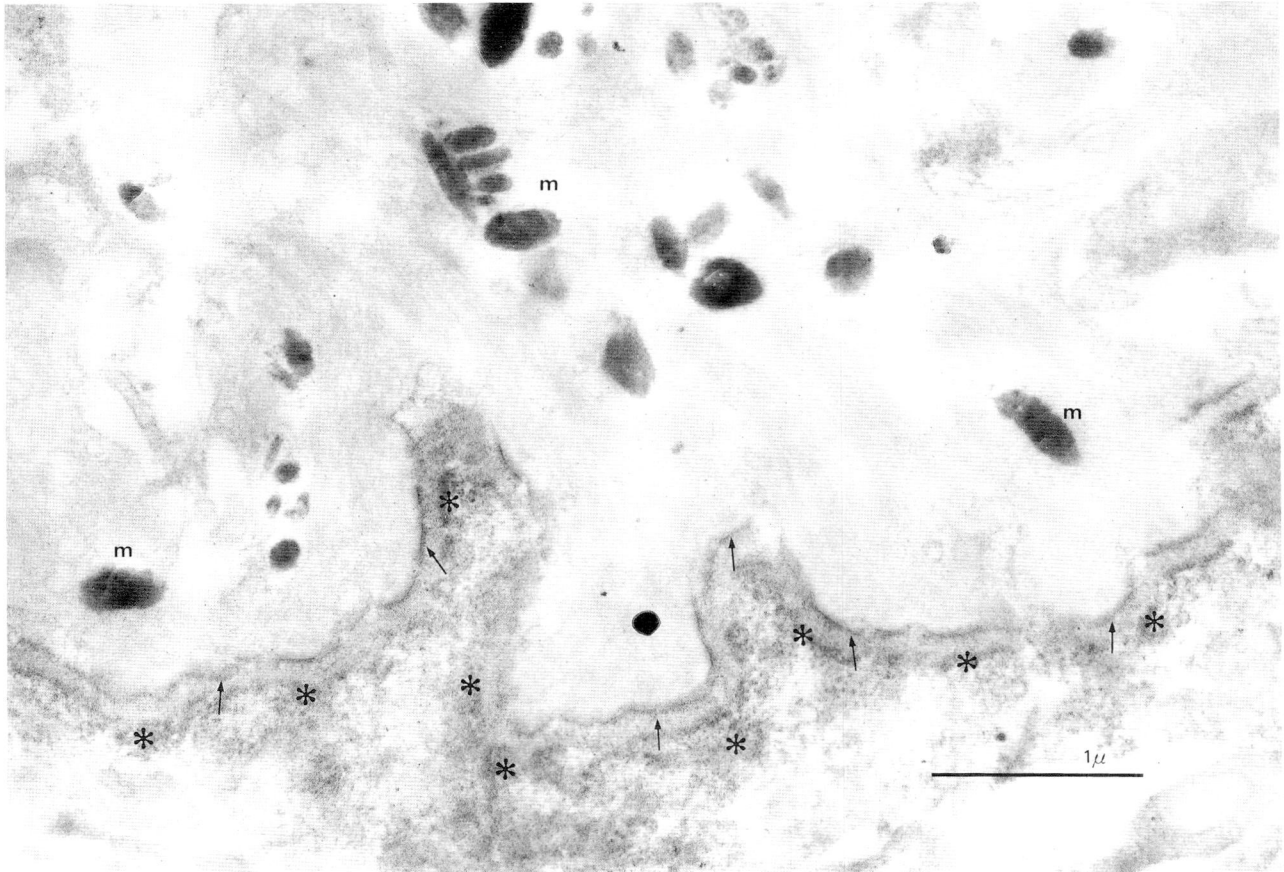

Fig. 4. Electron microscopic findings with immunoperoxidase staining.
Deposition of reaction products at the subbasal lamina region(*), and in the lamina lucida immediately below the cytomembrane of basal cells (arrows). m: melanin granules. (× 40,000)

Dermatitis herpetiformis

INTRODUCTION
Dermatitis herpetiformis Duhring (DH) was named by Luis Duhring in 1884[338] and characterized by chronic itchy bullous eruption. This disease frequently occurs in middle age. Subepidermal bulla, granular IgA deposits at dermal papillae, atrophy of small bowels, and the remarkable effect of DDS were thought to be specific for this disease[339]. Many of the patients become worse after taking gluten and have gluten-sensitive enteropathy; almost all of them have HLA-B8. The aetiology of this disease is unknown[340].

FINDINGS
The clinical features of this disease are well-demarcated erythema with small bullae (1), burning and intense itching. The histopathology is characterized by subepidermal bullae and neutrophil infiltration. Neutrophil microabscess at the papillary tip is thought to be the initial change (1).

Immunofluorescence microscopy shows granular IgA deposits at the papillary tip (2a, b) and associated complements such as C3 and/or properdin[341].

Immunoelectron microscopy demonstrates granular IgA deposits in relation to the microfibrillar bundle-elastic fibre system (3).

DIAGNOSIS (table I)
Today, granular IgA deposits at the papillary tip are thought to be specific for this disease[339]. Thus immunohistopathology employing immunofluorescent microscopy is the most important for diagnosis[342]. The other diagnostical findings are subepidermal bullae with neutrophils and a good response to DDS therapy. Immunoelectron microscopy may be helpful for the diagnosis[343]. The aetiology is not yet known, but this disease might be related to a connective tissue abnormality as a result of the immunoelectron microscopy findings[343].

BIOPSY AND KEY POINTS
The normal appearing skin of the patient with this disease is the best for immunohistopathologic biopsy. The skin at the margin of the lesion is also usable, but the skin biopsied from bullae should not be used for immunohistopathological diagnosis.

TABLE I   SUMMARY

Immunofluorescence	Granular IgA deposits at papillary tip
Circulating antibody against papillary tip	Not found
Immunoelectron microscopy of IgA binding sites	Microfibrillar bundle-elastic fibre system
Clinical features	Erythema with small bullae, itching and burning
Histopathology	Subepidermal bullae with neutrophil infiltration
HLA-B8	90%
Small bowel	Villi atrophy
Gluten	Sensitive in many cases
DDS	Effective

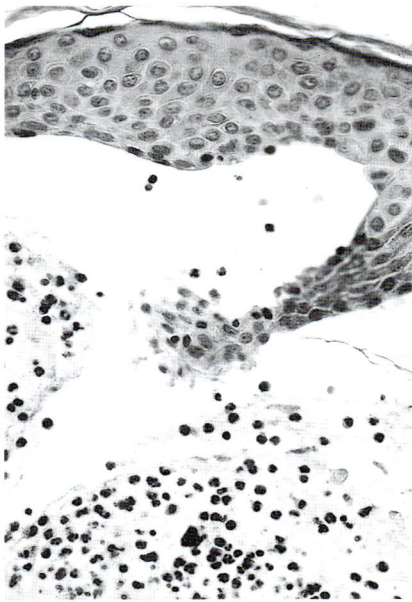

Fig. 1. Bullous lesion (H E stain). Subepidermal bullae with neutrophil infiltration. (× 400)

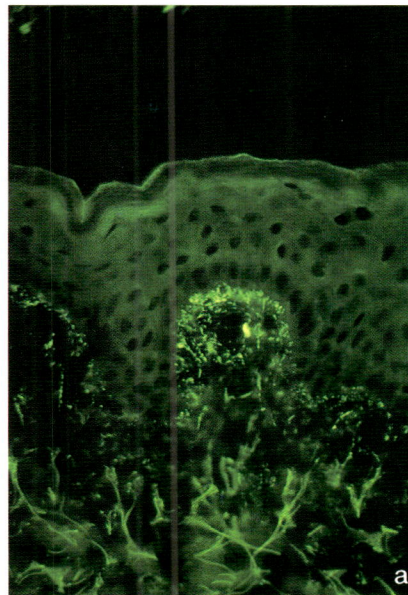

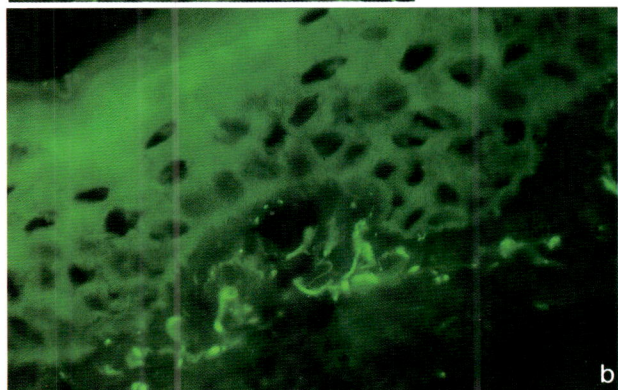

Fig. 2. Normal appearing skin (FITC-labelled method) with granular (a) (× 220) and fibrillar (b) deposits of IgA. (× 400 Courtesy of Dr. Katz, S.I.)

Fig. 3. Normal appearing skin (PAP-IEM counter-staining (−)). Dark granular reaction products indicate IgA deposits. (× 70,000)[343]

Collagen diseases and related disorders

Lupus erythematosus

INTRODUCTION

Systemic lupus erythematosus (SLE) is a systemic inflammatory and degenerative disease with multi-organ involvement and many immunological disturbances. The skin, kidney, heart, joints and central nervous system are frequently involved. The overproduction of diverse autoantibodies and depressed cellular immunity are among the common findings in this disease. The basic background of these immunological features may be in acquired polyclonal activation of B lymphocytes and twisted T lymphocytes.

Cutaneous changes are highly characteristic, but also show multiple, delicate features which must surely reflect the cellular and sub-cellular changes that occur with these immunological disturbances.

Utilizing immunohistological methods, a good amount of evidence has been obtained. The significance of LE cells, anti-nuclear factors, lupus band test, vascular changes, and lymphocytic infiltrates is described in this chapter.

THE SIGNIFICANCE OF FINDINGS

LE cells and anti-nuclear factors (ANF). Since the first description of LE cells by Hargraves in 1948, a positive finding of LE cells has been one of the most important diagnostic criteria for SLE. A number of studies have revealed that LE cells (**1**) are neutrophilic leucocytes which phago-

cytose a homogeneous inclusion body composed of DNA-protein complex (**2**) and antibodies (**3**). These inclusion bodies are immune complexes containing antigen, antibody, and complement. Figure 2 shows a green-stained (methyl-green pyronine solution) inclusion body in a LE cell which suggests the presence of DNA components. Human IgG can also be demonstrated in the same inclusion body as shown in figure 3. Anti-DNP protein antibody is known to play a critical role in LE cell formation.

ANF (antinuclear factor) is a general name for antibodies without species-specificity against nuclear components. These include DNA, RNA (messenger, transfer, ribosomal, small nuclear, heterogenous nuclear, etc.), several proteins with or without enzyme activities, histone and some other cell components. These antinuclear antibodies are summarized in Table I. Anti-ds-DNA antibody can often be found in severe cases of SLE and is well known to correlate with severe renal changes. Anti-nRNP antibodies are observed frequently in mild cases of Raynaud's disease, while anti-Sm antibodies appear in severe cases. Together with other autoantibodies against subcellular components, these antibodies might have some critical biological effects on the central dogma of cell activities.

To detect and standardize these ANF immunohistologically, it is particularly important to select appropriate substrates. Some cultured cell lines, such as KB cells or HEP-2 cells, are available and widely used[344]. It is important to read carefully the delicate pattern of fluorescent antigens. The relationship of the fluorescent pattern to ANF is summarized in Table II.

Lupus band test (LBT). In the diseased tissue of SLE and discoid LE (DLE), liquefaction degeneration of the basal cells (**4**) with oedematous changes and thickened subepidermal basement membranes (**5**) are characteristic features. In 1963, Burnham, et al.[345] found conspicuous granular deposits of immunoglobulins and complement at the epidermal-dermal junctional zones in accord with thickened PAS-positive basement membranes. These findings are highly characteristic of SLE and DLE, and can be found in over 90% of the diseased areas. A year later, Cormane[346] detected

TABLE I   ANTI-NUCLEAR ANTIBODIES IN SLE SERA

A. ANTIBODIES AGAINST DNA
  1. Anti-ds-DNA antibody
  2. Anti-ss-DNA antibody
  3. Against both ds-DNA and ss-DNA

B. ANTIBODIES AGAINST NON-HISTONE PROTEIN OR RNA PROTEIN COMPLEXES
  1. Anti-Sm antibody
  2. Anti-SS-A/Ro antibody
  3. Anti-SS-B/La antibody
  4. Anti-U1-RNP antibody
  5. Anti-PCNA antibody
  6. Anti-HMG 17 antibody
  7. Anti-Ki antibody
  8. Anti-Ma antibody
  9. others

C. ANTIBODIES AGAINST INTRA-NUCLEAR ANTIGENS
1. Anti RNA polymerase 1 Subunit antibody
2. others

PCNA*: proliferating cell nuclear antigen
HMG**: High mobility group

Fig. 1. LE cell in May-Giemsa staining. (× 400)

Fig. 2. LE cell in methyl-green pyronine staining. The inclusion body is positive for DNA-component. (× 600)

Fig. 3. LE cell in immunofluorescent reaction for human IgG. The inclusion body is positive for IgG. (× 400)

Fig. 4. Eosin-haematoxylin staining of SLE skin. Conspicuous liquefaction degenerations of basal cell layer are characteristic of SLE skin. (× 400)

Fig. 5. Thickened subepidermal basement membrane stained positive for PAS reaction. (× 400)

Fig. 6. Immunofluorescent staining for IgG shows thickened granular pattern at dermo-epidermal junction. (× 200)

Fig. 7. Peroxidase-labelled antibody method for IgG shows brownish-coloured granular deposits at junction. (× 200)

Fig. 8. Peroxidase-labelled antibody method for IgG under electron microscope. IgG are found as electron dense aggregates on collagen fibrils beneath the basal lamina. (× 20,000)

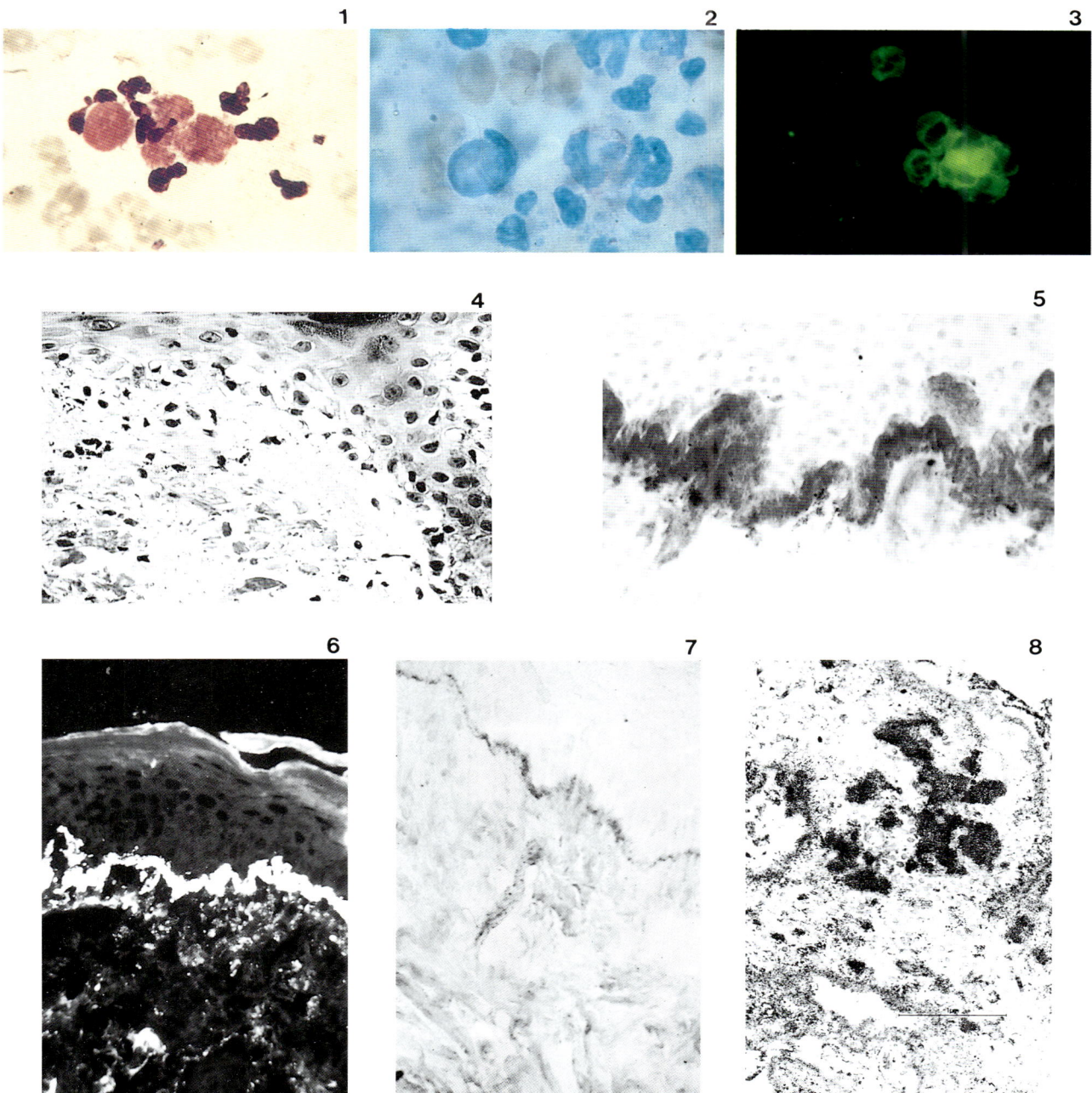

79

such deposits in the normal-appearing tissue of SLE, but not in that of DLE. These depositions in the normal skin of SLE are called lupus band test positive. They are found in 60% of SLE. Morphologically, they are differentiated into fine granular, coarse granular, lumpy, or thready patterns. These deposits are composed of IgG, IgM, IgA, IgE, Clq, C3, C4, C5, C3bINH, Factor B, ß1h-globulin, properdin, fibrin, albumin, plasminogen and fibronectin[347, 348] (6). With the peroxidase-labelled method, they can be visualized as brownish-granular deposits·at the junction (7). Under an electron microscope, these deposits are demonstrated as electron dense aggregates on the collagen fibrils beneath the basal lamina[349] (8). They are at present considered to be deposits of immune complexes, because such deposits can be found in the skin of Arthus' phenomenon. Antigens such as DNA are demonstrated in some cases of SLE, but immune complexes have not yet been confirmed in most cases. In addition, such deposits can be found occasionally in PSS[350], MCTD, linear sclero- derma[350], lichen planus, allergic vasculitis[351, 352], and the graft-versus-host reaction[353].

Davis and Gilliam[354] studied these deposits in a patient follow-up study spread over 10 years, and found that the patients with positive LBT of the IgG class had poorer prognosis than LBT-negative patients.

Immunopathology of the vasculatures. Blood vessels of various sizes in SLE skin show several histological changes, such as oedema, destruction, swelling, thickening (9) or obstruction with mucinous deposition and homogenization of collagen fibres. Immunopathologically, granular deposits of immunoglobulins (IgG, IgM, IgA) (10), complement, fibrin and fibronectin are found on the vascular walls. Granular deposits of immunoglobulins can be observed not only on the vascular walls, but also in the collagen matrix (11). Sometimes these vascular deposits are continuous with those on the dermo-epidermal junction (12). By electron microscopy using the peroxidase-labelled antibody tech-nique, these deposits are visible as dense aggregates on collagen fibrils outside the vascular basal lamina[349] (13).

Vascular deposits of immunoglobulins and complement are also reported in the skin of Schönlein-Henoch purpura, cryoglobulinaemic purpura, livedo vasculitis, lichen planus, granuloma annulare, pemphigus and other diseases.

Cellular infiltrates in the skin. Lympho-histiocytic infil-tration is common and a characteristic feature of SLE and DLE. Histiocytes are activated and found mainly in the dermo-epidermal zones and in the perivascular and periad-nexal areas. The dermis of DLE shows a more dense patchy infiltration than that of SLE (14). Some perivascular lymphoid cells display the presence of immunoglobulins (15).

Using newly-acquired monoclonal antibodies against the epitopes of lymphocytes, analysis of infiltrated lymphocytes can be carried out easily. Suppressor/cytotoxic T cells are predominant infiltrates in SLE[355], while helper/inducer T cells are frequently demonstrated in DLE[356]. Their signifi-cance in local lesions is still unknown. In both SLE and DLE, most exocytotic lymphocytes in the epidermis are suppressor/cytotoxic T cells.

TECHNICAL POINTS
Fresh, unfixed frozen sections are available for LBT and studies for immunoglobulin or complement deposits in the skin. The tissue specimens should be taken, free from artifacts, from relatively new lesions.

To estimate a prognosis, it is helpful to perform LBT on sections of normal-appearing skin from the flexor surface of the forearm. As for ANF study, cryostat sections of rat or mouse epithelial tissues are well-known substrates for immunofluorescence and enzyme immunoassay. If the SLE sera do not have a positive result, the ANA test on acetone-fixed mouse liver or kidney, on acetone-fixed monolayered cells (KB cell, HeLa cell, Hep 2 cell, etc.) should be performed.

TABLE II ANTI-NUCLEAR ANTIBODIES AND IMMUNOFLUORESCENCE PATTERN

1. Peripheral or shaggy pattern
   Antibody against ds-DNA, etc.

2. Homogeneous pattern
   Antibody against DNA, DNP, histone, etc.

3. Speckled pattern
   Antibody against nRNP, Sm, SS-B, centromere, etc.

4. Nucleolar pattern
   Antibody against nucleolus

Fig. 9. A thickened, hyalinized and necrotising blood vessel of livedoid skin stained in eosin-haematoxylin solution. (× 400)

Fig. 10. Direct immunofluorescent method for IgG shows granular deposits on the vascular walls and epidermo-dermal junction. (× 200)

Fig. 11. Direct immunofluorescent method for IgG reveals granular deposits not only at the junction and vascular walls, but also widely in the collagen bundles. (× 200)

Fig. 12. The granular deposits at the junctional zones are continuous with those on the vascular wall. (× 400)

Fig. 13. Electron-dense aggregates of IgG are found in the collagen fibrils just outside the blood vessel. Peroxidase antibody method for IgG. (× 20,000)

Fig. 14. Densely-packed lymphoid infiltration in DLE skin stained in eosin-haematoxylin solution. (× 200)

Fig. 15. B lymphocytes in DLE lesion show fluorescent IgG by immunofluorescent direct method for IgG. (× 200)

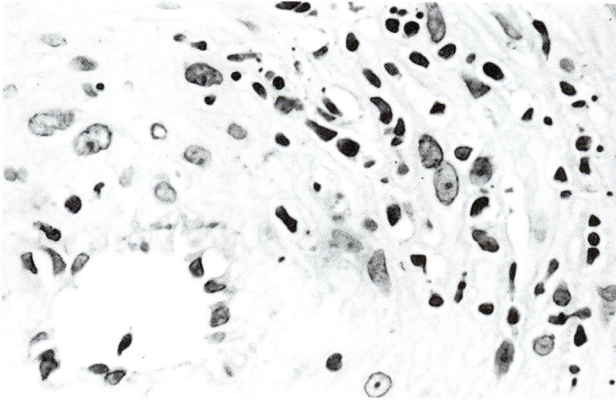

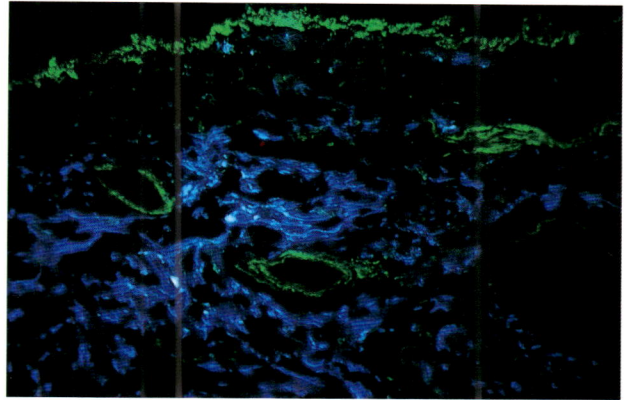

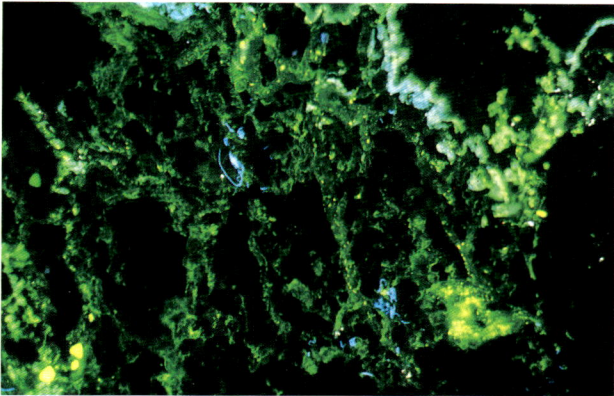

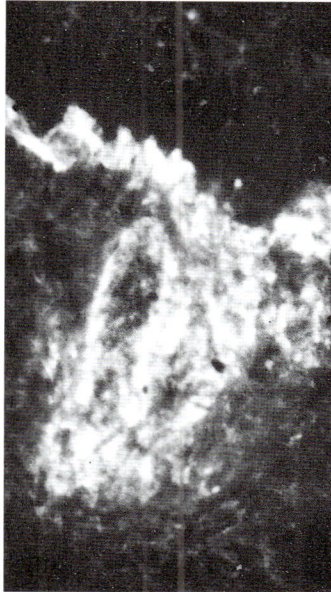

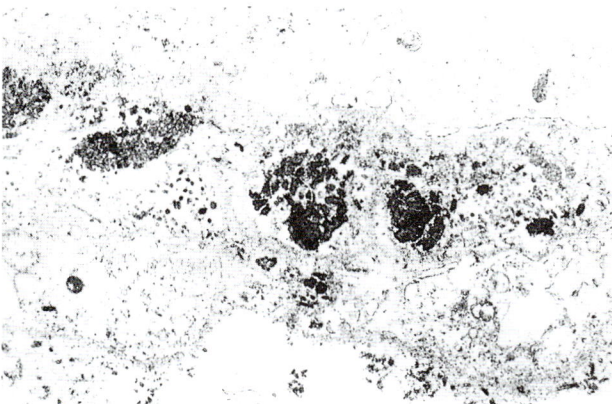

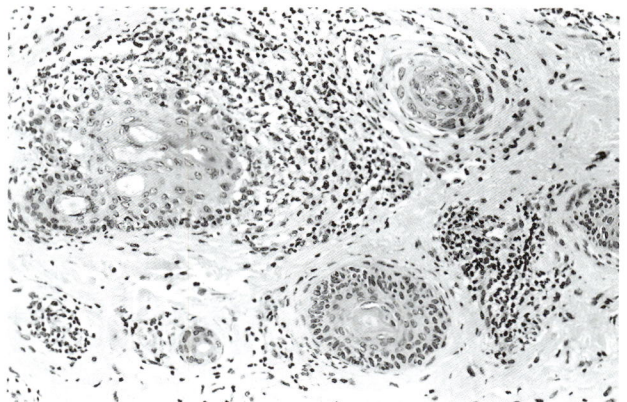

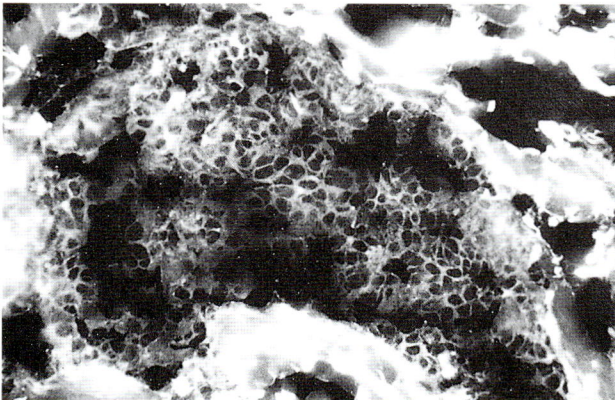

Scleroderma

INTRODUCTION

Scleroderma is an intractable disorder with a characteristic skin sclerosis. It is considered that abnormalities of connective tissue metabolism or the immunological system play an important role in its pathogenesis. Although the classification of scleroderma has not been unified, this paper is written according to the comprehensive classification shown in Table I[357], i.e., systemic types (progressive systemic sclerosis (PSS), mixed connective tissue disease (MCTD), and acute diffuse scleroderma having diffuse sclerosis with poor prognosis); cutaneous types (scleroderma in plaques, scleroderma in bands and linear scleroderma); and intermediate types (generalized morphoea and subcutaneous morphoea). Immunohistological characteristics will be discussed for each type of disease.

FINDINGS AND RELEVANCE TO DERMATOLOGY

In general, skin lesions in scleroderma were considered not to show any immunohistological changes, which were frequently seen in lupus erythematosus. Since Winkelmann[358] proposed the disease entity mesenchymal scleroderma — which is almost identical to MCTD as described by Sharp et al.[359] — immunological studies for lesional skin have proved to be of some value in scleroderma. It is now well recognized that a variety of immunological changes are observed in different types of scleroderma and such changes are important for the diagnosis[360].

In the case of PSS, by immunohistological techniques such as immunofluorescence, deposition of immunoglobulin and complement components is found to be negative in both lesional and non-lesional skin. However, antinuclear antibodies are frequently detected in the sera of patients. Among these, anti-Scl-70 antibodies (Og antibodies) are the most important and are found in approximately 30% of patients with PSS. These antibodies are considered to be extractable nuclear antigen (ENA) antibodies.

In the case of MCTD, IgG and IgM deposition at the basement membrane zone and the small blood vessels in the dermis or IgG deposition in the nuclei of keratinocytes are frequently observed (1). Deposition of IgG in the nuclei of keratinocytes is closely related to the presence of anti-RNP (ribonucleoprotein) antibodies in the sera of patients and is seen in normal skin as well as lesional skin. There has been controversy for years as to whether this change is a real in vivo phenomenon or an in vitro artifact. It is rather difficult to believe that the large molecules of IgG can penetrate through the viable keratinocyte cell membrane and bind to the antigen in the nuclei. It seems more likely that this change is due to an in vitro reaction during the biopsy or staining procedures, although this concept has not been fully supported by the experimental data to date[361, 362].

In the case of localized or cutaneous morphoea, immunohistological changes have not been well described. IgM deposition at the basement membrane zone is often seen in localized scleroderma, mainly in linear scleroderma or generalized morphoea, and antinuclear antibodies are often easily detectable when cultured cells are used as the substrate[363] (2). Furthermore, immunoelectron microscopic studies have shown that IgM is deposited in subbasal lamina, where lupus erythematosus also show immunoglobulin deposition[364]. Table II shows the summary of our data. These results strongly suggest that immunohistological studies are of considerable use for the classification of scleroderma. Immunological examinations should therefore be routinely performed to aid diagnosis.

TECHNICAL POINTS

Unfixed cryostat sections are preferable for immunofluorescence study. Paraffin-embedded sections are not suitable for the peroxidase-anti-peroxidase method (PAP). For immunoelectron microscopy 2–4% paraformaldehyde or PLP fixation is recommended.

TABLE I   SCLERODERMA CLASSIFICATION

SYSTEMIC

1. Acrosclerotic form
   = Barnett & Coventry Type 2
   = Progressive systemic sclerosis (Goetz)
   = Systemic scleroderma of acrosclerosis type (Ishikawa)
   = Acroscleroderma (Jablonska)
      (CRST Syndrome)

2. Mesenchymal inflammatory scleroderma (Winkelmann et al.)
   = Mixed connective tissue disease (Sharp)
   = Systemic scleroderma with mild skin changes (Ishikawa)
   = Barnett & Coventry Type 1

3. Acute diffuse scleroderma or malignant scleroderma
   = Systemic scleroderma with generalized skin changes (Ishikawa)
   = Barnett & Coventry Type 3

4. Subcutaneous morphoea
   = Shulman syndrome

5. Generalized morphoea

Cutaneous

Morphoea

   localized morphoea
   in plaques
      (in drops)
   in bandes
   linear scleroderma
      scar and hemiatrophy
   widespread or multiple morphoea

Generalized morphoea
   diffuse scleroderma
   subcutaneous morphoea

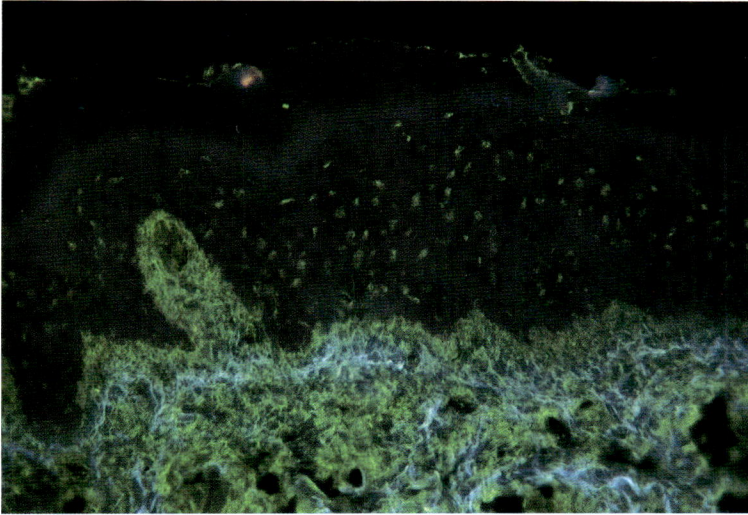

Fig. 1. IgG deposition in the nuclei of keratinocytes (direct immunofluorescence).

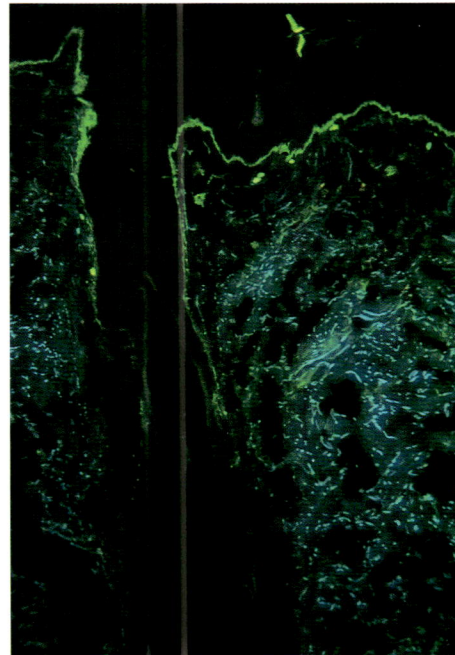

Fig. 2. IgM deposition at the basement membrane zone (direct immunofluorescence).

TABLE II   IMMUNOHISTOLOGICAL FINDINGS IN LESIONAL SKIN AND CIRCULATING ANTI-ENA ANTIBODIES IN VARIOUS TYPES OF SCLERODERMA

Diagnosis	No. of cases	Deposition in lesional skin				Circulating antibodies	
		IgG	IgA	IgM	C3	RNP	Scl-70 (0g)
PSS	6	2	0	0	0	0	5
MCTD	9	8	2	7	0	5	0
Localized scleroderma	15	0	0	8	0	N.T.	N.T.
scleroderma in plaques	3	0	0	1	0		
scleroderma in bandes	3	0	0	2	0		
linear scleroderma	4	0	0	3	0		
generalized morphoea	5	0	0	2	0		

N.T.: Not tested.

83

Behcet's disease

INTRODUCTION

Behçet's disease (BD), described by Hulusi Behçet (1937)[365], is a systemic disorder in which there are mainly oral, ocular, cutaneous and genital lesions. In addition to these symptoms, BD frequently associates visceral involvement, such as vascular lesions, intestinal lesions, neural involvement and arthritis. Although the aetiology of BD is obscure, there are some aetiological theories such as viral infection[365,366], bacterial infection[367], bacterial infectious allergy[368,369], autoimmunity[370,371], and toxic reaction to heavy metals[372]. Recently it has been suggested that HLA-BW51 is closely associated with BD[373].

Epidemiology. It has been reported that the disease appears mostly in the third decade in people who live in the mediterranean areas Korea and Japan. The ratio of male to female occurrence of BD is considered to be 3:1[374,375]. According to a national Japanese epidemiological study, a total of 5,512 patients with BD (4.6 per 100,000 population) were registered throughout Japan to the end of March 1983. In Hokkaido Prefecture the highest prevalence rate was noticed, at 12.5 per 100,000 population with a male to female ratio of 1:3, thus predominant in women[376].

Clinical manifestation. BD is a multisystemic disease with mucocutaneous, ocular, articular, intestinal, vascular and neurological involvement. In the skin, erythema nodosum (EN)-like eruptions, acneiform eruptions and painful thrombophlebitis occur mainly on the trunk and legs, and pustules tend to appear after micro-trauma and/or stimulation. On the oral and genital mucosae, small punched-out ulcerations, referred to as aphthous ulcers, often appear. In the ocular lesion, iritis with hypopyon, retinal and vitreous haemorrhages, and papilloedema recurrently occur in some cases. The result is blindness. In addition to these symptoms, the vascular symptoms, such as aneurysm, peripheral gangrene, vascular thrombosis and superficial phlebitis occur; and neural symptoms and gastrointestinal tract cholinic ulcers appear. Sometimes the disease develops to severe clinical conditions.

HISTOLOGICAL AND IMMUNOHISTOLOGICAL (IF) FINDINGS

Mucosal lesions. In aphthous ulceration, numerous mononuclear cells and polymorphonuclear cells (PMNs) were seen infiltrating towards the surface of the ulcer (**1a, b**). At the margin of the oral epithelium adjacent to the ulcer, some inflammatory cells were found in close association with epithelial cells (**1b**).

The direct IF studies showed deposits of IgG, IgA, IgM and C3 on the surface of the ulcer (**2a**) and IgM was deposited in the mononuclear cells infiltrated around the epithelial cells (**2b**). The infiltrates in the epithelial layer were composed of macrophages exhibiting OKM-1$^+$ (monocytes and granulocytes, Orthoclone Diagnostic Systems, U.S.A.) and HLA-DR$^+$ (monomorphic determinants, Becton Dickinson Monoclonal Center Inc., U.S.A.) (**2c**) and helper T cells exhibiting Leu 3a$^+$ (helper/inducer T cells) (**2d**). Moreover, there were also natural killer (NK) cells showing Leu 7$^+$ in the infiltrates.

The findings suggest that the infiltrates around the epithelial cells show direct lymphocyte cytotoxicity and/or antibody-dependent cell-mediated cytotoxicity (ADCC) against the epithelial cells of the oral mucosa[377,378].

Cutaneous lesions. In EN-like eruption, almost all of the infiltrates around the vessels in the deep dermis and interseptal fatty tissue were composed of mononuclear cells, showing septal panniculitis (**3a, b**). In the early stage of the lesion (one or two days after the appearance), neutrophilic infiltrate has been reported around the vessels in the deep dermis[379].

Direct IF studies showed deposits of IgM and C3 in the endothelium of the vessels (**4a**). When FITC-conjugated anti-streptococcus group D rabbit serum (Bacto-FA Streptococcus Group D; Difco Lab., U.S.A.) was used, positive fluorescence could be observed in the endothelium of the vessels in EN-like lesions (**4b**). The findings suggest the presence of immune complexes including IgM, complement and antigens related to streptococcus in lesion vessel walls[380]. The infiltrates around the vessels were predominantly associated with Leu 3a and HLA-DR, which were suggested to be helper T cells and macrophages. NK cells had also infiltrated. However, NK cells were not observed in the sections biopsied from patients with EN[381]. The findings of NK cell infiltration seemed to be correlated with the increase in the number of NK cells in the peripheral blood of patients in the active stage of the disease[382].

DIAGNOSTIC SIGNIFICANCE

The clinical manifestations are crucial for making the diagnosis of BD. The histological features of EN-like eruptions are undifferentiated from those of EN and/or erythema induratum. The histologic picture of aphthous ulceration is not characteristic either. However, the infiltration of NK cells and the deposition of streptococcus-related antigen in the lesions of BD is of interest immunohistologically.

TECHNICAL POINTS

1. To achieve an immunological reaction in the lesion of BD, the skin should be biopsied from early stage lesions.
2. To avoid non-specific staining, it is recommended that the FITC-conjugated antibody sera be adjusted to less than 2.0 the fluorescein/protein (F/P)-ratio using DEAE (diethylaminoethyl) cellulose column chromatography.
3. When the anti-streptococcus antibody serum (Bacto-FA Streptococcus Group D) is used, it is recommended that the F/P-ratio be adjusted to less than 2.0 and that the serum be absorbed with normal skin because the antibody cross-reacts with normal epidermal cells.

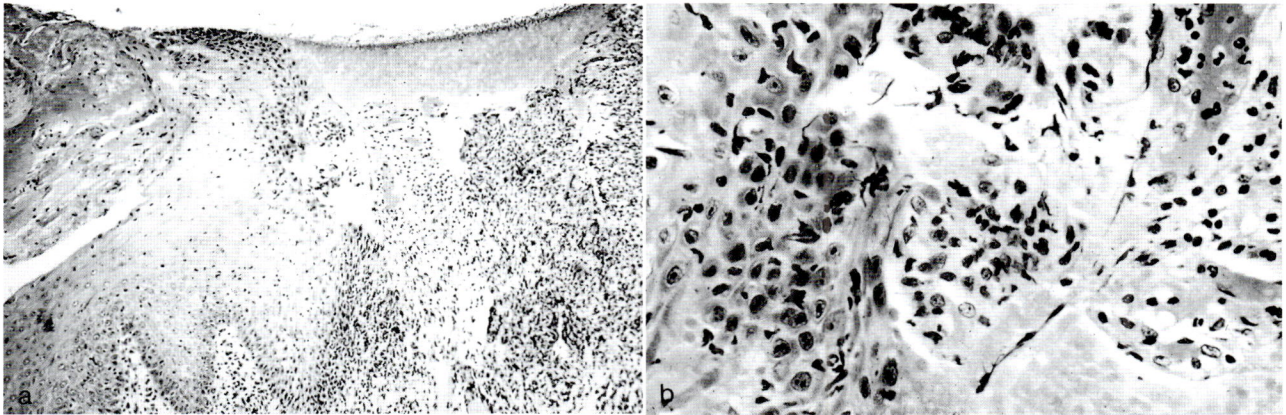

Fig. 1. Histological features of aphthous ulceration.
a. Aphthous ulceration oral mucosa. (HE, × 100)
b. High magnification of the margin of epithelium adjacent to
the ulcer (× 400). Note inflammatory mononuclear infiltrate
around the epithelial cells.

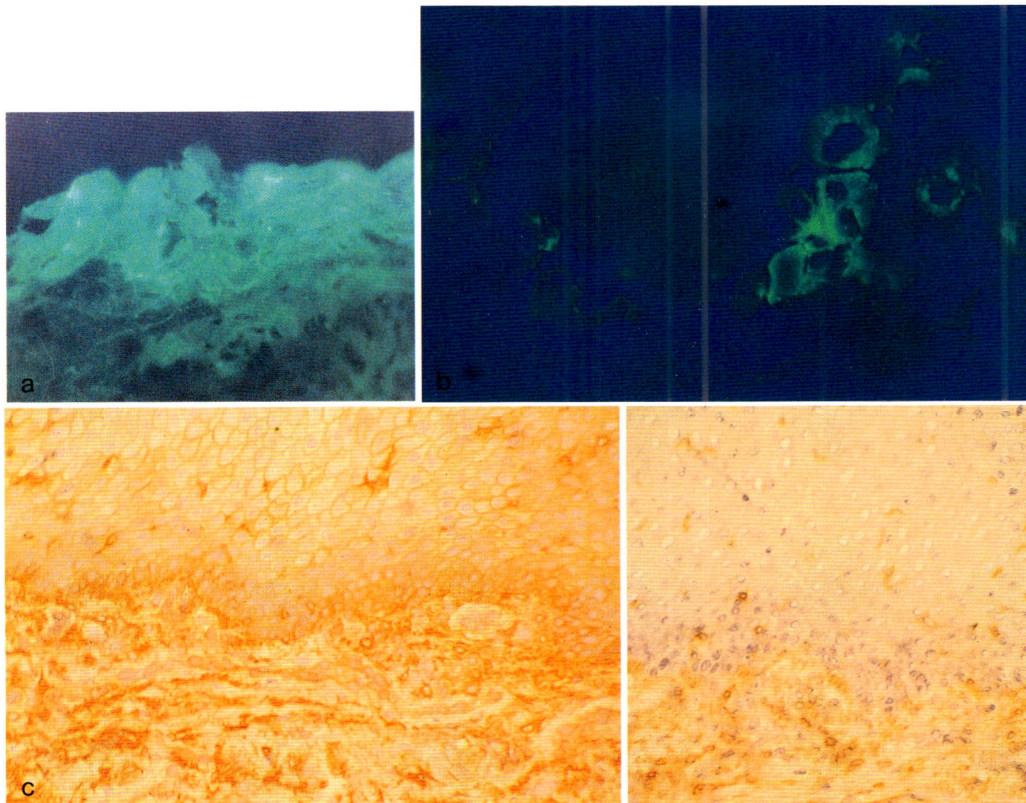

**Fig. 2. Immunohistological features of aphthous
ulceration.**
a. Deposits of IgG on the surface of the ulcer. (IF staining,
× 100)
b. Smear cells from the surface of aphthous ulcer. (IF staining,
× 1,000). Note IgM-bearing mononuclear cells around
epithelial cells of oral mucosa.
c. HLA$^+$ infiltrates in the epithelium. (Avidin-biotin complex
(ABC) method, × 400). Mononuclear cells with HLA-DR$^+$ can
be seen in the epithelium and proprial layer of aphthous ulcer.
d. Infiltration of mononuclear cells with Leu 3a$^+$. (ABC
method, × 400). Leu 3a$^+$ cells (helper T cells) are infiltrated
around the ulcer.

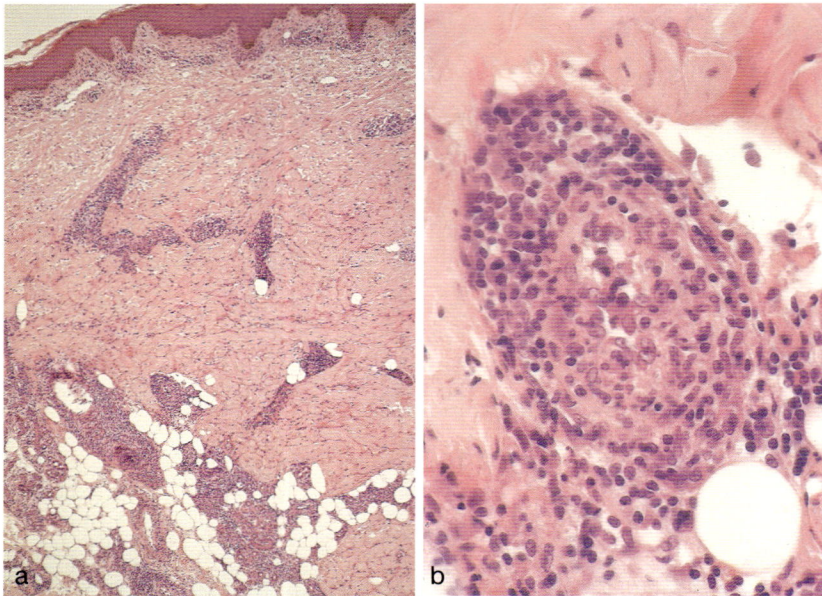

Fig. 3. Histological features of erythema nodosum (EN)-like eruption.
a. Lymphoid cell infiltrates around vessels in the middle and deep dermis. (HE, × 100)
b. High magnification (× 200). Lymphoid cell infiltrates around a vessel in the subcutaneous fat layer.

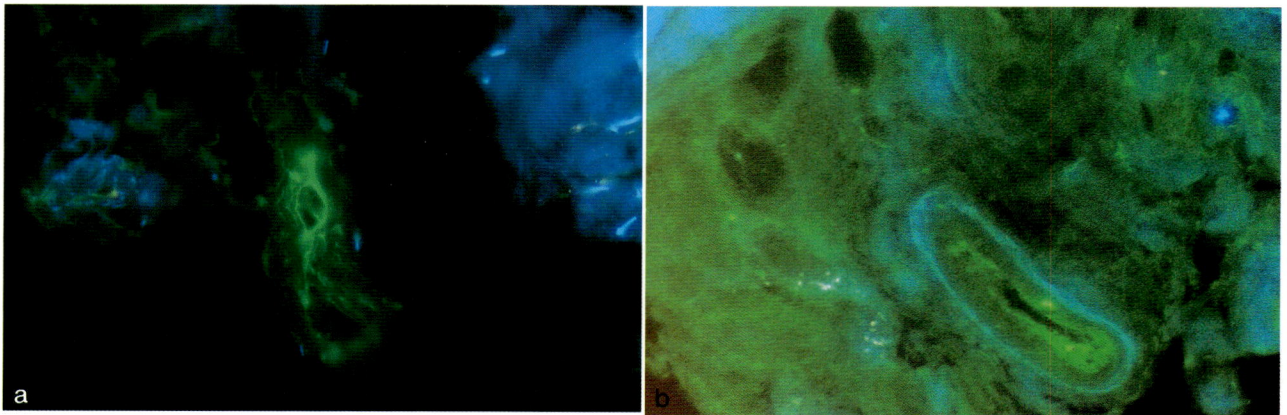

Fig. 4. Immunohistological features of EN-like eruption.
a. IgM deposit in the vessel wall of the deep dermis. (IF staining, × 200)
b. Positive fluorescence in the vessel wall of the deep dermis using FITC-conjugated anti-streptococcus group D rabbit serum. (IF staining, × 200)

TABLE I   HISTOLOGICAL GRADING SYSTEM FOR CUTANEOUS GvHD

GRADE	HISTOLOGICAL CHANGES
1.	Focal or diffuse vacuolar degeneration of the epidermal basal cells and Malpighian cells.
2.	Basal cell vacuolation, focal or diffuse spongiosis and dyskeratosis, or eosinophilic degeneration of epidermal cells.
3.	Clefts and spaces after necrosis of basal cells and Malpighian cells, often resulting in separation at the dermal-epidermal junction.
4.	Loss of epidermis.

Data from Glucksberg, H. *et al.*: Transplantation **18**:295, 1974.

Graft-versus-host (GvH) reaction in animals

INTRODUCTION

Graft-versus-host (GvH) reaction occurs from the immune responses of donor T lymphocytes to histocompatibility antigens of the recipient when immunocompetent cells are transferred to the allogeneic recipient incapable of rejecting them. GvH reaction causes the pathological manifestations termed GvH disease (GvHD), which is commonly seen in patients receiving allogeneic bone marrow transplantation.

CLASSIFICATION AND CLINICAL MANIFESTATION

GvHD can be classified as acute or chronic GvHD. The former usually appears between ten and forty days after bone marrow transplantation, while the latter develops several months or even years after the transplantation, with or without the preceding acute GvHD. The skin, gastrointestinal tract and liver are most commonly involved. A number of studies have demonstrated the development of cutaneous manifestations during the course of GvHD which are similar to a variety of naturally occurring skin diseases[383]. The cutaneous manifestations similar to toxic epidermal necrolysis (TEN) or lichen planus (LP) have been described clinically and histologically to have been present in acute GvHD. Chronic GvHD is characterized by the development of skin lesions that closely resemble LP, scleroderma, Sjögren's syndrome and cutaneous LE. Thus, our understanding of GvHD may lead to insights in the underlying pathophysiology of skin diseases mediated by autoimmune mechanisms.

AETIOLOGY

Recent experimental approaches using F_1 mice have suggested that acute GvHD is caused by donor T lymphocytes with suppressor/killer phenotype ($T^{s/k}$) which react to class I major histocompatibility complex (MHC) antigens of the recipient, whereas chronic GvHD is mediated by the T lymphocytes with helper phenotype (T^h) which react to class II MHC antigens[384]. It is well known that class II-negative keratinocytes express this antigen normally in GvHD. Because GvHD also develops following syngeneic or autologous bone marrow transplantation, differences in histocompatibility antigens are not a prerequisite for the development of GvHD. Glazier et al. reported the development of GvHD-like syndrome upon withdrawal of Cyclosporin-A (CsA) therapy in syngeneic bone marrow transplant recipients[385].

We recently demonstrated that autoreactive cloned T^h (specific for self class II antigens) induce histological changes identical to those seen in human GvHD, following intradermal inoculation in naive syngeneic recipients[386]. In epidermis in which cutaneous GvHD had been induced, expression of I-A (class II antigens) by keratinocytes was observed (1). The histological changes varied from LP-like (2) to TEN-like lesions (3), depending on the dosage of the T cells transferred, but were in accord with Grades 2–4 of the criteria for human GvHD (Table I). These autoreactive T^h have been shown to kill not only class II-positive target cells but also class II-negative bystander target cells in the presence of class II-positive stimulator cells, probably via the release of lymphotoxin (LT) and IFN-[387]. This evidence would suggest that TEN and LP are caused from the activation of class II-reactive T^h capable of releasing LT and IFN-.

TECHNICAL POINTS

Epidermal sheets from the footpads of mice were separated from the dermis by incubation in 0.02% EDTA for two hours at 37°C. The epidermal sheets, fixed in acetone for twenty minutes, were stained for IA-bearing cells using an indirect immunofluorescence method.

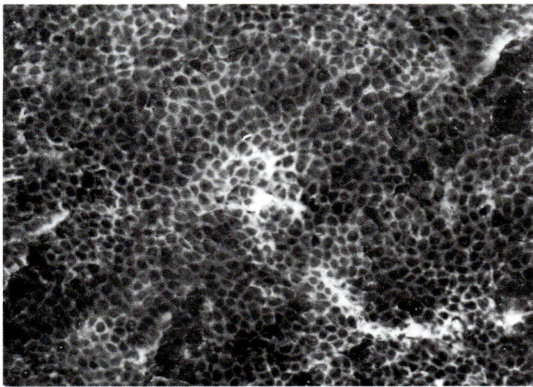

Fig. 1. Immunofluorescence of I-A-positive cells in epidermal sheets from murine footpads. At 72 hours after local transfer of autoreactive cloned T cells, the keratinocytes express I-A at the cell membrane. (× 80)

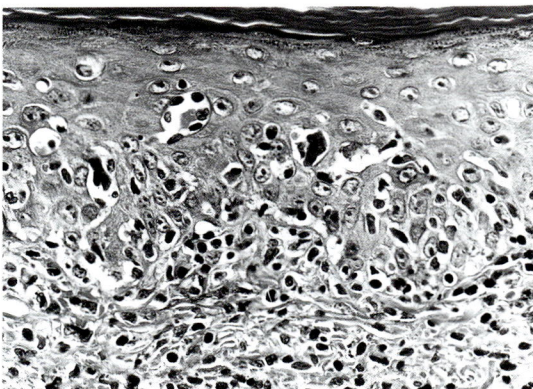

Fig. 2. Histology of murine footpad at 72 hours after local transfer of autoreactive clone T cells, showing Grade 2 cutaneous GvHD with basal vacuolar degeneration as the result of epidermal lymphocytic infiltration. Civatte bodies and satellite cell necrosis are observed. (× 50)

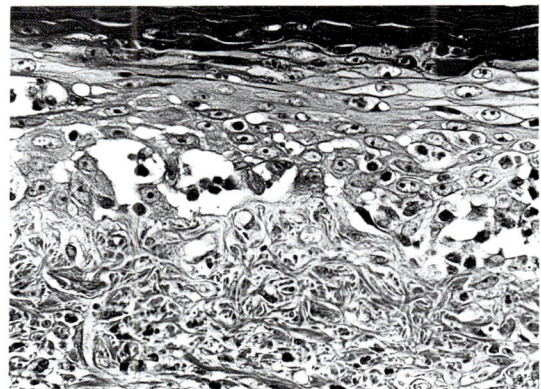

Fig. 3. At 72 hours after local transfer of autoreactive cloned T-cells, eosinophilic degeneration of epidermal cells and epidermal necrosis are seen. (× 50)

Human GvH reaction

INTRODUCTION

Graft-versus-host reaction (GvHR) is initiated by immune responses of donor T cells towards allogeneic histocompatibility antigens of the recipient[388]. This reaction results in graft-versus-host disease (GvHD), which affects various organs, particularly the skin, liver and gastrointestinal tract. GvHD is a major complication in allogeneic bone marrow transplantation[389].

Lichen-planus-like eruption (LPLE) is known as a clinical manifestation in an early phase of chronic GvHD, and the initial lesions are most often observed in the oral mucosa[390]. Therefore oral LPLE is very important, not only for early diagnosis of chronic GvHD but also for the study of the pathogenesis of GvHD. This lesion is also noteworthy as a model for lichen planus (LP) as the clinical manifestations and pathologic features are very similar[391]

Recent immunohistochemical techniques, especially the use of monoclonal antibodies (MoAb) directed against lymphoid subgroup antigens, allow analysis of infiltrated lymphocytes in skin lesions of GvHD. Previous immunohistochemical studies on cutaneous acute and chronic GvHD have indicated that infiltrated lymphocytes in these lesions are more numerous in OKT8+ cells (cytotoxic/suppressor-T cells) than in OKT4+ cells (helper/inducer-T cells)[392, 393]. Our recent study[394] on LPLE in GvHD has also shown a similar pattern of infiltrated lymphocytes. This suggests that cytotoxic T cells play a major role in cutaneous or oral mucosal GvHD.

FINDINGS

1. Clinical and pathological features. LP-like reticulated white striae are observed in lower lip and buccal mucosa. These lesions show a LP-like tissue reaction with satellite cell necrosis (SCN) characteristic of GvHD (**1**).
2. Infiltrated lymphocytes are stained by the indirect horseradish peroxidase-labelled antibody method in the serial sections of oral lesions in GvHD using MoAb. Leu-2a+ cells (cytotoxic/suppressor-T cells) predominate in upper lamina propria, the basal cell layer and the epithelium above the basal cell layer (**2**).

It is reported that IL-2 receptor is expressed on the surface of activated lymphocytes *in vitro*[395]. Some infiltrated lymphocytes in the areas of SCN, upper lamina propria and the basal cell layer bear this receptor (**3a**). Almost all of these cells correspond to Leu 4+ cells stained in adjacent sections (**3b**).

HLA-DR antigen is detected on keratinocytes in agreement with the findings of cutaneous GvHD[392, 396] (**4**), and the antigen expression is induced in keratinocytes by γ-interferon *in vitro*[397]. Therefore, such HLA-DR expression in the oral lesions of LPLE in GvHD might be of significance in antigen presentation or cell-mediated cytotoxicity involving keratinocytes.

Immunoelectron micrographs show the severe damage of keratinocytes with the disappearance of cytoplasmic organelles and degenerated tonofilaments to which Leu-2a+ cells are attached (**5a**), while the structure of keratinocytes attached to Leu 3a+ cells was preserved (**5b**). This finding indicates that Leu2a+ cells might be cytotoxic and might directly damage keratinocytes.

These findings suggest that cellular immunity mediated by cytotoxic T cells plays a major role in the pathogenesis of oral LPLE in GvHD.

METHODS

Punch biopsies (3 or 5 mm) are taken from oral mucosal lesions (buccal mucosa or lower lip) under local anaesthesia, and each of the tissue specimens is cut into two. One is promptly fixed in periodate-lysine-4% paraformaldehyde (PLP) for between four and six hours at 4°C. The other is fixed in 10% formalin for haematoxylin-eosin staining. The immunostaining is performed by the indirect horseradish peroxidase-labelled antibody method as previously reported. Briefly, serial 6μ thick cryostat sections are washed in PBS, immersed in 10% nonimmune goat serum in PBS for ten minutes, and then reacted overnight with MoAb at 4°C. After extensive washing, the sections are immersed in 0.3% methanol-hydrogen peroxide solution for thirty minutes in order to block endogeneous peroxidase activity. The sections are washed in PBS and then reacted overnight with horseradish peroxidase-labelled F(ab')₂ anti-mouse IgG at 4°C. After excess antibody reagents have been washed off with PBS, the sections are incubated in 0.2% diaminobenzidine (DAB) solution in 0.05 M Tris-HCL buffer, pH 7.6, containing 20 mM hydrogen peroxide and 10 mM sodium azide for five minutes, and then counter-stained with methyl green.

Cryostat sections adjacent to those used for light microscopy are selected for electron microscopic study. After sequential overnight incubations at 4°C with MoAb and horseradish peroxidase-labelled F(ab')₂ anti-mouse IgG. The sections are fixed in 0.5% glutaraldehyde in PBS for five minutes, treated with the DAB solution without hydrogen peroxide for fifteen minutes and then with the DAB solution containing 10 mM hydrogen peroxide for five minutes. The sections are postfixed with 2% osmium tetroxide, dehydrated in graded ethanols and embedded in Epon. Ultrathin sections, lightly stained with lead citrate, are examined with a Hitachi H-300 electron microscope.

TECHNICAL POINTS

1. The tissue specimens are promptly fixed in PLP.
2. The indirect horseradish peroxidase-labelled antibody method is better for the immunoelectron microscopic observation of cryostat sections than the peroxidase anti-peroxidase method (PAP) using immune complexes of large molecules.
3. Both the first antibodies and the horseradish peroxidase-labelled second antibodies are applied to cryostat sections for between eight and twelve hours at 4°C in order to permeate the tissue sections thoroughly.
4. The used second antibody consists of a mixture of antibodies against all four subclasses of mouse IgG.
5. Ultrathin sections are lightly stained with lead citrate for the observation of ultrastructure.

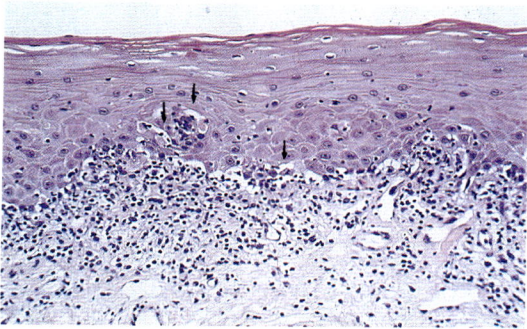

Fig. 1. Histology of reticulated white lesion of lower lip. Arrows show SCN. (Haematoxylin-eosin staining, × 100)

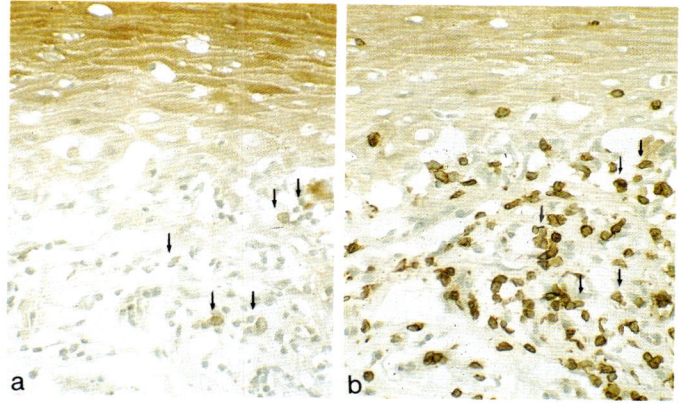

Fig. 2. T cell subsets of lichen planus-like oral lesion in GvHD. Leu-2a⁺ cells predominate in the lesion. (a) Leu2a; (b) Leu3a. (a, b × 125)

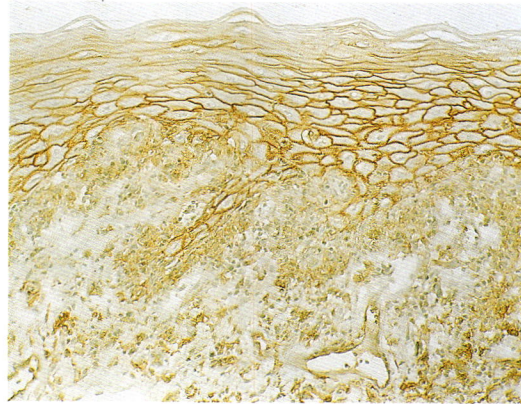

Fig. 3. Some of the infiltrated lymphocytes are reactive with anti-IL-2 receptor antibody (↑) (a). Nearly all of these cells correspond to Leu-4⁺ cells (↑) in adjacent sections (b). (a, b × 200)

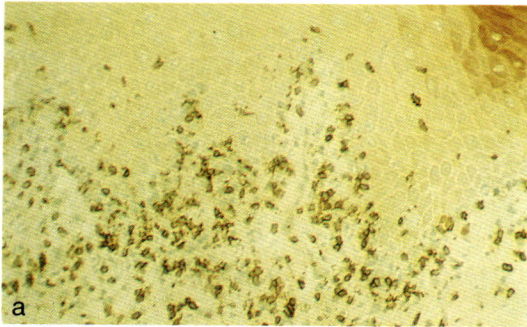

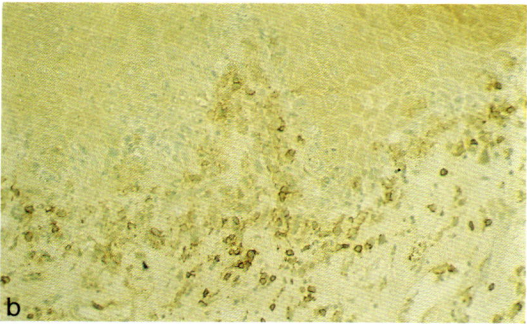

Fig. 4. All keratinocytes in the LPLE express HLA-DR antigen, particularly those in the cell membrane. (× 125)

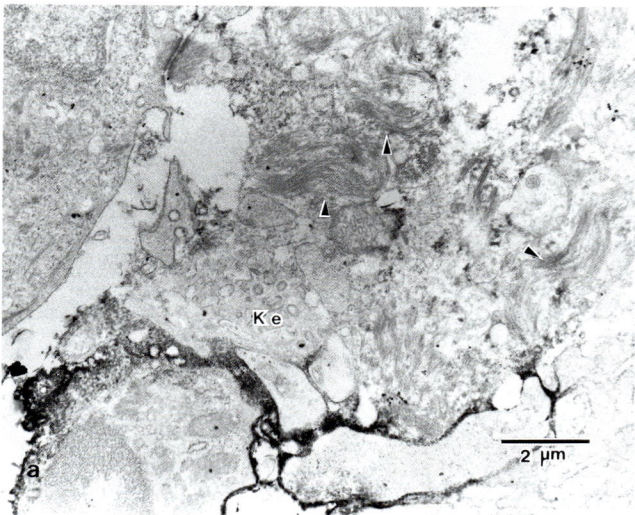

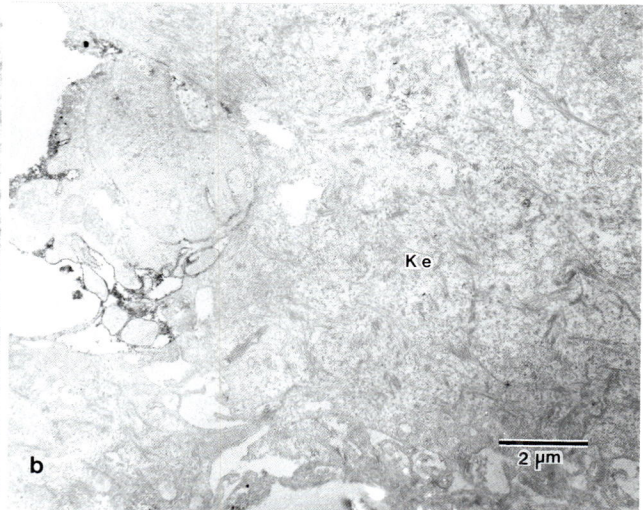

Fig. 5. An immunoelectron micrograph illustrates severe damage of the keratinocyte to which a Leu-2a⁺ cell is attached (a), while the structure of the keratinocyte attached to Leu-3a⁺ cell is preserved (b). Arrows show degenerated tonofilaments. Ke: keratinocyte.

89

Pityriasis rosea (Gibert)

INTRODUCTION

Viral or infectious aetiology for pityriasis rosea (PR) has been suggested, due to the typical short clinical course beginning with a single herald patch that is followed a week or so later by disseminated secondary eruption. There is no direct evidence, however, that definitely supports this hypothesis.

Histological studies have shown the presence of eczematoid or parapsoriatic changes[398, 399]. Ultrastructurally, cytolytic degeneration of keratinocytes adjacent to Langerhans cells is present in the epidermis[400]. From the immunological viewpoint, Takaki et al.[401] demonstrated IgM antibodies against keratinocyte cytoplasm in serum and in lesional skin, but Mobacken et al.[402] failed to disclose any such antibodies or immune complexes. We described the immunohistopathological characteristics of the lesions of PR, which strongly suggest an important role played by cellular immunity in the pathomechanism of PR[399].

FINDINGS

Large numbers of lymphoid cells in the perivascular infiltrate reacted with anti-pan-T cells, anti-helper-inducer subsets, and anti-HLA-DR monoclonal antibodies, while the epidermotropic mononuclear cells consisted of helper-inducer and suppressor-cytotoxic cells without any predominance pattern (**1**). In addition to epidermal Langerhans cells, some of the dermal infiltrating cells were reactive to the monoclonal antibody OKT6. Moreover, there was localized expression of HLA-DR antigen on the keratinocytes (**2**).

These immunohistological characteristics are very similar to those in allergic contact sensitivity reactions. Therefore it is suggested that cellular immune reactions take place in the lesional epidermis of PR.

TECHNICAL POINTS

The cryostat sections of snap-frozen biopsy specimens were stained by the avidin-biotin-peroxidase complex method[399, 403].

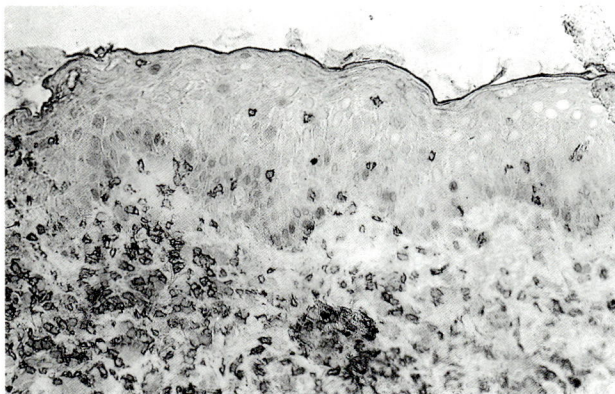

Fig. 1. Leu-1⁺ cells in pityriasis rosea.
Leu-1⁺ cells were found in exocytotic cells as well as in the perivascular infiltrate. (× 120)

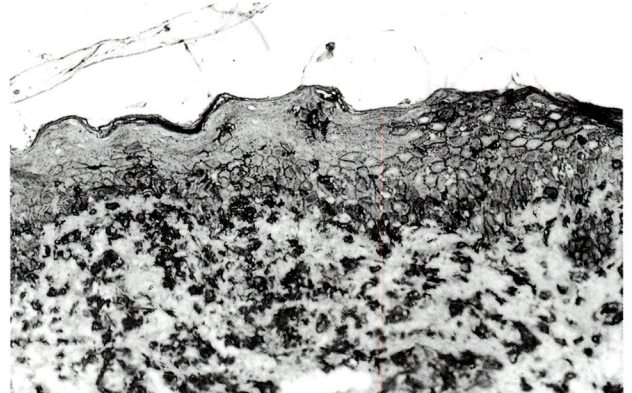

Fig. 2. HLA-DR⁺ cells in pityriasis rosea.
Most of the infiltrating cells expressed HLA-DR antigen. Localized expression of HLA-DR antigen on the keratinocytes. (× 120)

Erythema exudativum multiforme

INTRODUCTION

Erythema multiforme exudativum is considered to be one of the skin reactions caused by multifactors, such as herpes simplex virus, mycoplasma pneumonia, haemolytic streptococci and drugs. The initial eruptions are pinhead-sized oedematous papules, which gradually spread to form iris lesions. The centre of the lesion is slightly pale and depressed and the peripheral border is elevated. A bulla is occasionally seen in the centre. There is usually a mixture of new and old lesions. Hands, fingers, elbows and knees are usually symmetrically affected. Patients do not usually complain of pruritus, rather they complain of slight tenderness.

FINDINGS

Histological findings are divided into three types: the dermal, the epidermal, and the mixed dermal-epidermal[404]. In the dermal type, which is shown in the initial papular eruption or the active elevated border of the iris lesion, a perivascular mononuclear cell infiltrate, mixed with a small number of polymorphonuclear leucocytes and nuclear debris, is seen in the upper dermis. Slight vascular changes, such as endothelial cell swelling, are often noted (1). In the epidermal type, which is shown in the central depressed area of the iris lesions, diffuse epidermal necrosis is observed. In the peripheral area of the iris lesions, mononuclear cell infiltrate, with individual cell necrosis of the epidermis (the mixed dermal-epidermal type) is seen along the dermo-epidermal junction. Immunohistologically, deposition of immunoglobulin (IgG, IgM) and complement components is frequently seen on the blood vessels in the upper dermis of the early lesions of the dermal type[405-7]. In some specimens, such depositions are also seen in the dermo-epidermal junction[407]. Herpes simplex virus antigens have been demonstrated in the epidermal cells[408].

DIAGNOSTIC SIGNIFICANCE

The deposition of immunoglobulin and complement components on the blood vessels and along the dermo-epidermal junction are not specific findings for this disease, rather they are those commonly seen in cutaneous vasculitis. The findings of such depositions and the increased numbers of patients with this disease[405,407] suggest that this disease develops via the type III allergic reaction.

TECHNICAL POINTS

The lesion should be biopsied early. It is impossible to demonstrate immunoglobulin and complement component deposition in old lesions.

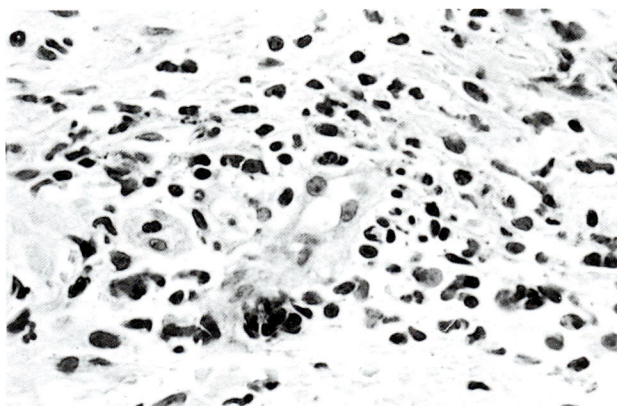

Fig. 1. Dermal type. Mononuclear infiltrate contains a small number of polymorphonuclear leucocytes around the slightly swollen endothelial cells in the upper dermis.

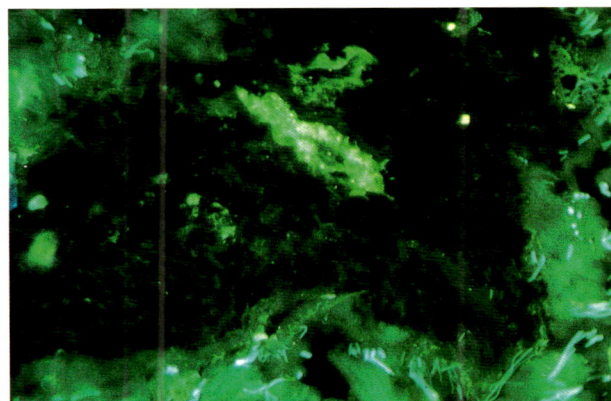

Fig. 2. Deposition of C3 on the blood vessel wall in the upper dermis. In some cases, IgM or IgG deposition is noted concomitantly.

Urticarial vasculitis

INTRODUCTION

Since McDuffie et al.[409] described four cases of hypocomplementemia with cutaneous vasculitis and arthritis in 1973, several subsequent reports have been published. Gammon and Wheeler[410] reported similar cases as urticarial vasculitis in 1979. Recently Monroe et at.[411], Callen and Kalbfleisch[412] and Sanchez et al.[413] summarized these cases and analyzed the clinical, laboratory and immunopathological features. Urticarial vasculitis can be divided into two subsets, idiopathic and symptomatic; the latter, a skin manifestation of general disorders such as collagen disease.

Urticarial vasculitis is characterized by the following clinical findings: recurrent and prolonged urticarial lesions containing purpura, pigmentation and occasionally bullae. Urticarial lesions persist for between 24 and 72 hours. Patients have a burning, slightly itching or painful sensation which is complicated by general symptoms such as polyarthralgia, abdominal or chest pain, and low grade fever. In addition, patients have elevated erythrocyte sedimentation rates and positive C-reactive protein. One of the most common findings is persistent hypocomplementemia. Histological findings from the lesions show leucocytoclastic vasculitis.

FINDINGS

The most prominent finding is the infiltration of numerous polymorphonuclear leucocytes which contain fragmentation of leucocytes with nuclear debris around dermal vessels and among collagen bundles (1). Other common histopathological findings are endothelial cell swelling, extravasation of red blood cells and fibrinoid deposits on vascular walls. By direct immunofluorescence, granular deposits of IgG and complement around the perivascular spaces of the papillary dermis (2) and at the dermo-epidermal junction can be identified. Normal-appearing skin without urticarial lesions sometimes displays immunoglobulin and complement in perivascular spaces or at the dermo-epidermal junction.

PATHOGENESIS

The pathogenesis of urticarial vasculitis is unknown. Immune complexes of unknown nature may be involved in the vascular wall and upper dermis. It has been suggested that persistent hypocomplementemia is the result of activation and consumption of complement due to immune complex formation in the cutaneous lesions.

TECHNICAL POINTS

The skin biopsy must be taken from both fresh and prolonged urticarial lesions or erythema multiforme-like lesions with purpura, pigmentation, vesicles and bullae. Normal-appearing skin may also be usable, as immunoglobulin and complement are often demonstrated in vascular walls or at the dermo-epidermal junction. Unfixed frozen sections are recommended for immunohistological procedures.

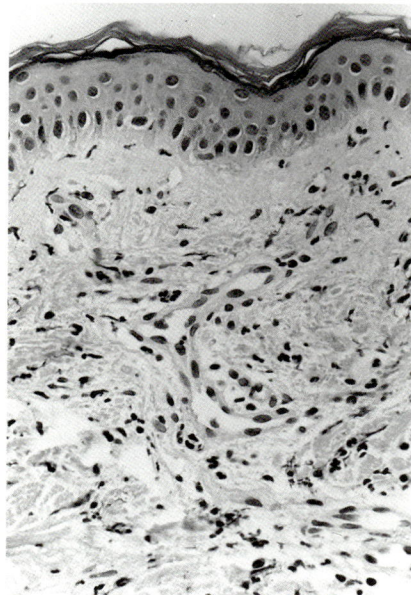

Fig. 1. Infiltration of polymorphonuclear leucocytes with nuclear debris around perivascular spaces and among collagen bundles. (HE stain × 200)

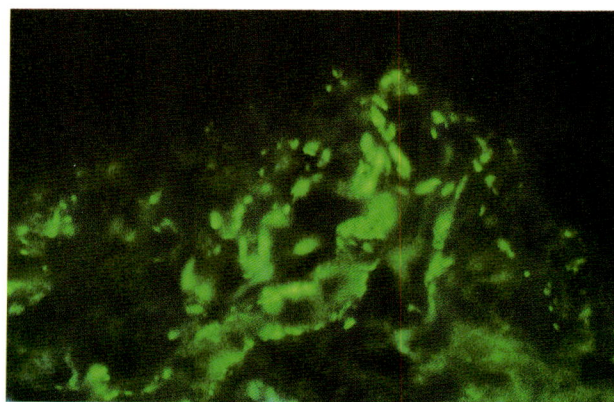

Fig. 2. Granular deposition of IgG on the vascular walls and in the perivascular spaces of the papillary dermis. (Direct IF stain × 400)

Schönlein-Henoch purpura

DEFINITION

Schönlein-Henoch purpura (S-H purpura) is an inflammatory disease resulting from leucocytoclastic vasculitis in the upper dermis, occurring predominantly in children. It is frequently associated with articular, gastro-intestinal and renal manifestations.

Some authors regard this term as synonymous with other forms of small blood vessel cutaneous vasculitis associated with systemic manifestations. But the association of palpable purpura with arthritis, gastro-intestinal symptoms, nephritis and the characteristic immunohistological findings which will be mentioned later, is usually striking enough to regard it as a syndrome.

IMMUNOFLUORESCENT FINDINGS

In the active stage, granular IgA deposits are usually detected in the small blood vessel walls in the upper dermis of skin taken from fresh purpuric lesions or clinically uninvolved predilection sites of S-H purpura (**1**). In cutaneous blood-vessel walls, deposition of alternative complement pathway components frequently occurs and IgM deposits are present in about one-third of the patients, while IgG deposits are rarely detected.

Granular IgA deposition, which is sometimes associated with deposition of secretory component, is also demonstrated in the glomerular mesangium of the kidney in patients with

CLINICAL AND PATHOGENETIC SIGNIFICANCE OF IgA DEPOSITS IN CUTANEOUS BLOOD VESSEL WALLS IN S-H PURPURA

Immunofluorescent study of skin biopsy specimens is very useful in the diagnosis of S-H purpura because IgA deposition in small blood vessel walls is invariably demonstrable in all patients with active S-H purpura.

Furthermore, this test is a sensitive indicator of disease activity in S-H purpura since IgA deposits are not found in patients with inactive S-H purpura.

Patients with S-H purpura usually demonstrate a selective elevation of serum IgA globulin[414]. Cryoglobulins containing IgA and properdin, and high levels of IgA immune complexes containing both IgA 1 and IgA 2 subclasses are found in sera of patients with S-H purpura[415, 416]. A selective increase in the number of circulating IgA-producing cells[417], B-cell activation with high spontaneous immunoglobulin synthesis[418], and a defective Con A-inducible suppression of *in vitro* immunoglobulin synthesis[418] are also noted in S-H purpura.

These findings suggest that the manifestation in S-H purpura in skin, kidney, joints and gastro-intestinal tract may occur as a result of activation of the alternative complement pathway by IgA immune complexes which become deposited in the small blood vessel walls of these involved tissues.

TECHNICAL POINTS

In S-H purpura, skin biopsy specimens for direct immuno-fluorescent study should be taken from fresh purpuric lesions because, in the involved skin, IgA-immune complexes are promptly phagocytized by polymorphonuclear leucocytes migrating into the lesions.

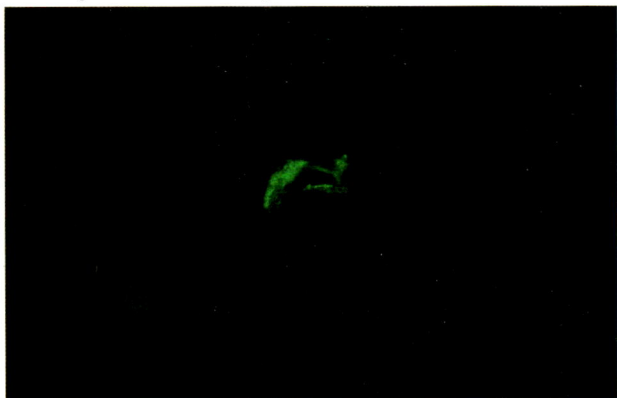

Fig. 1. Granular IgA deposits in the small vessel walls in the papillary dermis of involved skin in Schönlein-Henoch purpura. (× 400)

Fig. 2. Granular IgA deposits in the glomerular mesangium of the kidney in Schönlein-Henoch purpura nephritis. (× 200)

Fig. 3. Immunofluorescent photomicrograph showing granular deposits of secretory component in the glomerular mesangium of the kidney in Schönlein-Henoch purpura nephritis. (× 200)

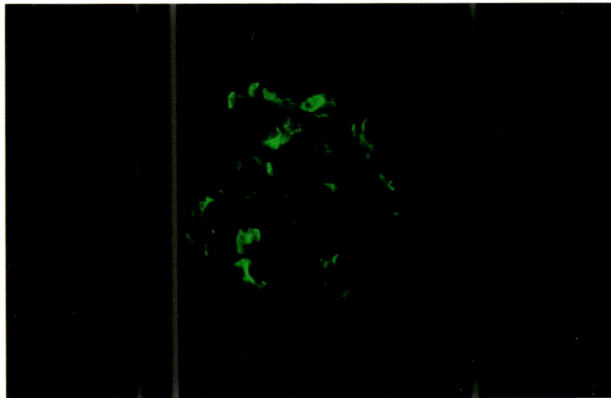

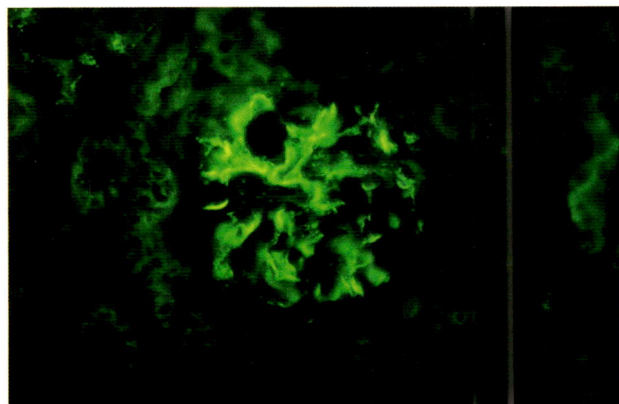

If the purpuric lesions present are all old, it is recommended to use uninvolved skin areas adjacent to the lesions as an alternative biopsy site.

No fixatives should be used on cryostat sections for direct immunofluorescence as these agents may cause serious interference with the immuno-fluorescence of IgA deposits.

Vasculitis allergica cutis (Ruiter)

INTRODUCTION
Vasculitis allergica cutis (Ruiter) is a necrotizing vasculitis affecting the small blood vessels of dermis and subcutaneous fat tissue; it is localized in skin without systemic manifestations (organ injury). The symptoms vary, including erythema, purpura, papule, small vesicles, ulcers and subcutaneous nodes, and new and old lesions are intermixed. It often occurs in the hind-limbs[419] of adults.

FINDINGS
Histopathologically, degeneration is seen in all layers of the dermis and in small blood vessels of subcutaneous fat tissue. The endothelial cells of blood vessels show swelling and degeneration, and on the vessel walls there is precipitation of fibrinoid substance. Infiltration of leucocytes with nuclear dust and haemorrhaging are observed, and a few eosinophils and lymphocytes may be seen (1). Occasionally, necrosis of epidermis occurs to form an ulcer. Changes in the large vessels are not seen as in periarteritis nodosa. By direct immunofluorescence, precipitates of IgG, IgM and C3 are seen on the walls of the small blood vessels at and around the lesions[420, 421] (2, 3).

DIAGNOSTIC SIGNIFICANCE
The cause of this disease is not known, although immunological mechanisms are being considered as a result of the similarity to necrotizing vasculitis and of findings through the immunofluorescent methods. This disease is also related to cases of decrease in serum complement values, increase in circulating immune complexes, and positive cases of cryoglobulin[422]. Immunoglobulin precipitates seen by immunofluorescence do not always correspond to the heavily-affected lesion areas observed by optical microscopy; this varies with time.

BIOPSY TECHNIQUE
Since there are various clinical symptoms, it is important to perform several biopsies from areas with different symptoms. The individual papule is small, so excision of the whole papule is possible. In the ulcer, the biopsy is taken from the periphery together with adjacent normal skin.

TECHNICAL POINTS
The work is performed immediately after biopsy on frozen sections without fixation.

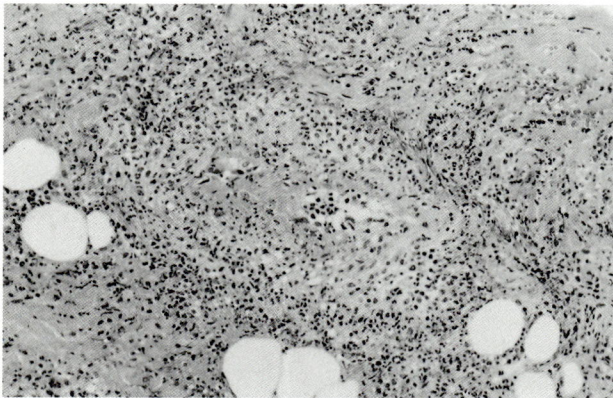

Fig. 1. Necrotizing vasculitis with small involved vessels. (H & E × 200)

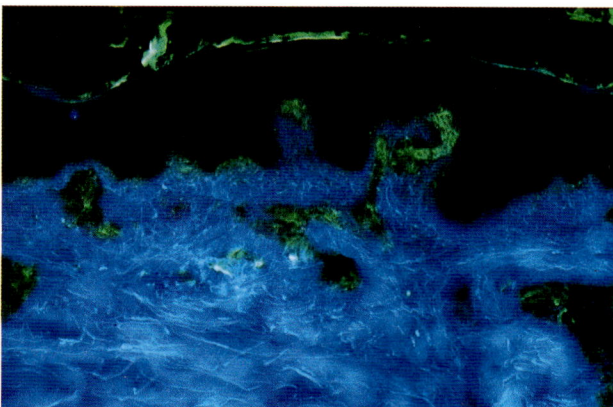

Fig. 2. Direct immunofluorescent method for IgM shows deposits on vascular walls. (× 100)

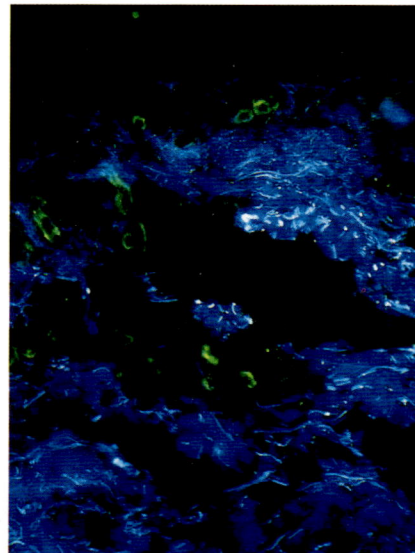

Fig. 3. C3 deposits on and around dermal vascular walls. (× 100)

Erythema elevatum diutinum

INTRODUCTION

Erythema elevatum diutinum (EED) is characterized by persistent, elevated erythematous plaques, 0.5 to several centimeters in diameter, which are preferentially located on fingers and extensor surfaces of lower legs, buttocks, elbows and knees. The lesions are often painful. This disease clinically resembles granuloma annulare or erythema multiforme but differs histologically from these two in that it shows an unusual type of leucocytoclastic vasculitis.

HISTOPATHOLOGY

Perivascular infiltrate consisting mainly of neutrophils with nuclear dust is a characteristic finding. Small vessels in upper to mid-dermis are surrounded by periodic acid Schiff-positive hyaline material which is similar to fibrinoid in its staining reactions but unlike leucocytoclastic vasculitis. Fibrinoid degeneration of the actual vessel walls is not significant. In late stages, the fibroblasts are perivascularly proliferated and associated with the synthesis of new collagen fibres (1a, 2a).

IMMUNOPATHOLOGY

Immunofluorescent microscopy occasionally depicts perivascular deposition of immunoglobulins (mainly IgG and IgM) and complement components (2). C3 appears to be the major participant, as is shown in other types of vasculitis[423]. Deposition of fibrin and fibrinogen is also seen around vessel walls.

DIAGNOSTIC SIGNIFICANCE

Positive immunopathological findings may be of help in the diagnosis, although these findings are not specific to EED. The presence of immuno-deposits in skin and increased Clq binding activity suggests a pathogenetic role of immune complexes in this type of vasculitis[424]. Although antigen involvement is unknown, bacterial antigens, particularly streptococcal antigens, are suggested to be of pathogenetic significance, according to Wolff et al.[425] deposition of C3 was found at the site of intracutaneous injection of streptococcal antigens.

TECHNICAL POINTS

Appropriate sites and biopsy timing are necessary for detecting tissue-bound immuno-deposits. Lesions should be biopsied in the early stages as the presence of remarkable inflammatory reactions generally gives a false-negative result due to the phagocytosis of immune complexes by infiltrating neutrophils.

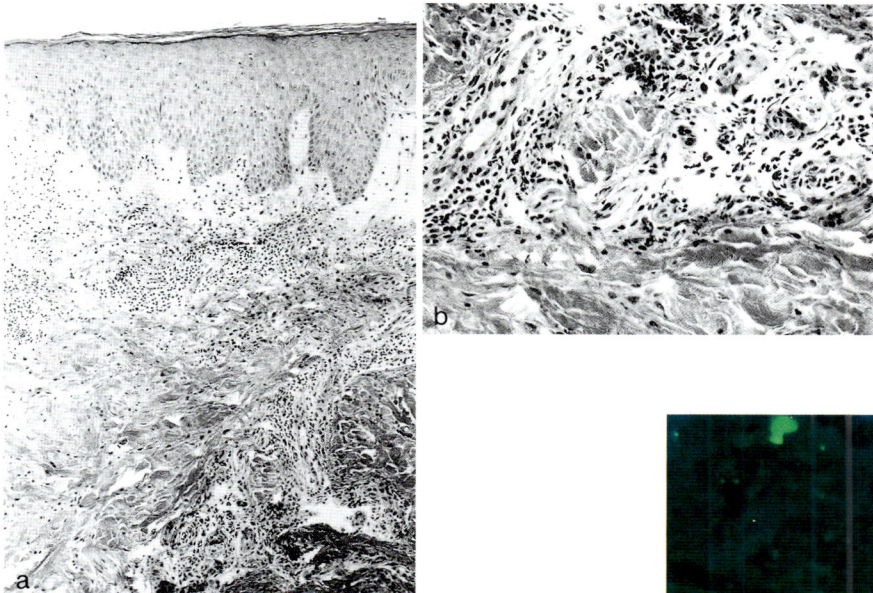

Fig. 1. Histologic features (HE staining).
a. Perivascular inflammatory infiltrate in upper and mid-dermis. (× 75)
b. Higher magnification showing infiltration of neutrophils and mononuclear cells. (× 350)

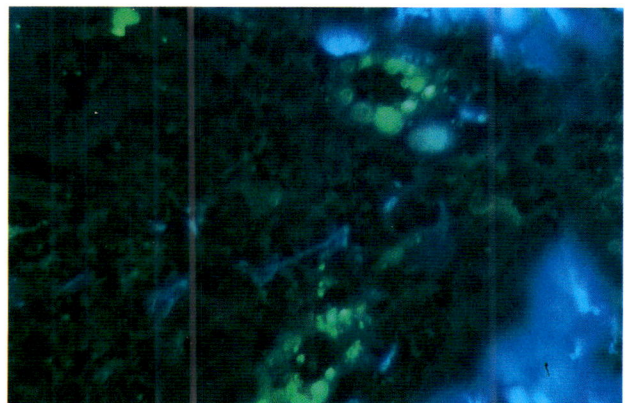

Fig. 2. Direct immunofluorescent staining showing perivascular deposition of C3 in mid-dermis. (× 200)

HB vasculitis

CONCEPT AND FINDINGS

Since the report of Gocke et al.[426] in 1970, vasculitis, which was thought to be evoked by hepatitis B virus, was known as HB vasculitis. They demonstrated circulating immune complexes containing Australia (Au) antigen and immunoglobulin in the same sera of four out of eleven patients with polyarteritis nodosa. Moreover, in one of these four patients Au antigen, IgM and ß1c-globulin were deposited in the blood-vessel wall of a muscle. Thereafter deposition of Au Ag was further demonstrated on the synovial membranes of a patient with arthritis as a prodromal manifestation of acute viral hepatitis[427] and HBe Ag deposition was found on the glomerular capillary walls of two hepatitis B virus carriers with glomerulo-nephritis[428].

Deposition of HBs Ag has also been found in skin. Dienstag et al.[429] found the deposition of HBs Ag as well as IgM, C3 and fibrin on lesional skin vessel walls in two patients with urticarial prodrome of acute viral hepatitis B. The pathological examination showed necrotizing venulitis in the involved urticarial skin. HBs Ag-antibody complexes were also identified in the cryoprecipitate of one patient's tissue.

We also showed the involvement of HB virus in cutaneous leucocytoclastic vasculitis[430]. Our patient was a 34-year-old woman, who experienced recurrent episodes of urticarial skin eruptions on the extremities for two years prior to her first visit to our clinic in 1980. Some of the eruptions, which usually lasted for several hours, remained as purpura. She sometimes felt slight fatigue and arthralgia. On admission, the physical examination showed no abnormality except for skin eruptions. Routine laboratory urine tests, blood cell count, liver function and serological tests showed no abnormality except for positive rheumatoid factor and high IgE level (1730 IU/ml). The total haemolytic complement level (CH 50) was normal. Further serological study revealed positive HBs Ag (X4096), negative HBs antibody, negative HBe Ag, positive HBe antibody and positive HBe antibody (above X 8192). These data indicated that she was a so-called asymptomatic HB virus carrier. Both urticarial and purpuric lesion biopsy specimens showed leucocytoclastic vasculitis in dermis (1). Direct immunofluorescent study of an urticarial lesion using FITC-conjugated anti-human IgM, Clq, C3 and fibrinogen (Behring Inc. F/P ratio approximately 2.0) diluted ten-fold, showed deposition of these molecules on dermal vessel walls. Furthermore, deposition of HBs Ag was demonstrated on lesional dermal vessel walls by immuno-fluorescence using FITC-conjugated monoclonal antibody against HBs Ag (F(ab)2, F/P ratio 1.13) (2)[431,432]. The specific fluorescence was blocked by the monoclonal antibody unconjugated with FITC. Circulating immune complexes containing HBs Ag and IgG were also detected in the serum by radioimmuno-assay[433].

The amounts of immune complexes correlated relatively well with the patient's clinical course (3). These results indicate the importance of circulating immune complexes deposited on vascular walls in the pathogenesis of necrotizing vasculitis.

SIGNIFICANCE

Since HB vasculitis is associated with the serum sickness-like prodromes[434] of hepatitis B, such as urticaria, poly-arthalgia and arthritis, the diagnosis indicates the initiation of hepatitis B. Persistent HB virus infection as is seen in asymptomatic HB virus carriers is considered to be essentially the same as hepatitis B (transient HB virus infection). The only difference is in the fact that it takes much longer for hepatitis to develop than acute hepatitis B. Thus HB vasculitis also suggests persistent HB virus infection.

It is possibly due to the seroconversions such as HBs antibody and HBe Ag → HBe antibody, which occur prior to the onset of hepatitis B, that HB vasculitis occurs in a prodromal stage of hepatitis B. By deposition of circulating immune complexes containing HB Ag, immunoglobulin and complement on local vascular walls, a type III allergic reaction occurs which causes necrotizing vasculitis.

METHODS

The subjects for biopsy are those patients with serum sickness-like prodrome of hepatitis B or HB virus carriers with urticarial eruption or purpura. Lesional sites should be biopsied. HBs Ag, immunoglobulin and complement have not been detected at non-lesional sites[435].

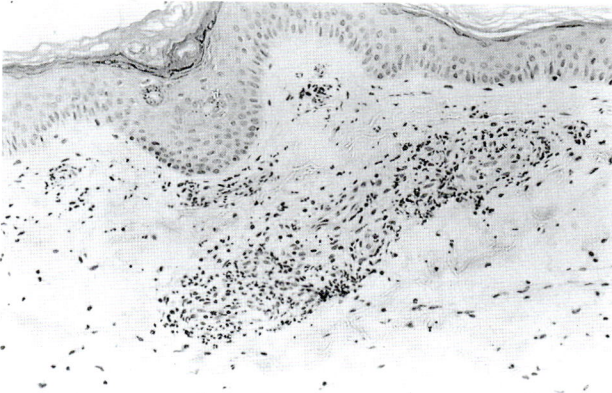

Fig. 1. The specimen obtained from an urticarial lesion of our patient. Leucocytoclastic vasculitis is seen in upper dermis. (HE, × 50)

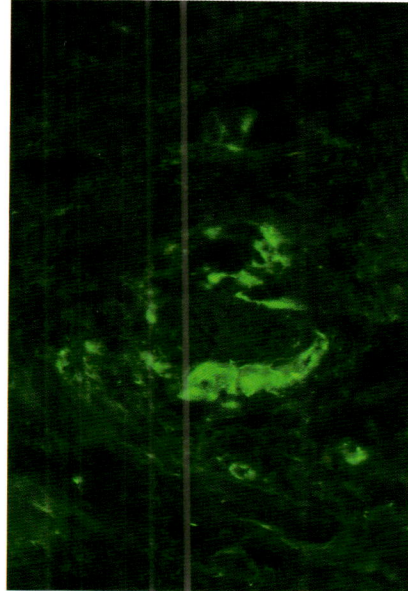

Fig. 2. Direct immunofluorescent study using FITC-conjugated monoclonal antibody against HBs Ag. Skin specimen from an urticarial lesion of our patient. Vascular walls in upper dermis are specifically stained. (× 127)

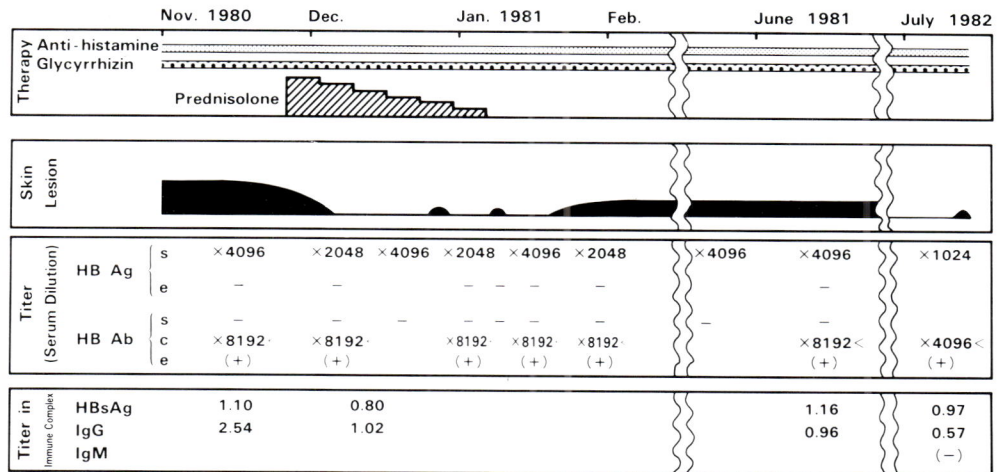

Fig. 3. Clinical course of our patient.

Livedo vasculitis

INTRODUCTION

Livedo vasculitis[436,437] has been identified as being similar to atrophie blanche, livedo reticularis with summer ulceration, livedoid vasculitis and periarteritis nodosa cutanea. The main histological finding is focal continuous vasculitis from deep to superficial dermis and is expressed as segmental hyalinizing vasculitis[437] (1). This disease has been categorized as allergic vasculitis caused by immune complexes[438,439], because the early vascular lesion shows multi-nuclear leucocyte infiltration with nuclear debris and fibrinoid degeneration. The thick, hyalinized and organized vascular walls suggest that a chronic-persistent vasculitis may occur.

FINDINGS

Direct immunofluorescent methods denote the deposits of immunoglobulins, complement and fibrinolytic materials such as fibrin, fibrinogen and plasminogen, on vascular walls in the deep dermis. The deposits present a granular pattern (2) or linear-annular pattern linked with fine granules on the thick walls (3). Immunoglobulin or complement reveal the deposition of immune complexes. And fibrinogen or plasminogen suggest that an abnormal fibrinolytic process occurs and the inflammation persists.

TECHNICAL POINTS

As blood vessels in deep dermis are the most important, biopsy samples must be taken at great depth, including subcutaneous fat. In the early lesions with strong inflammation, immunoglobulin and complement are highly positive. On the other hand, in lesions with ulcer, it is difficult to find an active vascular lesion. In the scar-like lesions with hyalinized vascular walls, deposits of immunoglobulin or fibrinolytic materials are often observed. The finding that the vascular walls with organic change may effect the persistent inflammation of vasculitis is of great interest.

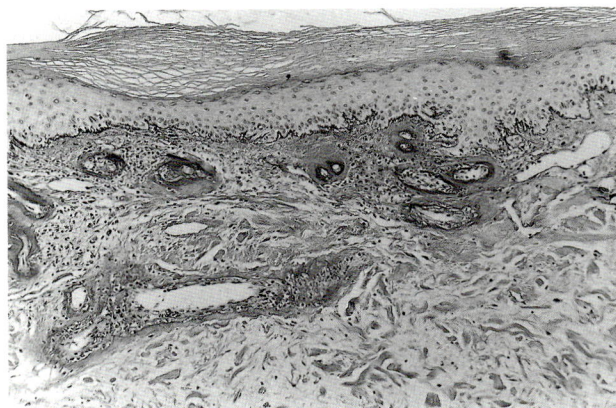

Fig. 1. PAS stain. (× 100)

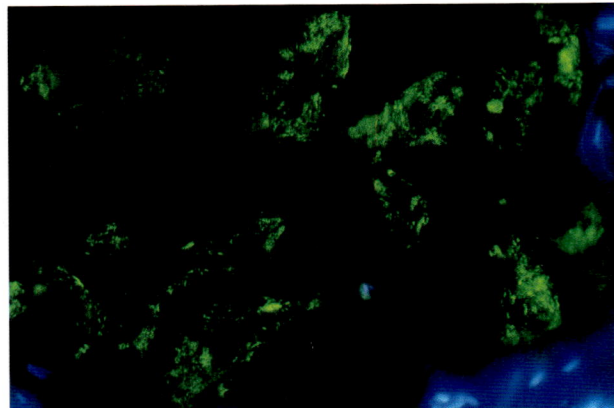

Fig. 2. Immunofluorescent microscopy, Plasminogen. (× 200)

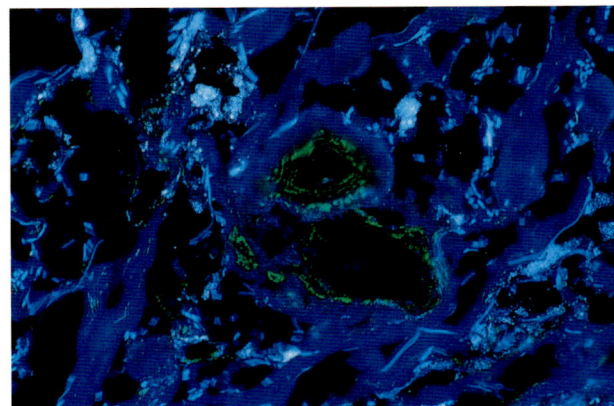

Fig. 3. Immunofluorescent microscopy, IgG. (× 200)

Wegener's granulomatosis

INTRODUCTION

Wegener's granulomatosis is a systemic vasculitis with poor prognosis. In the beginning, a necrotizing granuloma occurs in the nose and advances to the general organs. The histological triads are necrotizing granulomatous lesions of the upper respiratory organs or lungs, systemic necrotizing vasculitis and glomerulonephritis. About half of the patients have skin lesions. Some are more like eruptions, necrotic papules or nodules, vesicules, urticarial rash, and erythema multiforme – whereas others are like lesions[440], oedema, purpura, telangiectasia and pyoderma gangrenosum. The aetiology is unknown but is considered, as in vasculitis, to be caused by immune complexes[441].

FINDINGS

Histological findings present thrombus and fibrinoid degeneration of blood vessels in deep dermis to subcutaneous fat. There is severe infiltration of neutrophils, lymphocytes and histiocytes (**1, 2**). Direct immunofluorescence denoted the granular deposits of immunoglobulin, complement and fibrinogen on various sized vascular walls (**3**). It is suggested that immune complexes are deposited on the vascular walls and neutrophil infiltration follows. Then the destruction of walls occurs and advances to granulomatous lesions.

Histologically, it is difficult to classify periarteritis nodosa, but there is a more severe granulomatous reaction seen in Wegener's granulomatosis. It has been reported that immune complexes with antibody excess have a tendency to form granuloma[442].

TECHNICAL POINTS

The lesions of necrotizing vasculitis can be found from purpuric nodules including fat tissue, which may advance to punched-out ulcer. In both the ulcer and reactive eruptions – oedema, erythema, purpura and papules, it is often easy to miss the main vascular lesion and positive immunofluorescent findings. It is very important to be selective when determining the time and area of biopsy sampling.

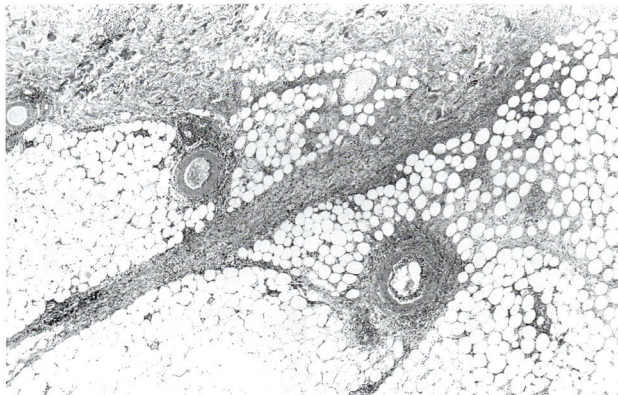

Fig. 1. H-E stain. (× 40)

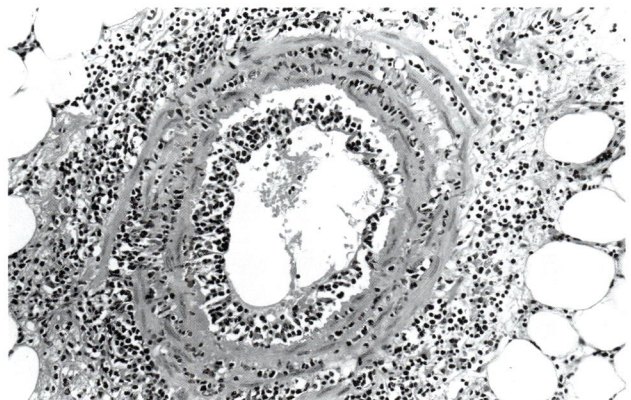

Fig. 2. H-E stain. (× 200)

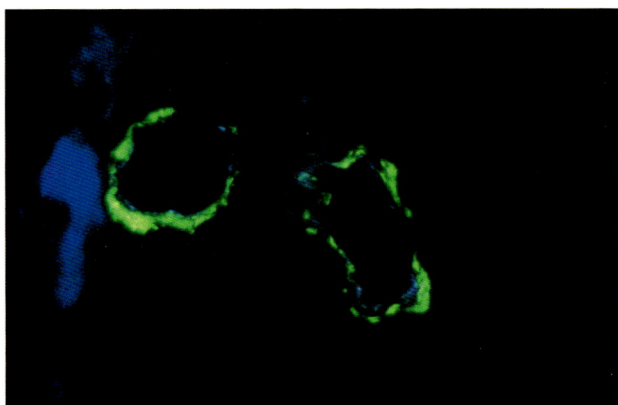

Fig. 3. Immunofluorescent microscopy, IgM. (× 100)

Experimental cutaneous vasculitis

INTRODUCTION

In the vasculitis group, which includes necrotizing vasculitis, leucocytic vasculitis and allergic vasculitis, serum immune complexes were detected and deposits of immunoglobulins and complement were demonstrated on vascular walls. It was suggested that circulating immune complexes were deposited on vascular walls or immune complexes were newly formed on the walls, followed by the inflammation of neutrophils which advanced to the destruction of blood vessels. As there may be abundant antigen in patients, it is very difficult to discuss the antigen side of immune complexes. In experimental models, to understand the inflammatory process and the deposition mechanism of immune complexes, a single antigen was used.

In dermatology there are many variations of vasculitis caused by immune complexes – Schönlein-Henoch purpura, Ruiter's vasculitis, urticarial vasculitis, erythema elevatum diutinum, livedo vasculitis, Wegener's granulomatosis and vasculitis associated with collagen disease. Many animal skin models of vasculitis, particularly the Arthus reaction, have been used because it is easy to observe and take samples without sacrificing the animal[443-447].

We have observed the Arthus reaction in the skin of albino rabbits and guinea pig using horseradish peroxidase [HRP] as the antigen[448-451]. HRP has a molecular weight of 40,000 and can be demonstrated by light and electron microscopy after reaction with diaminobenzidine. Most anti-HRP antibody is composed of IgG and can be observed by the immunofluorescence method. In order to prove that the deposits in tissue are immune complexes, it is necessary to detect both antigen and antibody at the same time. This is possible in HRP-anti-HRP complexes.

FINDINGS

Oedematous erythema or purpura occurred after intra-cutaneous injections of low dose HRP in HRP-sensitized animals (Arthus reaction). Polymorphonuclear leucocytes infiltrated the dermis, particularly around the small vessels, and vessel wall destruction and erythrocyte extravasation were seen. Following the diaminobenzidine reaction to determine the antigen side (HRP), fine brown granular deposits or aggregates could be seen on vascular walls and between collagen bundles by light microscopy (1). The immunofluorescence method revealed the deposition of IgG (anti-HRP antibody) and complement on vessel walls. These presented the same distribution as the antigen.

In active Arthus reaction serum antibody adhered to the injected antigen, and complements combined with antigen-antibody complexes. Neutrophils were mobilized to sweep complexes. This was followed by severe inflammation after phagocytosis. In reversed passive Arthus reaction, in which HRP solution was intravenously injected in a normal animal just after intracutaneous injection of anti-HRP antiserum, the inflammation was relatively mild and the tissue damage was less than in active Arthus reaction. Therefore, reversed passive Arthus reaction could be adequately observed by electron microscopy.

In vitro-prepared insoluble HRP-anti-HRP complexes which were injected into the dermis were presented as electron-dense aggregates by electron microscopy in figure 2. There were severe inflammatory reactions whereby the cells with a destroyed membrane released lysosomes (2).

In reversed passive Arthus reaction, immune complexes were deposited between endothelial cells and pericytes, on basement membranes, and within collagen bundles (3). Some of the immune complexes were phagocytosed by neutrophils or macrophages, and some of them adhered to the cell membrane of eosinophils (4). Some even attached to the cell membrane of keratinocytes (5). By electron microscopy, the distribution of more fine immune complexes can be demonstrated and infiltrated cells can be distinguished.

TECHNICAL POINTS

As diaminobenzidine hardly penetrated the usual samples for electron microscopy, it was necessary to make sections as thin as possible. The cryostat sections were used as samples for electron microscopy; the dyeing was better but the tissue damage was more severe. In our laboratory the samples were cut as thin as possible (0.2–0.4 mm) using a razor under a biological microscope.

As diaminobenzidine reacts with erythrocytes, lysosome in leucocytes and endogenous peroxidase, caution is necessary. The present methods are suited to the observation of immune deposits, which adhere to the cell membrane or are deposited outside the cells. A treatment acceptable of endogenous peroxidase and a comparison of the antibody-side of immune complexes should be sought.

Moreover, it is expected that a model of arteritis caused by immune complexes is necessary to determine the influence of degenerated vascular walls and to search for a factor which prolongs the inflammation.

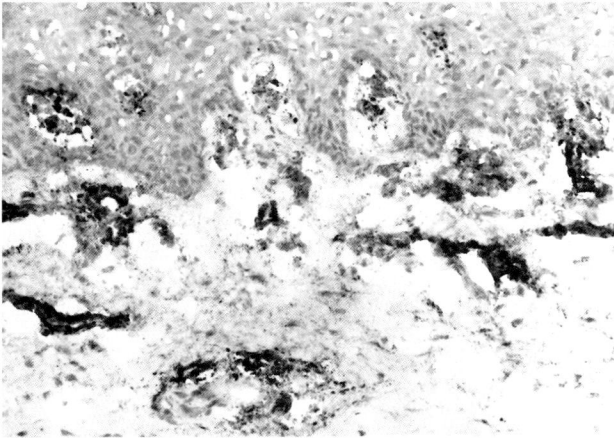

Fig. 1. Reversed passive Arthus reaction, cryostat section. (× 100)

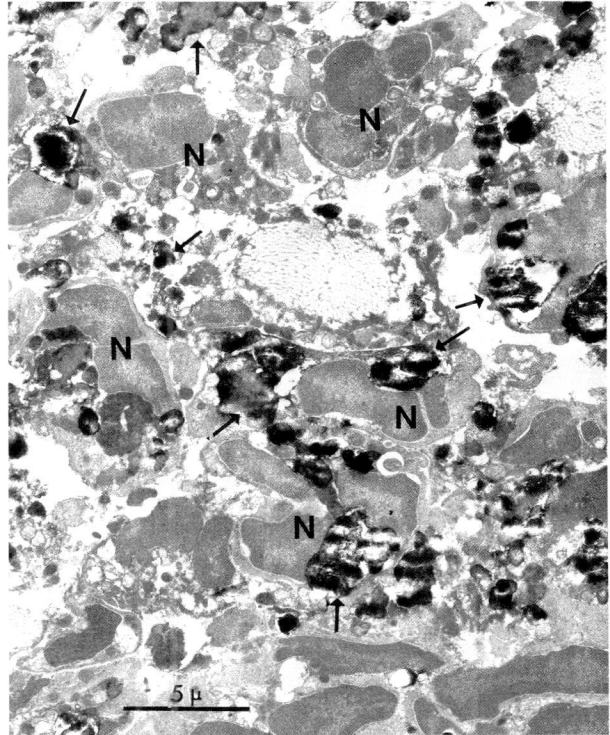

Fig. 2. HRP-anti-HRP complexes were injected in dermis, and observed by electron microscopy.
N: neutrophil; arrow: immune complex.

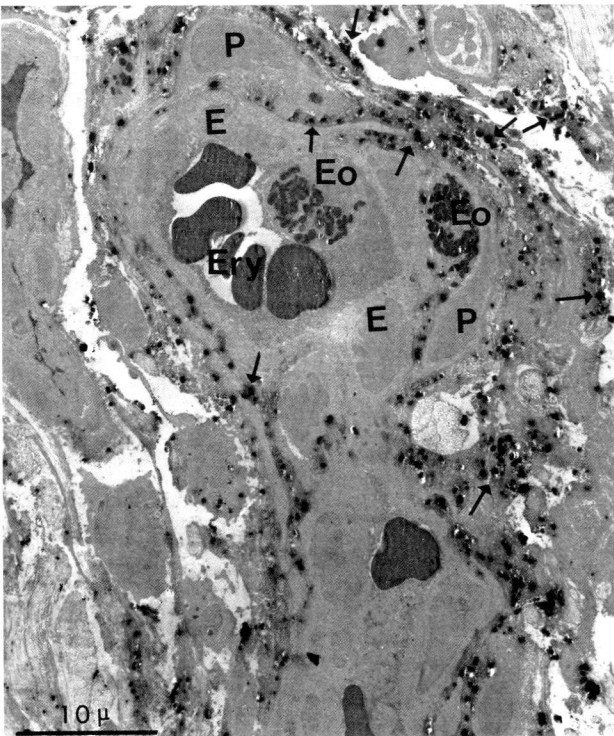

Fig. 3. Reversed passive Arthus reaction, by electron microscopy. E: endothial cell; P: periocyte; Eo: eosinophil; arrow: immune complex.

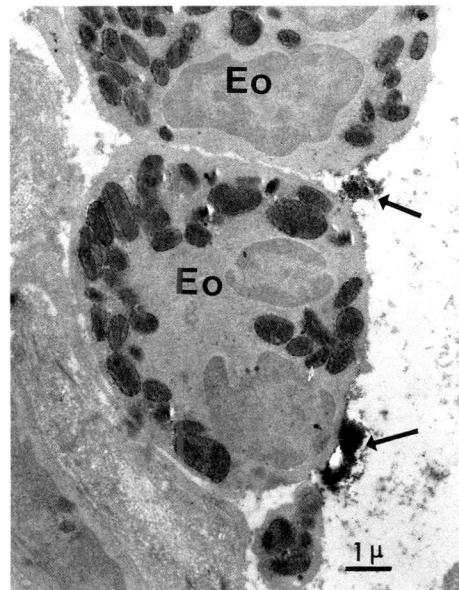

Fig. 4. Immune complex (arrow) adhered to the eosinophil cell membrane (Eo).

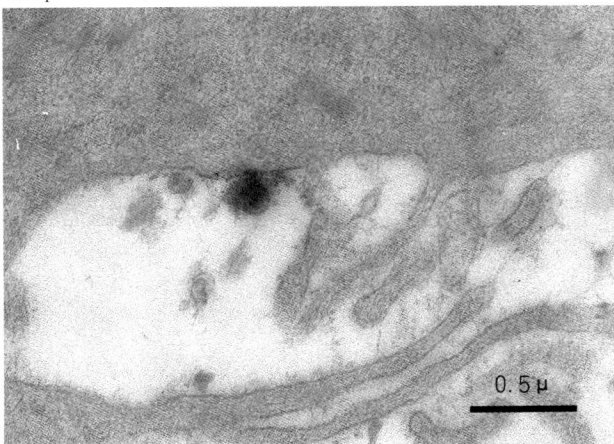

Fig. 5. Immune complex attached to the keratinocyte cell membrane.

D Eczematous diseases

Atopic dermatitis

INTRODUCTION
Atopic dermatitis, a hereditary eczematous disease, has its onset in early infancy, and frequently continues into childhood, adolescence, or adult years. Skin manifestations of the disease are classified into five types: (1) acute eczematous lesion, (2) lichenified patch, (3) prurigo lesion, (4) follicular eruption, and (5) dry eczema.

HISTOLOGICAL FINDINGS
All of the five types of clinical manifestations histologically show an eczematous change. The epidermis reveals moderate to marked acanthosis and varying degrees of spongiosis with mononuclear cell migration. The dermal infiltrate consists mainly of lymphocytes[452], but it also contains a fair number of histiocytes. The number of mast cells is often increased[453].

IMMUNOHISTOLOGICAL FINDINGS
Examinations using monoclonal antibodies show that the lymphocytes seen in the dermis consist predominantly of T cells[454, 455, 456]. Only a few B cells are found. The infiltrating T cells include a large number of helper T cells (1), and relatively few suppressor T cells (2). Langerhans cells are abundant in the acanthotic epidermis and in the dermal T cell infiltrates (3).

EVALUATION OF THE CELLULAR EVENTS
An immunohistological feature of the disease is the pattern of cell-mediated immune reaction. The presence of an increased number of helper T cells and Langerhans cells may reflect active antigen processing in the skin lesions. The absence of B cells is compatible with current concepts of the relative importance of B cells in humoral immunity and T cells in cell-mediated immunity. It is likely, then, that a cell-mediated immune reaction is implicated in the pathogenesis of atopic dermatitis.

LESION SELECTION FOR BIOPSY
The immunohistological features of skin lesions in this disease are frequently obscured by secondary changes due to the application of topical corticosteroids. It is therefore important to examine skin lesions which were not treated with topical steroids for at least two weeks prior to biopsy.

Fig. 1. Subacute skin lesion in AD. The majority of lymphocytes in the dermis and areas of spongiotic epidermis are helper T cells. (Leu-3a staining, × 75)

Fig. 2. Subacute skin lesion in AD. A majority of infiltrating lymphocytes are suppressor T cells. (Leu-2a staining, × 75)

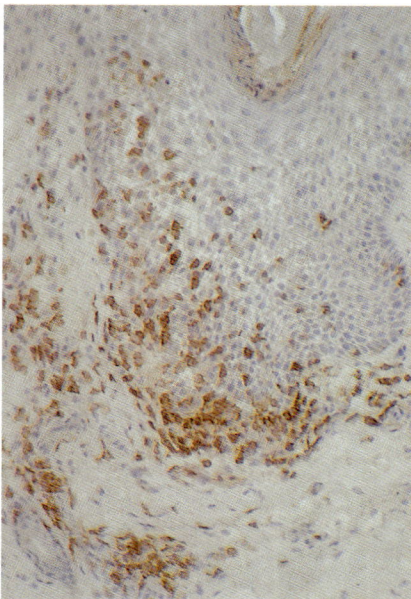

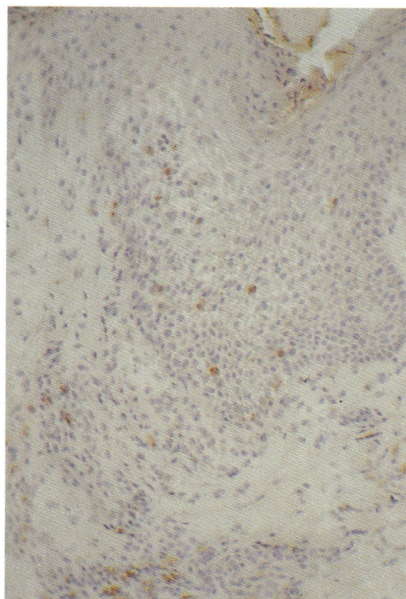

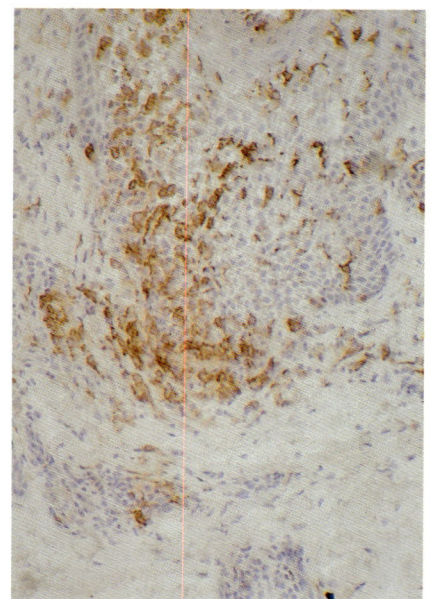

Fig. 3. Subacute skin lesion in AD. Many Langerhans cells are present in the slightly acanthotic epidermis, in spongiotic areas, and throughout the dermal infiltrates. (OKT-6 staining, × 75)

Contact dermatitis

INTRODUCTION

Allergic contact dermatitis is one of the disorders with a well understood pathomechanism, due to the large amount of research carried out on animals. Namely, hapten combine the carrier protein(s) of Langerhans cells and this binding allows antigen presentation genetically restricted to HLA-DR gene products. Further, this process activates T cells, making effector T cells. Therefore, the immunohistopathological analysis of allergic contact dermatitis is leading to an understanding of the pathomechanism of many inflammatory dermatoses of unknown aetiology. McMillan et al.[457] examined the immunohistopathology of positive patch tests and elucidated the characteristics of the surface phenotypes of infiltrating cells in allergic contact dermatitis.

FINDINGS AND THEIR SIGNIFICANCE

The major infiltrating cells are Leu-1[+], T11[+], Leu-3[+], Leu-2a[−], HLA-DR[+], T9[−], Leu-7[−], B1[−], J5[−] (**1**). The percentage of Leu-2a[+] cells in exocytotic T cells is the same as that of Leu-3a[+] cells. Occasionally T6[+] cells are observed in the dermis as well as the epidermis. Further HLA-DR antigen expression on the keratinocyte surface is also one of the common findings (**2**). According to Scheynius et al.[458], however, these immunohistopathologic findings are qualitatively very similar to those in irritant contact dermatitis.

TECHNICAL POINT

Cryostat sections of snap-frozen biopsied specimens were stained by the avidin-biotin-peroxidase complex method[459,460]

Fig. 1. Leu-1[+] cells in allergic contact sensitivity reaction.
Leu-1[+] cells are found in exocytotic cells as well as in the perivascular infiltrate.

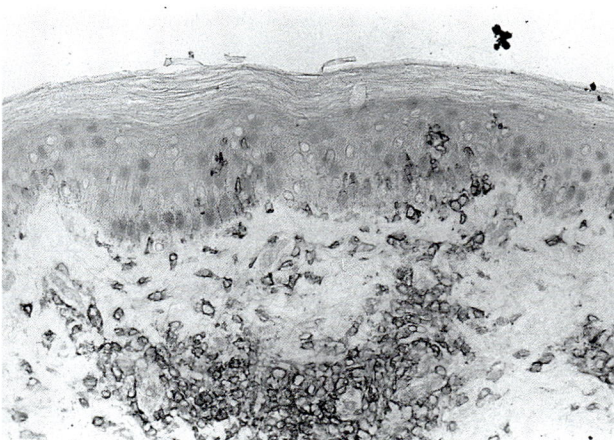

Fig. 2. HLA-DR[+] cells in allergic contact sensitivity reaction.
Most of the infiltrating cells express HLA-DR antigen. Moreover, there was localized expression of HLA-DR antigen on the keratinocytes.

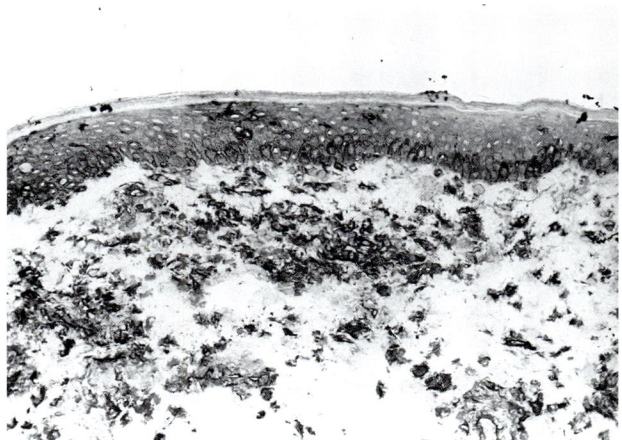

Distribution of antigen in allergic contact dermatitis

INTRODUCTION

In contact sensitivity, the most common antigens are chemical substances of low molecular weight, called haptens, such as nickel, chromium, *P. phenylene diamine*, and urushiol. The small haptens which induce contact sensitivity would not normally be antigenic, but it appears that these low molecular weight compounds can acquire sensitizing capacity when they traverse the body and become covalently conjugated to normal body protein carriers. According to the concept relating to the mechanism of contact sensitivity, the hapten applied to the skin enters the skin and there becomes a complete antigen by conjugation with the carrier proteins present there. The complete antigen acts to sensitize by stimulating T lymphocytes. The T cell recognition of the antigen is specific for hapten/carrier conjugate. These T cells, after being stimulated by the antigen, are retained in the draining lymph node where they proliferate and differentiate into various subpopulations of lymphocytes such as memory cells and effector cells. The subpopulations of sensitized lymphocytes then spread throughout the body, which consequently becomes hypersensitive. A second contact with the same hapten elicits an inflammatory skin reaction due to the interaction of the effector cells with the complete antigen.

One of the important questions is which structures in the body, especially in the skin, acquire the ability to induce contact sensitivity by combination with the hapten. A number of studies regarding the localization of allergens in the body following skin surface application have been carried out to answer this question. In the attempt to study the localization of allergens, researchers have used various simple chemical allergens which are easily obtained in radioactive form. For example, Eisen and Tabachnick[461] observed the distribution of dinitrobenzene groups in guinea pig skin by means of radio-autography and specific histochemical staining. Even through these methods details of histological localization of the allergens remain inadequate. Thus we have attempted to examine the distribution of 2,4-dinitrochlorobenzene (DNCB) applied to guinea pig skin surface by immunohistological methods using antiserum to 2,4-dinitrophenyl (DNP) groups as the tracer for DNCB.

FINDINGS

Cutaneous localization of DNP groups following skin painting with DNCB. In our investigation[462], the localization of DNP groups in the skin of guinea pigs following skin painting with DNCB was examined histologically using an immunofluorescence method. DNCB penetrated through the epidermis, the dermis, and then combined with skin components, particularly epidermis, within a few minutes of application. DNP groups were clearly detected in the areas corresponding to the cell membrane and cytoplasm of epidermal cells (1). The DNP groups were found on approximately 80% of the epidermal cells[463]. Our examination[464] using a scanning immunoelectron microscopy technique with bacteriophage T4 as the visual marker also showed DNP groups distributed on the surface of epidermal cells, particularly on that of keratinocytes (2). This indicates that DNCB binds to the surface components of epidermal cell membrane. High affinity of DNCB to epidermal cell components *in vivo* has been demonstrated in several studies. It has been shown that following DNCB painting of guinea pig

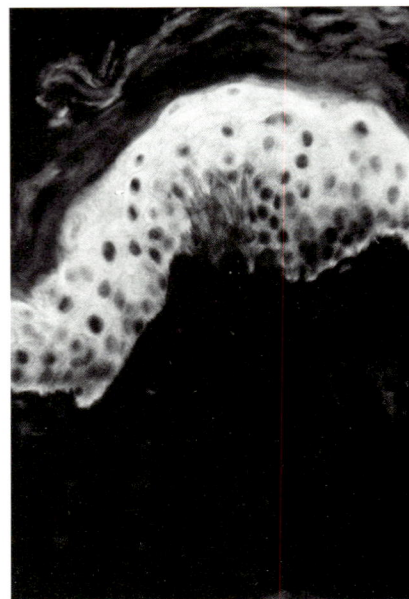

Fig. 1. Guinea pig skin section obtained three hours after painting with 5% DNCB in ethanol. Stained with fluorescent antibody to DNP groups. Fluorescence is distributed in the cell membrane and cytoplasm of Malpighian cells. (Paraffin section, × 300)[462]

skin roughly half of the material is present at the local skin site and in total about 99% is in the epidermis[461].

It has been postulated that Langerhans cells, which comprise a small subpopulation of epidermal cells, are essential for the induction of contact sensitivity to simple chemical allergens. Recent reports have focussed on the importance of the cells regarding the antigen presentation to immunologically competent lymphocytes. Findings which indicate that hapten-bound Langerhans cells may directly stimulate T cells have been reported[465]. These data suggest that T cells recognize the hapten molecules in association with Ia antigen on the surface of Langerhans cells. So, next we attempted to determine whether DNP groups are localized on epidermal Langerhans cells following skin painting with DNCB[466]. The epidermal cell suspensions prepared from DNCB-painted guinea pig skin were double-stained for Ia antigen and DNP groups. DNP groups were found to be distributed on the epidermal cells with Ia antigen (presumably Langerhans cells) (3).

The distribution of DNP groups in lymphoid tissues following skin painting with DNCB. We were also able to show by immunofluorescence that DNP groups are distributed on the cells in the peripheral lymphoid system of guinea pigs with DNCB-painted skin[467–9]. The majority of the cells (DNP cell) were found in the peripheral blood, spleen and thoracic duct at one to six hours after painting, but the maximum number was reached in lymph nodes draining the site of DNCB application at twelve hours post-painting (4, 5). Our results indicate that (1) DNCB reacts directly *in vivo* with cell membranes in the peripheral lymphoid system of guinea pigs following epicutaneous application of the agent, and that (2) DNCB in free unreactive form remains in the lymphoid system for at least twelve hours post-painting. Scanning immunoelectron microscopic study using anti-DNP antibody and bacteriophage T4 demonstrated that DNP groups are localized on the surface of the cells in the lympoid system and vary in the number and distribution of DNP groups (6)[470]. The DNP cell population was determined by the antibody and ferritin as a visual marker, for both T and B cells, and macrophages (7)[471].

104

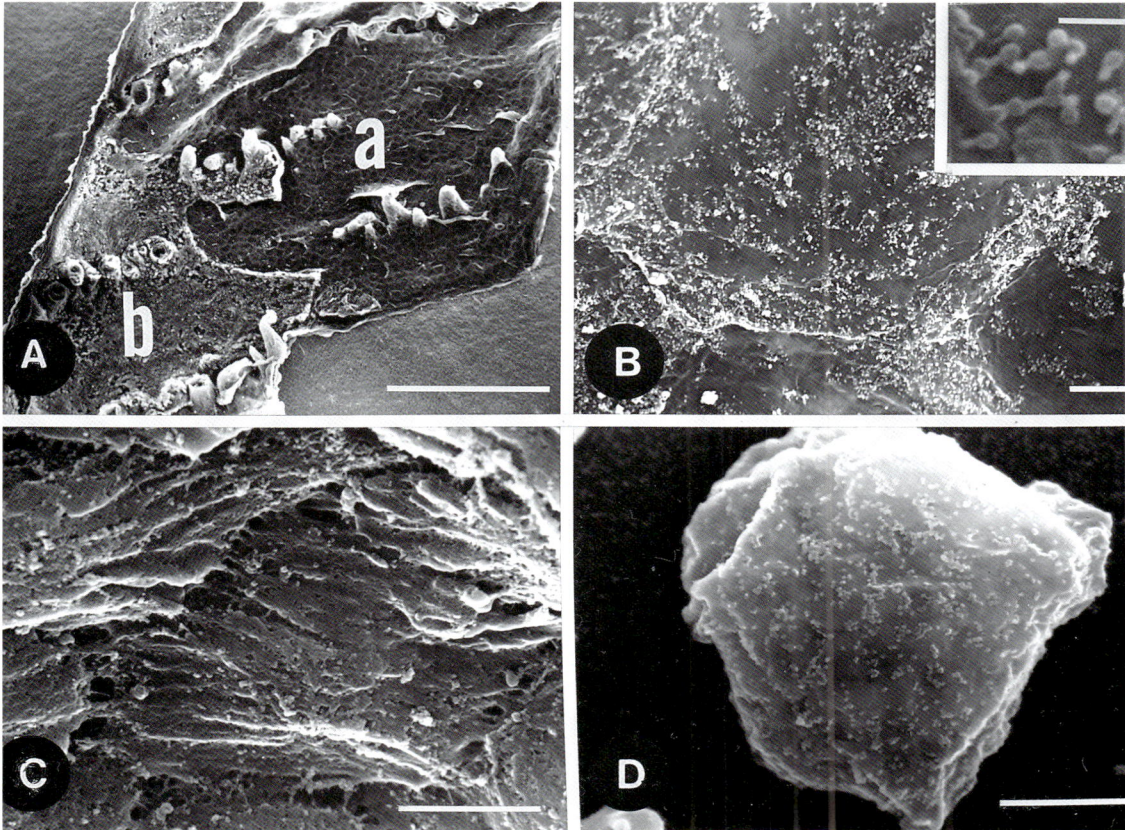

Fig. 2. (A) Scanning electron micrograph of epidermis dermal-side up obtained from DNCB-painted guinea pig ear skin and labelled using an indirect technique for scanning immunoelectron microscopy. Treated with rabbit anti-DNP IgG, followed by bacteriophage T4 conjugated with goat anti-rabbit IgG antibody. Horny layer is exposed in a part of the sheet (a), and (b) the surface of Malpighian cells can be seen in another part of the sheet. Bar = 0.5 μm

(B) Higher magnification of Part a of panel A. T4-anti-IgG are distributed over the surface of horny cells. The morphological identity of T4-anti-IgG is confirmed, due to the clearly distinguishable T4 hexagonal head and tail at higher magnification (inset, bar = 5 μm). Bar = 50 μm.

(C) Higher magnification of Part b of panel A. Diffuse distribution of T4-anti-IgG on the surface of Malpighian cells is observed. Bar = 50 μm.

(D) Scanning electron micrograph of epidermal single cell prepared from DNCB-painted ear skin, followed by treatment with anti-DNP and T4-anti-IgG. T4-anti-IgG is distributed over the cell surface. Bar = 50 μm.

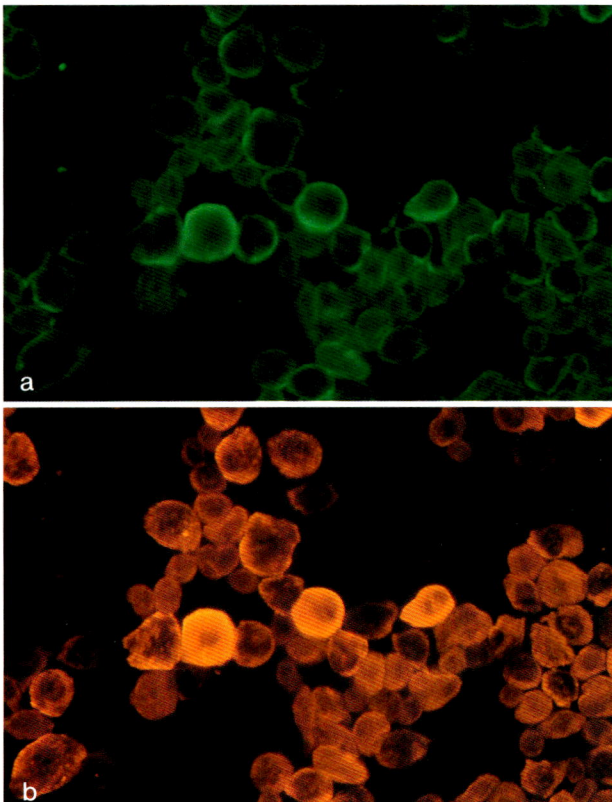

Fig. 3. (A) Single epidermal cells prepared from DNCB-painted ear skin of strain 13 guinea pig was exposed first to anti-Ia, followed by TRITC-anti-Gp IgG and then directly to FITC-anti-DNP. Rhodamine excitor demonstrates Ia-positive cells (orange). (× 400)

(B) Almost all epidermal cells are stained with FITC-anti-DNP in the same area as panel A, viewed under fluorescent light (green). The cells with Ia antigens exhibit DNP groups. (× 400)

It has been shown that trinitrophenyl (TNP) groups covalently couple to major histocompatibility antigens (H-2) on the cell surface of mouse spleen cells treated in vitro with trinitrobenzene sulfonate,.and that other proteins including immunoglobulins are also conjugated with the hapten[472]. Clement and Shevach[473] have shown that whereas most of the various histocompatibility antigens are TNP-derived in amounts proportional to the degree of membrane protein derivation as a whole at in vitro trinitrophenylation of guinea pig peritoneal exudate cells and splenocytes, only small amounts of TNP-modified strain II guinea pig Ia antigens are found, and no hapten-modified strain 13 guinea pig Ia antigens are detected. Analysis of hapten-lymphoid cell complexes formed in vivo has not yet been carried out, but it is reasonable to assume that similar conjugation also occurs in vivo. On the other hand, it has been known that autologous lymphoid cells coated with contact sensitizer

cause unresponsiveness when injected into normal animals[474]. Haptenated major histocompatibility complex determinants have been demonstrated as necessary for suppressor T cell induction[475]. These findings suggest that the lymphoid cells associated with DNP groups occurring in the lymphoid system following skin painting with DNCB may be tolerogenic in the induction of suppressor mechanism.

TECHNICAL POINTS
Both frozen and paraffin sections can be used for the immunofluorescence study on the localization of DNP groups in DNCB-painted skin[476]. For scanning immunoelectron microscopic studies, epidermal cell suspensions are mounted on the surface of a cover glass treated with 0.1% poly-L-lysine to insure uniformly distributed adherence without any loss of the distinctive cell shape. The cell suspensions are then prefixed with a 1% glutaraldehyde solution for ten minutes and treated with 0.15 M glycine.

Fig. 5. Sections prepared from guinea pig regional inguinal lymph node 24 hours after painting with DNCB. Stained with fluorescent antibody to DNP groups. Fluorescence is present in the cells in subcapsular, intermediate and medullary sinuses. (× 120)

Fig. 6. Scanning electron micrographs of cells in the draining lymph node taken from the intact guinea pig skin 12 hours after painting with DNCB. Labelled using an indirect technique of scanning immunoelectron microscopy. The cells were treated with rabbit anti-DNP IgG, followed by bacteriophage T4 conjugated with goat anti-rabbit IgG.
(A) Four white cells are seen. T4 anti-IgG is distributed over the cell surface of one cell. Bar = 10 μm.
(B) Under higher magnification, the cell shows a diffuse labelling pattern. Bar = 1 μm.
(C) Higher magnification micrograph of a labelled cell. The morphological identity of T4-anti-IgG is confirmed, due to the clearly distinguishable hexagonal head and tail of T4. Bar = 0.1 μm.

Fig. 7. Transmission electron micrographs of a macrophage in the draining lymph node taken from the guinea pig skin 12 hours after skin painting with DNCB incubated with EAC and then with ferritin-anti-DNP.
(A) Macrophage forms a rosette with EAC. Bar = 1 μm.
(B) Higher magnification of a portion of the cell (arrow in panel A). Ferritin is distributed over the cell surface. Bar = 1 μm.

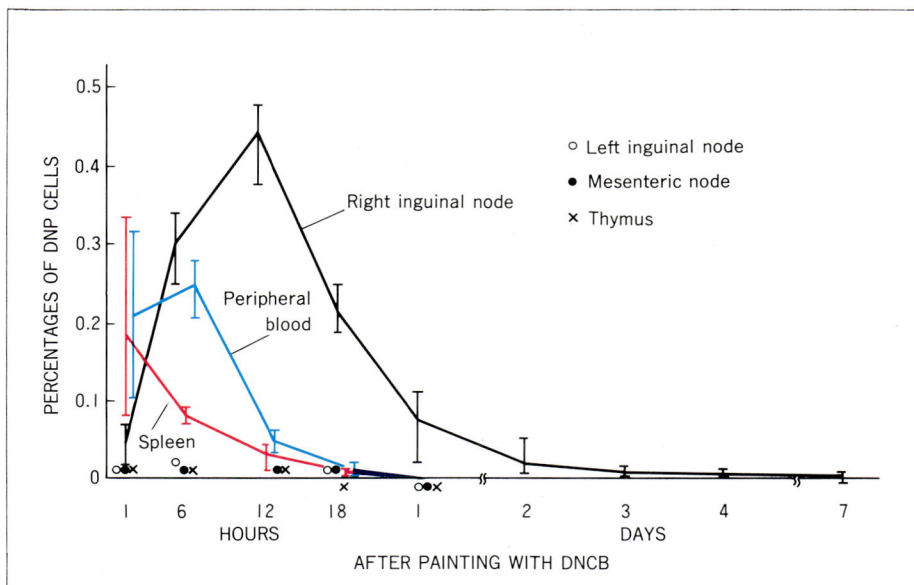

Fig. 4. Frequency of the cells with DNP groups in the lymphoid system at various time intervals after painting the right inguinal skin of normal guinea pigs with DNCB. Mean and frequency range from three to five animals.

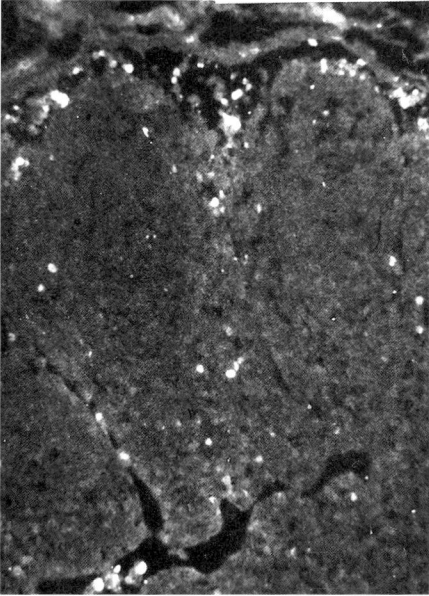

5

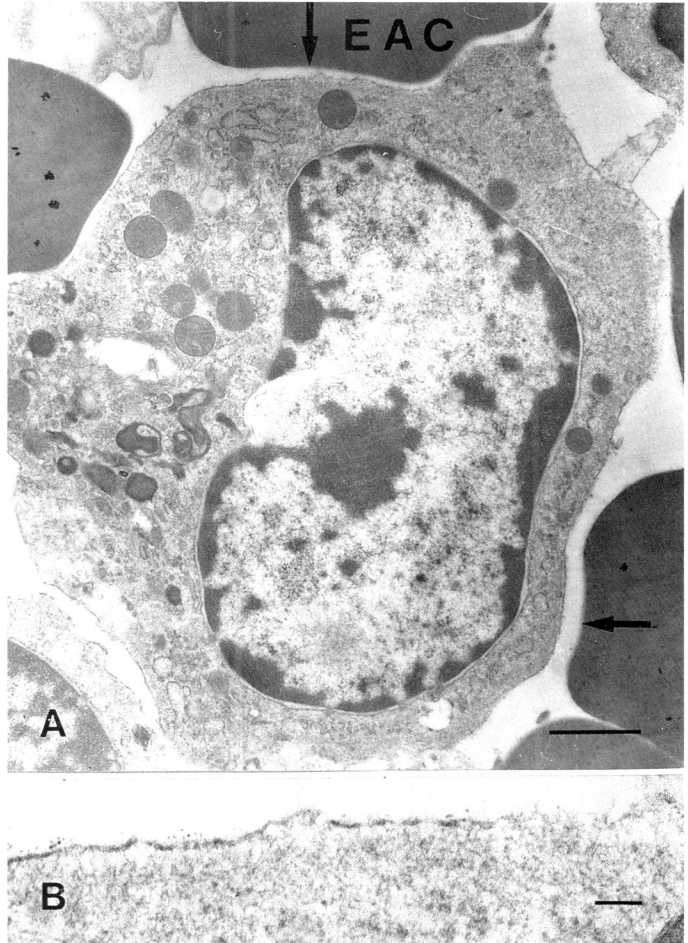

7

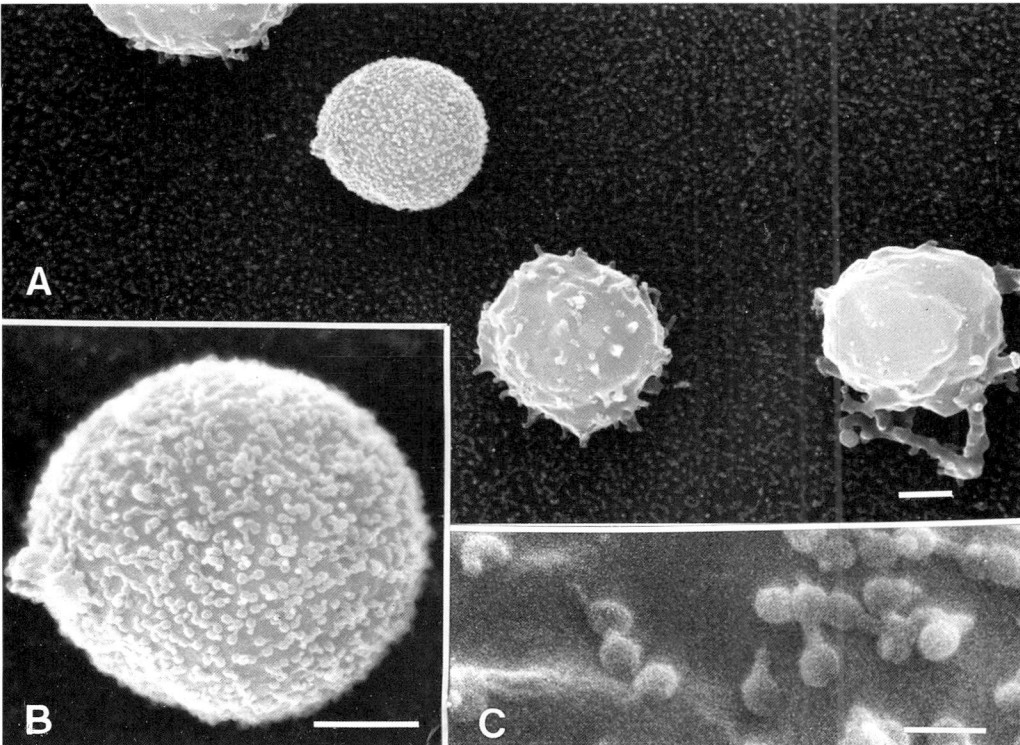

6

E Inflammatory keratosis

Psoriasis

INTRODUCTION

Psoriasis is a chronic erythematous disease, characterized by histological features showing epidermal proliferation with subcorneal microabscess and inflammation in the dermis. The lesions predominantly appear on the scalp, elbows, hip and knees. These sites are easily stimulated by rubbing. The clinical features are classified into four types: psoriasis vulgaris, erythrodermic psoriasis, pustular psoriasis and psoriasis arthropathica.

Major histocompatibility (MHC) in psoriasis. It is already known that the disease occasionally occurs in the same family, but the genetic pattern of psoriasis is still obscure. With regard to the MHC of psoriasis, it has been suggested that the disease is significantly associated with HLA-B13, B17 and BW37[477] and that there are two types of haplotype, HLA-A1, BW37, CW6 and DRW6 and HLA-A2, B13, CW6 and DRW7 in Japanese psoriatic patients[478].

Proliferation of epidermal cells. Histologically, there is capillary dilatation and oedema in the papillary dermis of initial lesions. In the fully developed lesions, the rete ridges of epidermis show regular elongation and markedly thickened parakeratotic horny layer with leucocytic accumulation (Munro's microabscess) and mononuclear lymphoid cells are infiltrated around the dilated capillaries in the upper dermis. In active lesions, the rate of epidermal cell proliferation is markedly accelerated in the S-phase of the cell cycle[479, 480]. It has been demonstrated that this marked acceleration of the cell kinetics is dependent upon the inbalance of cyclic AMP/cyclic GMP ratio in the cytoplasm of epidermal cells[481], due to the impairment of ß-adrenergic receptors on the cell membrane[482]. Therefore, it is speculated that leukotriene is produced from the epidermal cells by the hyperactivity of lipoxygenase in arachidonic cascade[483].

Inflammatory and immunologic reaction. In the initial lesions of psoriasis, mononuclear cells move from dilated capillaries in the dermal papillae, so-called 'squirting papillae', into the lower portion of the epidermis. Following the mononuclear cell infiltration, neutrophils are intermittently discharged from the dilated capillaries and reach the parakeratotic horny layer. Langhof and Müller (1966)[484] indicated that chemotaxis occurs in the psoriatic scales during the mechanism of Munro's microabscess. It has been demonstrated that psoriatic scales contain immunoglobulin and complement related to the anti-stratum corneum antibody which is present in the serum of patients with psoriasis vulgaris[485]. Beutner et al. and Jablonska et al.[486, 487] developed an autoimmune theory for the anti-stratum corneum in the pathogenesis of psoriasis.

Regarding the chemotactic factor which causes Munro's microabscess under the parakeratotic horny layer, it has been suggested that psoriatic leukotactic factor (PLF) is derived from C3 and C5[488]. We have demonstrated that PLF is mainly dependent upon the alternate pathway of the complement system, activated by the immune reaction associated with IgG and secretory IgA (sIgA) in the stratum corneum[489]. Immune complexes (IC), including IgG-IgA antibody, can be extracted from psoriatic scales[490]. It has been suspected that IC contain antigens related to keratin protein. IC are also detectable in the sera of psoriatic patients[491]. Regarding delayed-type hypersensitivity (DTH) in patients with psoriasis, it is supposed that the function of suppressor T cells is reduced in the peripheral blood[492].

Clinical features. The eruptions develop from pinhead-sized papules to various sizes of erythematous plaques with the characteristic thickened scales. In pustular psoriasis, groups of shallow pustules prominently develop on the erythematous base over the entire body or on the acral areas of the extremities.

Histological features. The histological picture from the biopsy of an early small papule shows a microabscess under the stratum corneum, exocytosis in the epidermis and infiltration of lymphoid cells around dilated capillaries in dermal papillae (**1a**). In the fully-developed psoriatic lesion, the epidermis shows regular elongation of the rete ridges, Munro's microabscess under the thickened parakeratotic horny layer, and thinning of the suprapapillary portions of the squamous layer (**1b, 1c**). Mononuclear cell infiltrates are noted to move up into the lower epidermis from the dilated capillaries in the upper dermis. In pustular psoriasis, a large pustular formation can be seen under the stratum corneum (**1d**). A spongiform pustule, designated as Kogoji's spongiform pustule, is present in the margin of the pustular site.

Immunofluorescent (IF) findings. In the early lesion, together with the accumulation of leucocytes under the stratum corneum, there are deposits of IgG, IgA and complement components. It has been found that the deposit of IgA includes a secretory component (S-component) which is suggested to be secretory IgA (sIgA) (**2a, b, c**). The deposits of S-component were detected at the dermal papillae of early lesions; a large amount of S-component deposition was noted at the D-E junction of the fully-developed psoriatic lesions (**2d**). Under the stratum corneum of the full-developed lesion in Munro's microabscess, large amounts of IgG, IgA and IgM were deposited and complement components, C1q, C3, properdin and Factor B (glycine-rich glycoprotein), were also detectable. On the other hand, in the early lesions, deposits of C3, properdin and Factor B were predominantly detected[490] and the complement reaction was suggested as an alternate pathway.

DIAGNOSTIC SIGNIFICANCE

The presence of Munro's microabscess under the stratum corneum, regular proliferation of the epidermal rete ridges and mononuclear infiltrate around dilated capillaries in the dermal papillae in the fully-developed psoriatic lesions are the histological characteristics. The deposits of immunoglobulin and complement in Munro's microabscess suggest the presence of phagocytized IC by macrophages and neutrophils which were accumulated by PLF.

TECHNICAL POINTS

(1) The frozen sections, cut using a cryostat 4 µm, should be fixed in cold acetone for five minutes.
(2) In order to avoid non-specific staining of the thickened parakeratotic horny layer, it is recommended that FITC-conjugated antibody sera be adjusted to a fluorescein/protein (F/P)-ratio of less than 2.0 by DEAE (diethylaminoethyl) cellulose column chromatography.

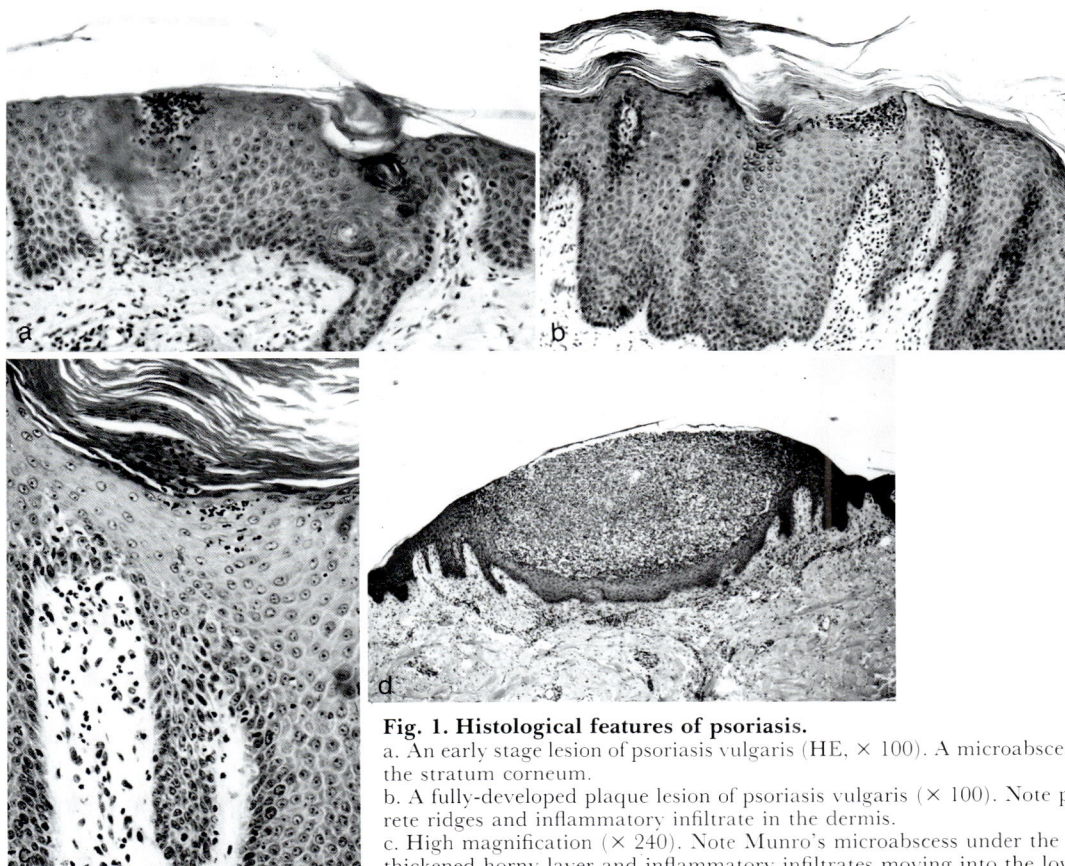

Fig. 1. Histological features of psoriasis.
a. An early stage lesion of psoriasis vulgaris (HE, × 100). A microabscess has been formed on the stratum corneum.
b. A fully-developed plaque lesion of psoriasis vulgaris (× 100). Note proliferated epidermal rete ridges and inflammatory infiltrate in the dermis.
c. High magnification (× 240). Note Munro's microabscess under the parakeratotic thickened horny layer and inflammatory infiltrates moving into the lower portion of the epidermis and in the dermal papilla.
d. Large subcorneal pustule of pustular psoriasis (× 100).

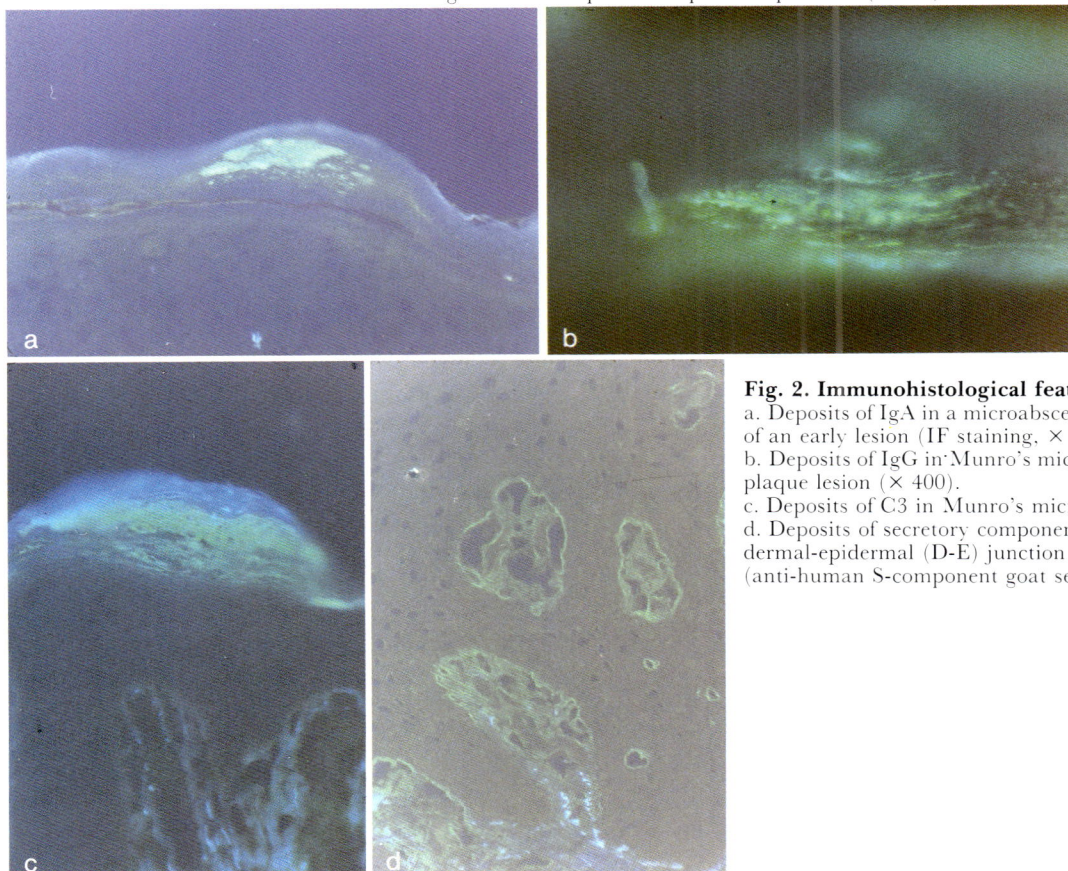

Fig. 2. Immunohistological features of psoriasis vulgaris.
a. Deposits of IgA in a microabscess under the stratum corneum of an early lesion (IF staining, × 120).
b. Deposits of IgG in Munro's microabscess in a fully-developed plaque lesion (× 400).
c. Deposits of C3 in Munro's microabscess (× 400).
d. Deposits of secretory component (S-component) in the dermal-epidermal (D-E) junction of a fully-developed lesion (anti-human S-component goat serum, × 200).

Pustulosis palmaris et plantaris

INTRODUCTION
Pustulosis palmaris et plantaris is a chronic disorder with sterile pustules occurring on the palms and soles.

FINDINGS
Clinically, the lesions may appear initially as multiple small vesicles on the palms and soles, which later become purulent with resultant brown macule formation. Pustular eruptions are occasionally observed in the extra-palmoplantar area; but this must be distinguished from acute generalized pustular bacterid[493] which shows pustular vasculitis, sterile pustules with underlying vasculitis[494]. Histologically, the primary eruption is an intraepidermal spongiotic vesicle with mononuclear cell infiltration. Neutrophil invasion occurs when the blister fluid comes in contact with the stratum corneum and then the subsequent formation of intraepidermal unilocular pustules occurs[495] (**1**).

PATHOGENESIS
Patients with this dermatosis are prone to focal infections such as tonsillitis or arthro-osteitis and impaired glucose tolerance[496]. As for the mechanism of the formation of sterile pustules, a leukotactic factor in the stratum corneum of pustulosis palmaris et plantaris, complement cleavage products (C3a and C5a), seems to be responsible[497]. Significantly high titres of complement-fixing anti-stratum corneum (SC) antibodies have been reported and anti-SC antibodies may be involved in the activation of complement with subsequent accumulation of neutrophils[498]. However, the significance of anti-SC antibodies still remains unclear. In any event, in view of the report that colchicine is effective in the treatment[499], there is no doubt that neutrophil chemotaxis plays a crucial role in pustule formation.

TECHNICAL POINTS
It is important to choose the biopsy site carefully and to select early lesions.

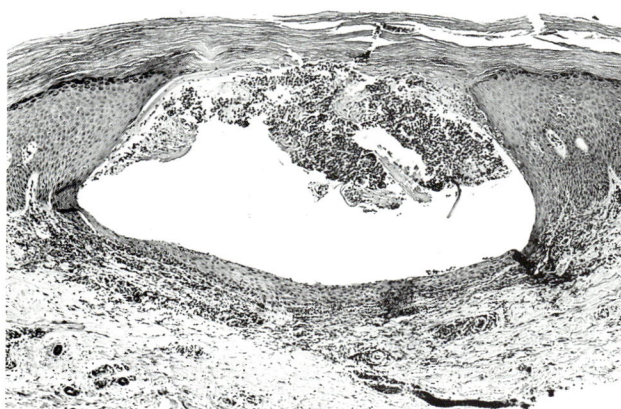

Fig. 1. Histological features.
An intraepidermal unilocular pustule. (× 100)

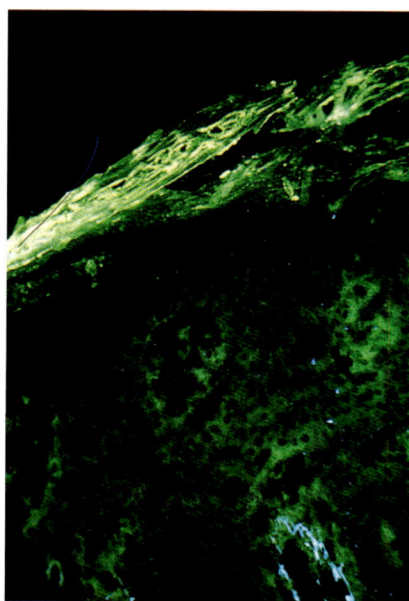

Fig. 2. Anti-SC antibodies.
Significantly high titres of complement-fixing anti-SC antibodies. (× 200)

Lichen planus

INTRODUCTION

Lichen planus (LP) is characterized by the presence of small, inflammatory keratostic flat papules localized mainly on the extensor surface of the four extremities, trunk and genital area. The aetiology of LP is still unknown, but some types are due to drug intoxication.

FINDINGS

Histological findings. The histological findings of eosin-haematoxylin staining have certain features in common: moderate hyperkeratosis, elongation of rete ridge, liquefaction degeneration of basal cell layer, flattened epidermis (so-called wiped out), presence of colloid body (hyaline body, Civatte body) and band-like infiltration of mononuclear cells in the upper dermis[500] (**1**).

Immunopathological findings. In the diseased skin of LP, an extensive deposition of IgM in the colloid body is detectable by the direct immunofluorescent technique (DIF). Occasionally, this deposit is composed of IgG, IgA, C3, C4, Clq and fibrin[501, 502] (**2**). Also, band-like or granular deposits of fibrin at the dermo-epidermal junction (DEJ) are highly prevalent (**3**). In some cases, the deposition of fibrin at DEJ is gradually continuous to the middle dermis[502]. The presence of IgM, IgG and C3 at the DEJ[503] and complement and fibrin at capillary walls[502, 504] have also been reported.

Using recently derived monoclonal antibodies against the epitopes of lymphocytes, analysis of infiltrated lymphocytes can be carried out easily. The majority of these are helper/inducer T cells reactive to OKT4. Their active significance in local lesions is still unknown (**4**).

DIAGNOSTIC AND PATHOGENETIC SIGNIFICANCE

The findings of DIF, as stated above, are also used to determine lesions of lupus erythematosus, fixed drug eruption and dermatomyositis, although cluster formation of hyaline bodies strongly suggests those of LP. These findings are particularly helpful for the determination of the differential diagnosis of LP on scalp and/or mucous membrane.

It is also important that the majority of the deposited substance at DEJ in LP is fibrin rather than immunoglobulin and/or complement, as in LE.

Recently, some reports have indicated immunological disturbances in LP, while the DIF finding of hyaline bodies might merely be caused by its sponge structure[505].

TECHNICAL POINTS

Fresh-frozen, unfixed tissue sections should be used for DIF. The tissue specimens should be taken from relatively new lesions, thus reducing the possibility of artifacts.

It is recommended that the LBT be carried out on sections from normal-appearing skin at the flexor surface of a forearm in order to estimate patient's prognosis.

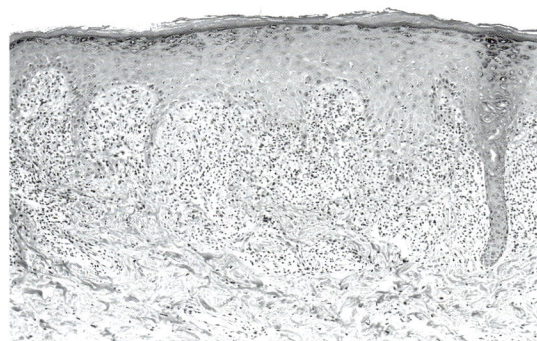

Fig. 1. Histological findings with eosin-haematoxylin staining. (× 200)

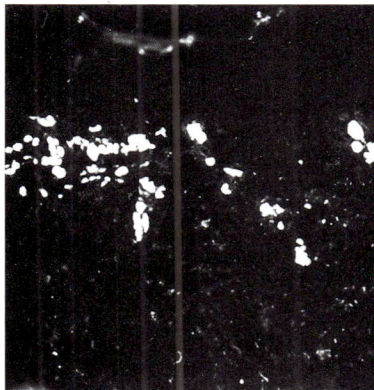

Fig. 2. Colloid body with direct immunofluorescent staining for IgA. (× 200)

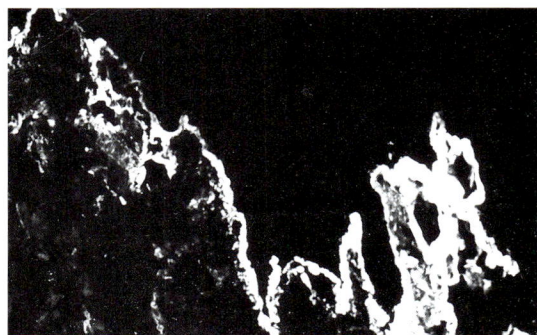

Fig. 3. Immunofluorescent staining for fibrin shows the band-like pattern at the dermo-epidermal junction. (× 200)

Fig. 4. Infiltrated lymphocytes positively stained by OKT4 antibody (avidin-biotin-peroxydase method). (× 400)

F Metabolic diseases

Amyloidosis

INTRODUCTION

The biochemical composition of amyloids is not uniform, differing in each clinical type. Each amyloid is derived from different precursor proteins which produce a characteristic clinical syndrome to which a clinical name is given. Amyloid deposits in the skin are seen not only in localized cutaneous amyloidosis, but also in systemic amyloidosis. In many cases of AL amyloidosis (precursor protein: light chain of immunoglobulin, primary systemic amyloidosis and systemic amyloidosis associated with multiple myeloma), characteristic cutaneous lesions develop. On the other hand, in secondary systemic amyloidosis (precursor protein: serum amyloid A protein) and in familial amyloid polyneuropathy (precursor protein: prealbumin) the skin lesions rarely develop, but small amyloid depositions are often histologically detectable even in skin which shows no clinical sign. Therefore, both rectum and skin biopsies have recently come to be regarded as an important way to diagnose amyloidosis histopathologically.

Regarding the classification of systemic amyloidosis, the following examinations are necessary laboratory tests of the serum M protein and urinary B-J protein, and the histochemical test of potassium permanganate reaction of Wright et al.[506]. Recently, antisera antibodies against amyloid proteins and amyloid precursor proteins have been produced and some are now commercially available. These antibodies have made it immunohistopathologically possible to diagnose and classify many cases of amyloidosis.

THE IMMUNOHISTOPATHOLOGICAL EXAMINATION FOR AMYLOID FIBRIL PROTEINS

Systemic amyloidosis. AL amyloidosis, AA amyloidosis and familial amyloid polyneuropathy are immunohistopathologically distinguishable. Antisera antibodies AA and AL show idiotypic specificity[507].

Antisera antibody against human AA amyloid protein, obtained by immunizing a rabbit with purified AA, was purchased from the DAKO Corporation, California (**1**). The amyloid protein from familial amyloid polyneuropathy was stained with anti-human prealbumin serum (**2**). For this examination, paraffin-embedded sections were used.

Localized cutaneous amyloidosis. Macular and lichen amyloidosis: Polyclonal and monoclonal antibodies against epidermal keratin cross-reacted with amyloid[508–12] (**3**). Many studies have suggested that cytoid bodies are the precursors of amyloids[506–13]. Eto et al.[511] used five different monoclonal antikeratin antibodies to study the immunological characteristics of skin amyloids and cytoid bodies. The amyloid was stained strongly with EKH4 (which stains the lower two to three layers in normal human epidermis), but only weakly stained or not at all with monoclonal antibodies AE1 (which stains the basal cell layer) and EKH1 (which recognizes all classes of intermediate filaments). EKH4 antibody also strongly stained the cytoid bodies in both lichen planus and discoid lupus erythematosus and the tumour cell of basal cell carcinoma, but did not stain the amyloid of nodular amyloidosis or primary systemic amyloidosis. On the other hand, some authors[512–14] report that polyclonal anti-epidermal keratin antibodies do not stain the amyloid in cutaneous amyloidosis. For this examination, paraffin-embedded sections were not usable.

Amyloidosis cutis nodularis atrophicans: Amyloid deposits are found throughout the dermis and surrounding the blood vessel walls. The clinical and histopathological findings of this amyloidosis are similar to those of systemic amyloidosis. Immunohistochemically, the antisera antibody against AL stained the amyloid[515] (**4**). For this examination, paraffin-embedded sections were used.

OTHER IMMUNOHISTOCHEMICAL FINDINGS

Amyloid p-component is immunohistopathologically detectable in amyloid in all types of amyloidoses and in isolated amyloid fibrils[516], and the binding between amyloid p-component and amyloid fibrils is strictly calcium-dependent. In localized cutaneous amyloidosis, immunoglobulin IgG, IgM, IgA, C1g, C3, C4, C5, and anti-basement membrane zone antiserum, obtained from a patient with bullous pemphigoid[517], were detected within the amyloid masses.

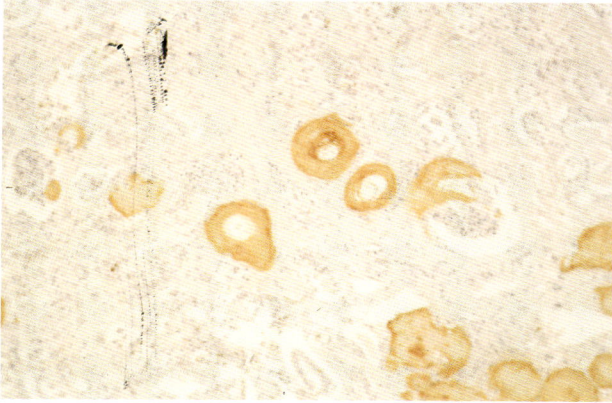

Fig. 1. Secondary systemic amyloidosis. Amyloid materials surround kidney blood vessels stained with anti-serum antibody against amyloid A protein. (PAP immunostain, courtesy of Professor M. Ohashi, Department of Dermatology, Nagoya University School of Medicine, Japan.)

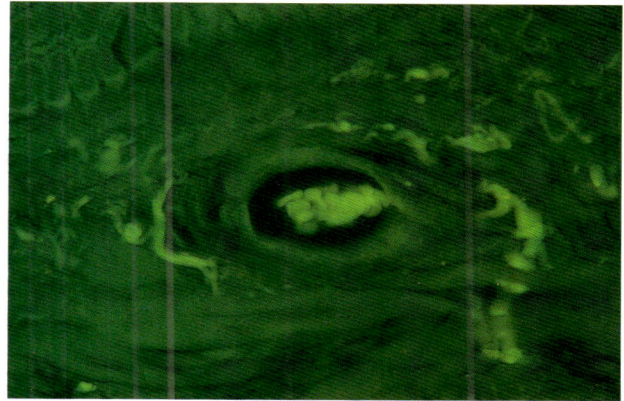

Fig. 2. Familial amyloid polyneuropathy. Amyloid materials surround elastic fibres stained with anti-serum antibody against prealbumin (immunofluorescent stain).

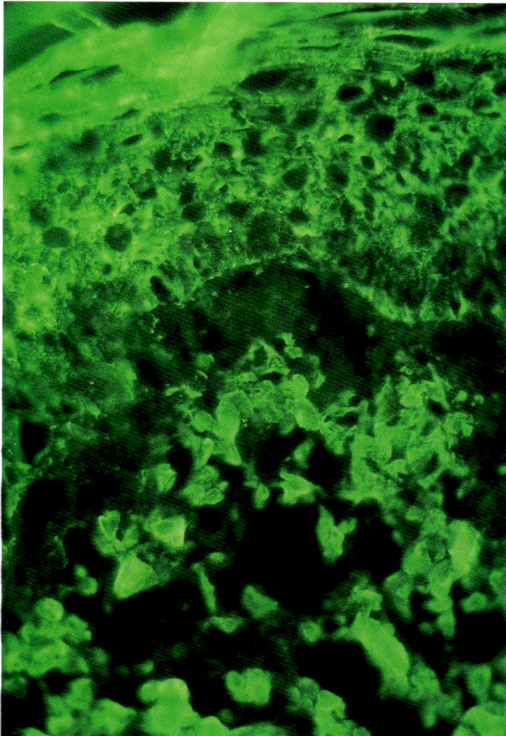

Fig. 3. Lichen amyloidosis. Amyloid materials in papillar layer stained with anti-serum antibody against keratin. (Immunofluorescent stain, from Maeda, H. *et al*: Br. J. Dermatol. **106**:345, 1982.)

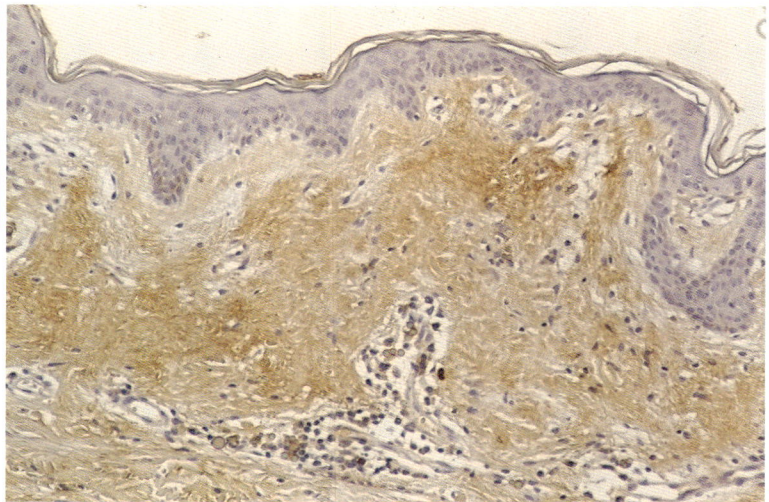

Fig. 4. Amyloidosis cutis nodularis atrophicans. Amyloid materials in dermis stained with anti-serum antibody against AL. (PAP stain, from Kitajima Y. *et al*: Arch. Dermatol. **122**:1425, 1986.)

Porphyria cutanea tarda

INTRODUCTION

All porphyrias with cutaneous manifestations are similar as regards immunohistological findings[518-21]. The findings are marked in erythropoietic protoporphyria (EPP), porphyria cutanea tarda (PCT) and variegate porphyria (VP). Generally, these findings are specific in the exposed areas. Theoretically, these findings do not appear in patients with porphyrias who were not exposed to sunlight, despite great metabolic abnormalities. Therefore, the findings are often affected by the occupation or life history of the patient. There are no specific techniques for an immunohistological approach in this field. Routine tissue preparation, fixation and embedding techniques are used.

FINDINGS

A deposition of immunoglobulin G (IgG) and fibrinogen is seen at the dermo-epidermal junction. The most characteristic finding is the deposition of IgG surrounding the small blood vessels in the upper dermis (1). Occasionally, immunoglobulin M (IgM), C3 and C4 are deposited in the same areas. The deposition of IgG in the dermo-epidermal junction is linear, while the deposition occasionally observed of C3, fibrinogen and albumin is granular. The deposition of IgG surrounding the small blood vessels in the upper dermis is diffuse and amorphous and is more prominent in patients with EPP than those with PCT. Bullae formation is often frequent in PCT. IgG, C3 and C4 are granularly deposited at the bottom of the bullous lesions. Fluorescence with anti-type IV collagen and anti-laminin antibodies is observed in the thickened basement membrane of the blood vessels in the dermis[522].

DIAGNOSTIC SIGNIFICANCE AND PATHOGENESIS

These findings are not necessary for the diagnosis of porphyrias. However, laboratory examinations for porphyrins should be done when the eruption is limited to the exposed areas and a deposition of PAS-positive materials is observed. A deposition of immunoglobulin coincides with PAS-positive materials.

A phototoxin reaction occurs through the synergistic effect between porphyrins, which differs according to the type of porphyria and the amount of sunlight. This results in leakage of intravascular substances and the degeneration of endothelial cells, that is vascular damage in the upper dermis[523]. Subsequently, it is suggested that the deposition of immunoglobulin occurs in the same areas where repair of blood vessels takes place. The process of repair is still not clear. Slight deposition of these materials is occasionally seen in the unexposed areas. This may suggest that even 400 nm of light can penetrate clothing and affect the dermis.

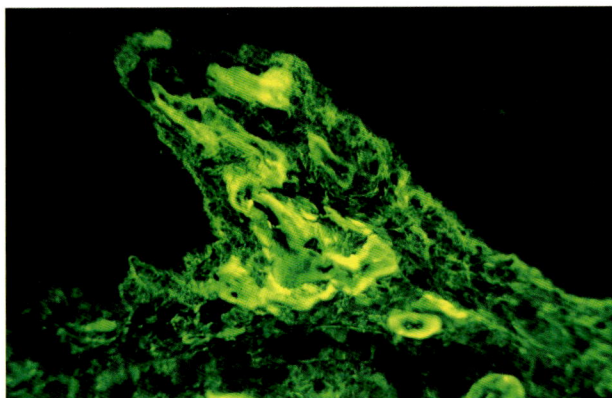

Fig. 1. Immunohistological findings in a patient with PCT (51-year-old, male). Deposition of IgG is seen at the dermo-epidermal junction and surrounding the small blood vessels. (Courtesy of Dr. S. Anan.)

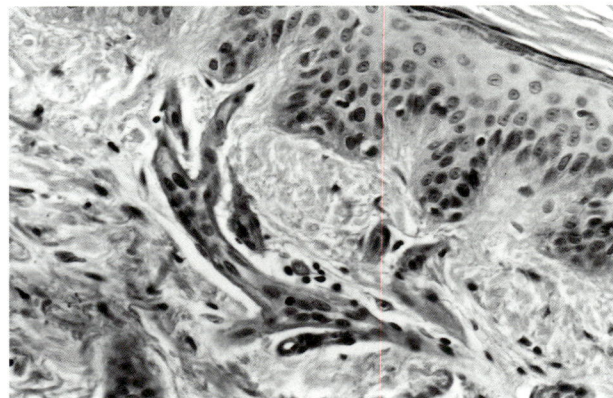

Fig. 2. Histopathological findings using PAS stain in a patient with PCT (72-year-old, male). PAS-positive materials are seen around the small blood vessels in the papillary and subpapillary dermis.

IMMUNOFLUORESCENCE FINDINGS

A granular or reticular pattern of complement C3 was deposited in part of what appeared to be the hyaline membrane of the hair bulb of anagen hair follicles (**1**). Deposition of complement C3 was also discovered in the internal layer (annular) of the connective tissue sheath at the lower 2/3 transient portion of the hair follicle. The deposition was linear and perpendicular to the long axis of the follicle, running along with the collagenous fibre (**1**). In the hair follicles, assuming the shape of a catagen follicle, the C3 deposition was striking in the thickened hyaline membrane (**2**). Complement C5 and C9 were also deposited there. No deposition of Clq, C4 or properdin were observed in the hair follicles of the scalp and no deposition of immunoglobulin (IgG, IgA, IgM, IgD and IgE) was found[524,525]. Bystryn et al.[526] reported the deposition of C3 in affected hair follicles of patients with alopecia areata and male pattern alopecia.

The deposition of IgG and IgM in the hair follicles and circulating antibody against hair follicles was reported by Nakajima[527].

DIAGNOSTIC SIGNIFICANCE

According to the authors' findings, there was no difference in the deposition of complement C3, C5 and C9 in the hair follicles of normal scalps and the scalps affected by alopecia areata. However, it appears that complement components are closely related to the hair cycle; the deposition of complement components in hair follicles of normal scalps occurred chiefly in the transient portion of the hair follicles. The behaviour of the deposition was reflected in the morphological state of the hair follicles in each stage of hair cycle, even in alopecia areata.

Bystryn et al.[526] and Nakajima[527] suggested that immuno mechanisms play a role in the pathogenesis of alopecia areata.

BIOPSY

The biopsy was taken from within the margin of lesion that is observable at each stage of the hair cycle.

TECHNICAL POINTS

(1) As specimens sectioned within a cryostat were easily separated from the glass slide when washed with phosphate-buffered saline (PBS), the cryostat section must be as thin as possible and completely dried.

(2) In order to observe the form of the follicle, the cryostat section must be made perpendicular to the long axis of the follicle.

(3) The sections observed under the fluorescence microscope were then stained with haematoxylin and eosin to observe the hair follicle histology under a light microscope.

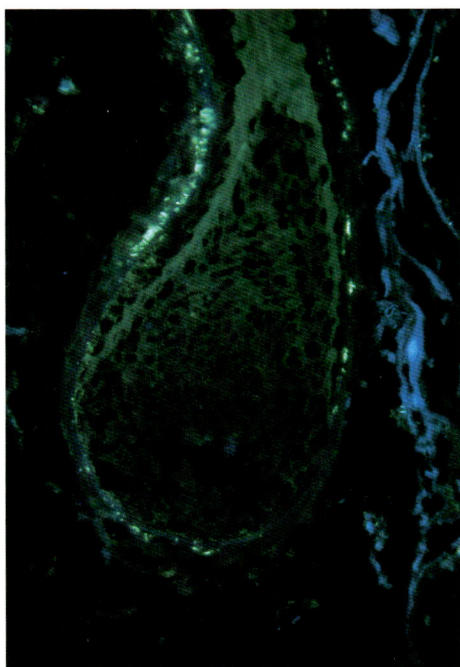

Fig. 1. IF staining showing granular deposition of C3 in the anagen-like follicle in alopecia areata lesion. (× 100)

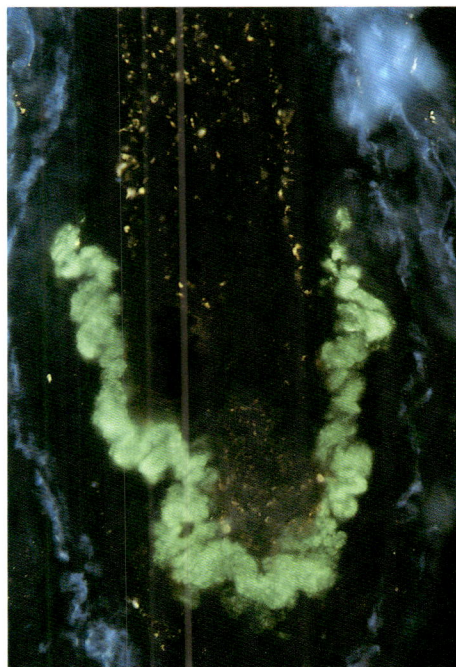

Fig. 2. IF staining showing heavy deposition of C3 in the thickened hyaline membrane in the catagen-like follicle in alopecia areata lesion. (× 200)

H Infectious diseases

Mycoses

INTRODUCTION

Clinical laboratory procedures in medical mycology demonstrate and isolate causative fungi found in various tissues and fluids. The fluorescent antibody (FA) technique (Coons *et al.*)[528] rapidly detects and identifies microorganisms and demonstrates antibodies in sera. This method can also be used for the rapid detection and identification of both viable and nonviable fungi in culture and in most types of clinical materials, including paraffin sections of formalin-fixed tissues[529,530].

A fungal infection can be diagnosed with confidence by direct microscopy if the aetiological agent produces diagnostically distinct forms in tissue and if it is present in the typical form; otherwise, the diagnosis is merely presumptive. Under such circumstances, use of the FA technique as an adjunctive diagnostic procedure, with its added dimension of serologic specificity, increases the accuracy of direct examinations. The FA technique can also be used as the initial procedure to examine specimens for the presence of fungi.

FINDINGS

Basically, the FA technique is an immunochemical staining procedure that permits microscopic visualization of antigen-antibody reactions. Such visualization is accomplished through the use of an antibody coupled to a fluorochrome.

After staining using the FA technique, fungal elements emit a brilliant greenish fluorescence, while the tissue components show a light bluish autofluorescence providing a beautiful contrast. It should be noted however, that the intensity of the specific fluorescence of the fungal cells is not equal; the strength of staining varies among individual cells within the same focus.

DIAGNOSTIC SIGNIFICANCE

The FA technique is at present considered a valuable adjunct to the histopathological diagnosis of fungal infections, particularly pathogens involved in opportunistic fungal and actinomycotic infections (Table)[531]. It should also be noted that the FA technique is ideal for detecting and identifying fungi in histologic sections previously stained with haematoxylin and eosin, or stained using the Giemsa, Brown and Brenn, or Gram methods. Fungi in sections previously stained by the periodic acid-Schiff, Gridley's or Gomori's methenamine-silver procedures cannot generally be stained by the FA procedure. Apparently, the oxidation of cell wall polysaccharides of fungi alters the antigenicity of the organisms so that they do not react with the labelled antibodies.

Prolonged storage of formalin-fixed tissues, either wet or in paraffin blocks, does not seem to affect the antigenicity of fungi. So this method is useful not only in diagnosing a current infection, but also for retrospective diagnosis of a fungal infection.

METHODS

Descriptions of the preparation of the fungal antigens, the production of antisera, the preparation of fluorescent conjugates, and the purification of conjugates are listed in laboratory guide books[531,532].

Direct FA technique. The labelled antibody solutions are applied to culture smears, clinical materials, or sections of tissue. After 30 to 40 minutes of incubation at 37°C, the preparation is rinsed, mounted generally with buffered glycerol saline (pH 7.8), and examined for stained fungal elements or antigen.

Indirect FA technique. A fluorescein-conjugate directed against the globulin of animal species producing the initial antibody is used to make the antigen-antibody reaction visible. In the first stage, unlabelled antibody serves as the antibody. In the second stage, the fluorescein-tagged anti-globulin combines with the antigen-antibody complex and thus illuminates the complex.

TECHNICAL POINTS

Direct application of FA reagents to deparaffinized tissue sections is usually satisfactory if the sections are thin (4–6 µm or less), if fungal elements are abundant, and if the tissue is not dense. When such desirable conditions are not possible, satisfactory results can be obtained if deparaffinized sections are digested in a 1.0% trypsin solution (pH 8.0) for one hour at 37°C, prior to the application of FA regents[530].

For FA staining of fungi in histologic sections previously stained with haematoxylin and eosin, or by the Giemsa or Gram methods, coverslips are removed by gently heating the slides to soften the adhesive prior to immersion in xylene. The preparations are then rinsed in phosphate-buffered solution (pH 7.2) and, if necessary, are digested in 1.0% Trypsin (pH 8.0) as are unstained, deparaffinized sections.

(Figures 5 and 6 courtesy of Dr. H. Kume, Department of Pathology, Kitasato University School of Medicine, Sagamihara, Japan.)

TABLE I   FUNGI AND ACTINOMYCETES THAT ARE CURRENTLY IDENTIFIED BY THE FLUORESCENT ANTIBODY TECHNIQUE

Actinomyces israelii	*Cryptococcus neoformans*
A. naeslundii	*Histoplasma capsulatum*
A. viscosus	(tissue forms of both varieties)
Arachnia propionica	*Pseudallescheria boydii*
Aspergillus spp. (to genus)	*Prototheca wickerhamii*
Blastomyces dermatitidis (tissue form)	*P. zopfii*
Candida spp. (to genus)	*Sporothrix schenckii*
Coccidioides immitis (tissue form)	

(Chandler, F.W., Kaplan, W., Ajello, L.: 'Color Atlas and Text of the Histopathology of Mycotic Diseases', Year Book Medical Publ., 1980[531])

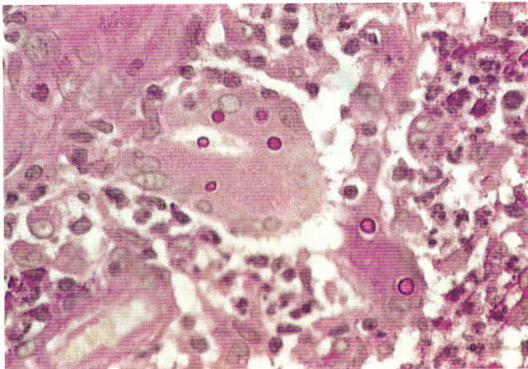

Fig. 1. Cutaneous sporotrichosis, periodic acid-Schiff stain. (Original magnification × 400)

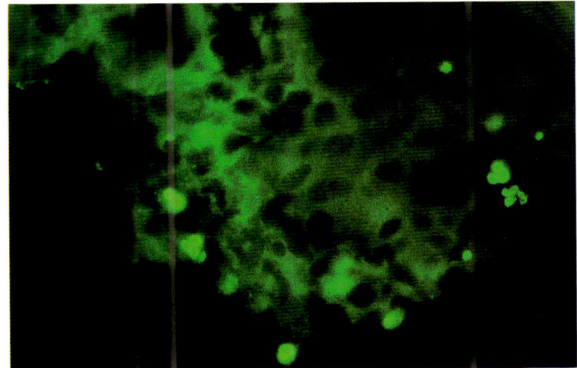

Fig. 2. Cutaneous sporotrichosis, direct FA technique. (× 400)

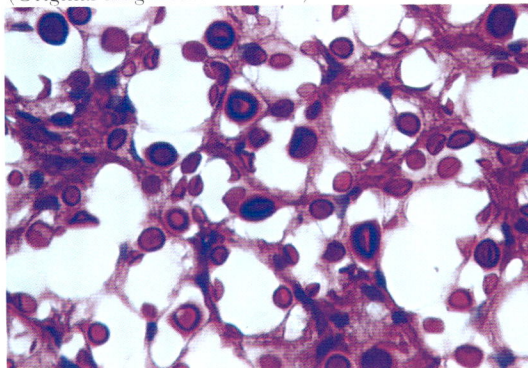

Fig. 3. Cutaneous cryptococcosis, periodic acid-Schiff stain. (× 600)

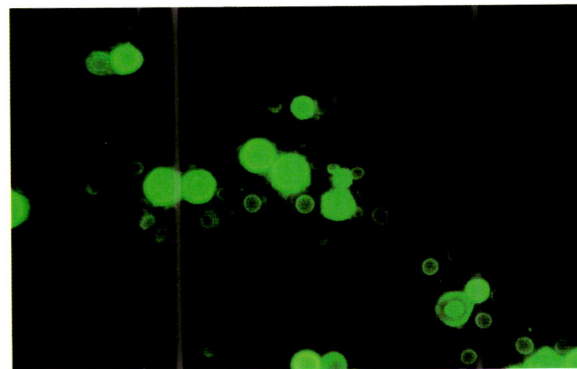

Fig. 4. Cutaneous cryptococcosis, direct FA technique. (× 600)

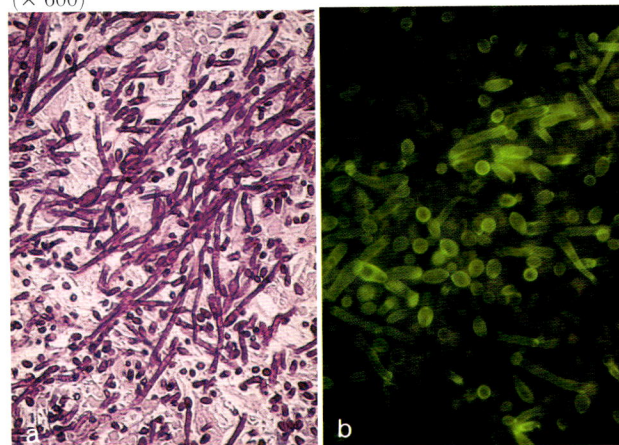

Fig. 5. Oesophageal candidiasis, periodic acid-Schiff stain × 400 (a) and indirect FA technique × 400 (b).

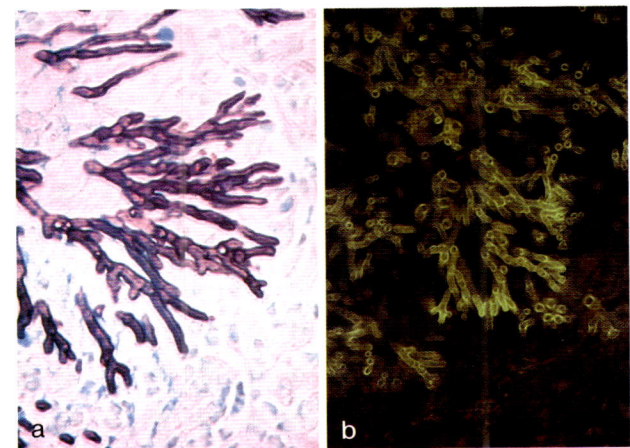

Fig. 6. Pulmonary aspergillosis PAS staining, × 400(a), indirect immunofluorescence method, × 400(b)

117

Spirochaetal diseases

INTRODUCTION
Syphilis is a treponematosis caused by *Treponema pallidum* (*T.p.*) and is well known as one of the sexually transmitted diseases (STD).

For the diagnosis of primary and secondary syphilis, it is necessary to demonstrate *T.p.* from the lesions. Although histologic patterns and clinical features may suggest a diagnosis of syphilis, they are not specific enough to establish the diagnosis. The serological tests for syphilis and the present illness are helpful in making a diagnosis but, occasionally, it is hard to ascertain whether the eruptions are syphilids or not.

T.p. can be found demonstrated in secretions from the lesions of syphilids by the dark-field examination, the Indian ink method, and the Parker ink method. Occasionally, however, it is difficult to determine *T.p.* in cases of secondary macules and in some types of papules[533, 534]. In these cases, it is crucial to demonstrate *T.p.* in the tissue sections. We usually use silver stains such as the Warthin-Starry method[535] and Gifu University method[536] to identify *T.p.* in the tissues, but these staining procedures have little specificity for *T.p.* Reticulum fiber and other tissue elements can also be stained, although satisfactory results are not always obtain-able; thus *T.p.* cannot easily be distinguished from other tissue elements.

The immunofluorescent staining method is considered to be superior because this method is specific for *T.p.* and generally gives the best results.

FINDINGS
The case is a 21-year-old male who noticed erythema, papules with slight itching over most of his body about three weeks prior to testing. The histopathological features of the pale-reddish slightly elevated erythema were slight inflammatory cell infiltrates and dilatation of capillaries in the upper and mid-dermis (**1**). Using immunofluorescent complement stain[537], we tried to demonstrate *T.p.* in the tissue section to establish a diagnosis. *T.p.* was observed in both the epidermis and dermis, principally in the basal layer and lower portion of the prickle cell layer (**2**).

DIAGNOSTIC SIGNIFICANCE
When the clinical features suggest a diagnosis of syphilis and the histological features show only non-specific changes, the immunofluorescent complement staining method to demonstrate *T.p.* is extremely valuable because it can be performed even after materials are embedded in paraffin.

TECHNICAL POINTS
When attempting this immunofluorescent complement staining procedure, it is recommended to note the following:

(1) Handle the specimen section carefully as it is only 2 μm thick.
(2) Try contrast stain.
(3) Observe immediately after staining.

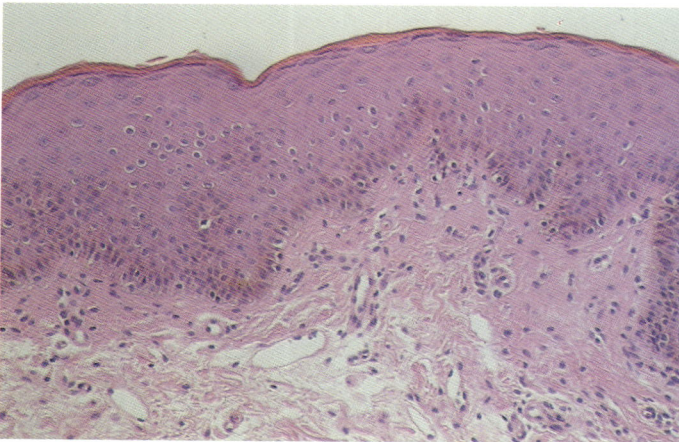

Fig. 1. Slight inflammatory cell infiltration and dilatation of capillaries noted in the upper and mid-dermis of slightly elevated erythema stained with HE solution. (× 50)

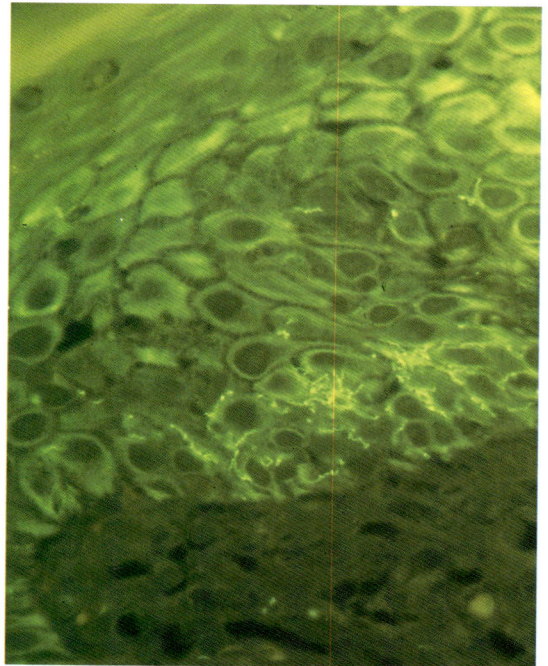

Fig. 2. The immunofluorescent complement staining method revealed many *T.p.* in the basal layer and lower portion of the prickle cell layer. (Exposure time 20 seconds × 132.)

Bacterial infections – impetigo and staphylococcal scalded skin syndrome

INTRODUCTION

Bullous impetigo occurs predominantly in infants and young children. Group 2 *staphylococci* grow in culture system using fluid in intact bullae. The exotoxin, exfoliatin, produces intraepidermal cleavage in the uppermost epidermis.

Staphylococcal scalded skin syndrome occurs mainly in newborns and infants, and rarely in adults. It begins with widespread erythema which rapidly progresses to flaccid bullae. Fluid of the bullae is sterile. Exfoliation may occur due to focal infection (e.g., purulent conjunctivitis, rhinitis).

PATHOLOGY

In both of these diseases, the cleavage plane of the bullae lies in the stratum granulosum (**1**). Electron microscopy shows that in the very early lesions, distension of intercellular spaces occurs prior to the alteration of desmosomes[538].

STAPHYLOCOCCAL SCALDED SKIN SYNDROME MODEL

Subcutaneous or intraperitonial injection of exfoliatin into newborn mice produces generalized erythema and exfoliation with intraepidermal cleavage at the level of the granular layer[539] (**2**). An indirect immunofluorescent study has shown that exfoliatin accumulates at the granular layer of both the exfoliated and non-exfoliated skin[540] (**3**).

PATHOGENESIS

The cell surface membrane of the granular layer cell has specific receptor sites for exfoliatin[541], suggesting that the receptor binding of exfoliatin is the initial step in the process of epidermal cell separation.

Exfoliatin is excreted through the kidneys[542]. It is known that the human kidneys are functionally immature in neonates and infants, and that most adult cases of staphylococcal scalded skin syndrome have an underlying disease, such as renal failure or immune deficiency. Thus, the interaction of renal insufficiency and immune suppression may play an important role in the aetiology of staphylococcal scalded skin syndrome.

MAKING THE SELECTION FOR BIOPSY

To confirm the histological and immunohistological features of the exfoliatin-induced epidermal cleavage, a biopsy should be taken from an early erythema, which extends into normal skin. In longstanding erythema, the epidermis is often dislocated from its primary site.

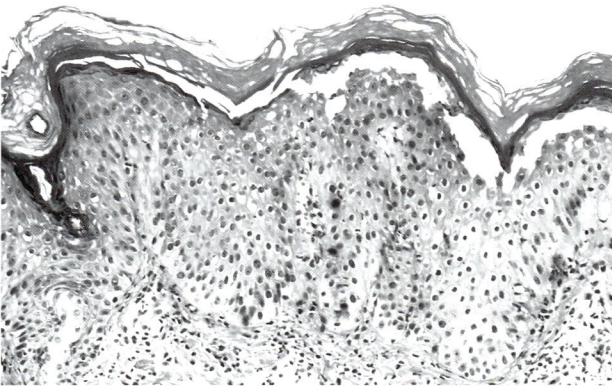

Fig. 1. Early lesion of bullous impetigo. Intraepidermal cleavage occurs within or immediately beneath the stratum granulosum. (HE, × 150)

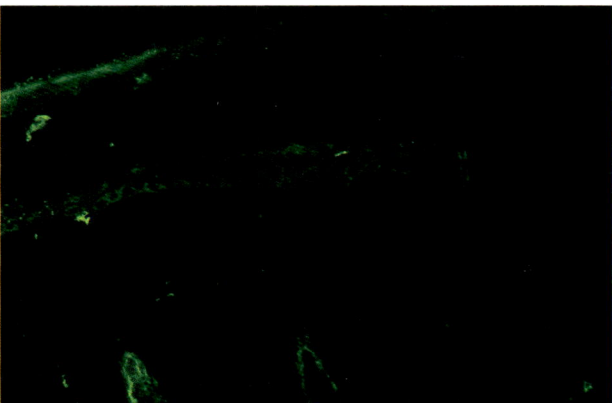

Fig. 2. Generalized scalded skin in a newborn mouse, induced by subcutaneous injection of exfoliatin. (Courtesy of S. Sakurai, M.D., Jikei Med. Univ.)

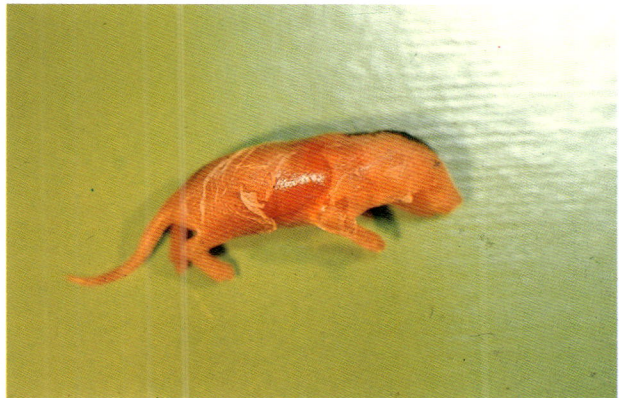

Fig. 3. Accumulation of exfoliatin at the subcorneal area of a flaccid bulla in a newborn mouse; induced by subcutaneous injection of exfoliatin. (Courtesy of I. Kondo, M.D., Jikei Med. Univ.)

Tsutsugamushi disease (Scrub typhus)

INTRODUCTION

Tsutsugamushi disease is a rickettsial disorder. The causative agent is *Rickettsis tsutsugamushi*, and the main vectors are leptus of *Trombicula akamushi* and *Trombicula pallidum*. This disease was once known as a relatively rare epidemic disorder in the North-East part of Japan, particularly in Akita, Yamagata, and Niigata Prefectures.

Tsutsugamushi disease is curable simply by the administration of tetracycline, but it can be lethal when the therapy is delayed[543], so an early diagnosis is extremely important. This disease exhibits peculiar clinical symptoms of high fever, eruptive small erythema, and a blister at the tick bite area which soon becomes necrotic and forms an eschar. The diagnosis, therefore, is not clinically difficult[544]. For the final diagnosis, however, direct proof of the existence of rickettsia in the patient's blood, or a significant rise in anti-rickettsial antibody titre in the patient's serum is necessary. This paper reviews methods of serological diagnosis of this disease in our hospital.

METHODS AND FINDINGS

Direct immunofluorescence test. Suzuki et al.[545] used a direct immunofluorescence test to detect the localization of rickettsia particles in body tissues.

Preparation of antibody. Rickettsia of each strain (Gilliam, Karp, and Kato) was injected into a guinea pig brain. Thirty days later, the animal was killed, and whole body blood was

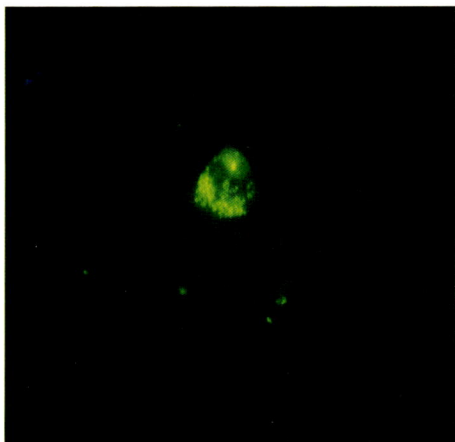

Fig. 1. Direct immunofluorescence test for blister fluid cell smear. Many rickettsia particles are seen in the histiocyte. (From Takahashi and Maie[544].) (× 400)

collected. Immunoglobulin G fraction of the blood was extracted, purified, and conjugated with FITC, then used for direct immunofluorescence test as the antibody.

Findings. Rickettsia particles in patients' tissues showed clear fluorescence. Tsutsugamushi disease is detectable at an early stage by examining cells from the blister which appears at the tick bite portion (**1**).

Indirect immunoperoxidase test. Suto et al.[546] measured anti-rickettsial antibody titre of patients' sera by the indirect immunoperoxidase test.

Preparation of antigen. Each standard strain of *Rickettsia tsutsugamushi* (Gilliam, Karp, and Kato) was inoculated into

cultured L cells. When the majority of cells showed degeneration from the cytopathic effect of rickettsia, the L cells were collected and gently centrifuged at 500 rpm for five minutes. Rickettsia particles were then placed in the supernatant. A very small amount of 0.3% bovine serum albumin PBS was added to this supernatant. Rickettsia particle smears were made by drawing the rickettsia suspension in and out of a micropipette and onto a glass slide. The smears were then air-dried, fixed with cold acetone for ten minutes, sealed in a cellophane bag and stored in a deep freezer ($-20°C$).

Preparation of substitute solution for peroxidase reaction. 0.3 gram of 3,3'-diaminobenzidine tetrahydrochloride and 1.0 gram of crystalline sodium acetate were dissolved in distilled water to make a total of 100 ml. The pH was adjusted to 6.2 using a 1N NaOH solution (about 2.5 ml). Then 0.7 ml of 3% hydrogen peroxide was added, and the solution stored in a dark bottle at room temperature.

Findings. The rickettsia smears were covered by patients' diluted sera and incubated at 37°C for twenty minutes, washed with (−)PBS three times, and then covered with peroxidase-labelled anti-human IgG (or IgM) rabbit antibody. After incubation at 37°C for twenty minutes, the smears were washed with (−)PBS and distilled water and then immersed in the substrate solution in a dark place at room temperature for ten minutes. After a brief wash with water, the smears were lightly stained with methylene blue solution for between two and five seconds, then washed with water, dried, covered with Diamox, mounted with a cover glass, and examined by light microscopy.

In the positive cases, each rickettsia particle showed a brown colour (**2**). The anti-rickettsial titre of serum and also the strain of the rickettsia were detected by this method.

TECHNICAL POINTS

It is very important to attempt to get thin rickettsia smears. Suto et al. obtained good thin smears by pipetting a very

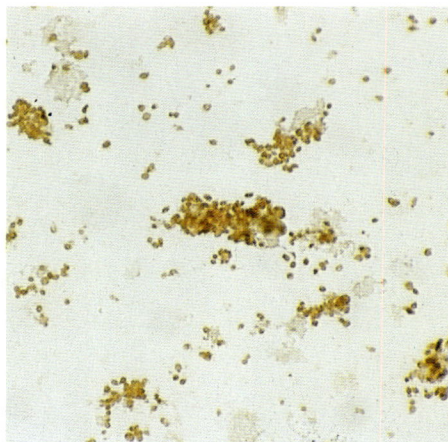

Fig. 2. A positive reaction for the indirect immunoperoxidase test. Each rickettsia particle shows brown colour. (Courtesy of Dr. T. Suto.) (× 400)

small amount of rickettsia suspension with a micropipette onto the glass slide and then drawing it up immediately.

The indirect immunoperoxidase test is more convenient than the indirect immunofluorescence test as the former does not require use of a fluorescence microscope, and the specimen can be stored a long time.

Abbreviations in the text:

PBS: Phosphate-buffered saline
FITC: Fluorescein isothiocyanate

Virus infections

5.1 Human papillomavirus infection

INTRODUCTION
Human papillomaviruses (HPVs) induce warts in skin and mucosa. Recently, the heterogeneity of HPVs was established by analysis of viral DNA using restriction enzyme analysis[547]. Warts can take on various types of clinical pictures, including common warts, plantar warts, digitate warts, flat warts and condyloma acuminatum. The HPV type is generally related to the clinical picture.

FINDINGS
Antisera raised against intact viral particles of a specific HPV are type specific, and will not react with other HPV types[548]. There is an anti-papillomavirus antibody (DAKO-B580, Dakopatts Co.), which is neither species specific nor type specific. This antibody is generated by immunizing rabbits with detergent-treated bovine papillomavirus Type 1, and is useful in the identification of cells that are infected with papillomaviruses. Using this antibody and cryostat sections the localization of the viral antigen can be determined by the indirect immunofluorescence method. The peroxidase-antiperoxidase (PAP) technique is more useful however, because paraffin-embedded sections can be employed.

Myrmecia warts contain many viral particles; the keratinocytes from above the basal layer are ordinarily filled with keratohyaline-like granules, and the nuclei contain virions (1). In common warts, the antigen is not often observed in the granular zone of verrucous lesions (2). In the case of common warts, when the epidermis is electron microscopically examined for viral particles, more than 90% of the cells do not present viral particles. When present, these particles are only in the stratum granulosum and stratum corneum. The amount of viral particles in wart tissues varies depending upon the clinical type. Myrmecia warts contain the most, with epidermodysplasia verruciformis, flat warts and condyloma acuminatum in decreasing order.

Antibody against wart-tissue antigen can be obtained by immunization of an animal with homogenized wart extract or semipurified wart virus antigen. In this case, antigen in the cytoplasm was also detected (3).

Recently, viral carcinogenesis of HPV has been reported. In these malignant tumour cells viral particles do not exist, only viral DNA exists. Anti-papillomavirus antigen is negative in malignant transformed cells, and only HPV DNA can be detected in cancer cells. With recent advances in the *in situ* hybridization techniques, viral genomes within the cells will be detectable[550].

TECHNICAL POINTS
To obtain tissue section adhesion, diluted 0.2% Poly-D-Lysine hydrobromide-(Sigma) dipped slides are recommended.

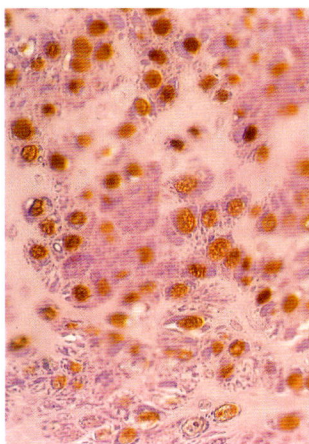

Fig. 1. Anti-papillomavirus antigen (DAKO B-580), PAP method in myrmecia wart.

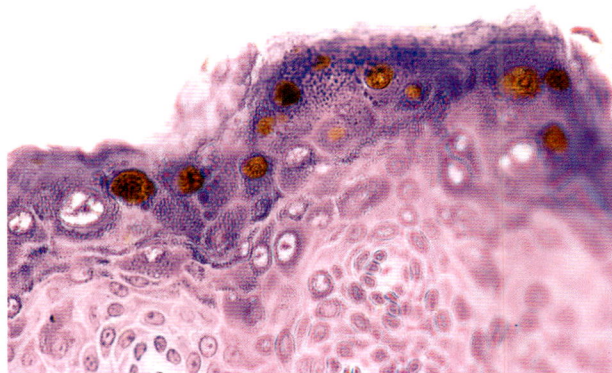

Fig. 2. Anti-papillomavirus antigen (DAKO B-580), PAP method in common wart.

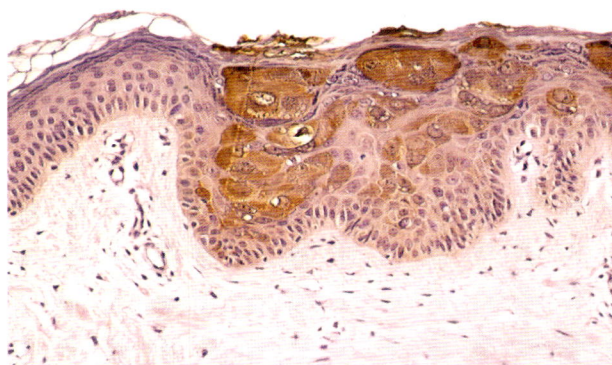

Fig. 3. Anti-wart-tissue antigen, PAP method in tinea versicolor-like lesion of epidermodysplasia verruciformis.

5.2 Herpesvirus infection

INTRODUCTION

Herpetoviridae has over forty viruses which show principally species-specific infection. Of these, six viruses such as type 1 and 2 herpes simplex (HSV), varicella-zoster (VZV), cytomegalo, Epstein-Barr and simian B, cause infection in man. In the field of dermatology, HSV and VSV infections are not unusual. HSV causes mild or serious diseases such as generalized infection in newborns, encephalitis, acute and recurrent herpes of oral lips, gingiva, genital organs, corneas and conjunctiva.

Recurrence is the result of reactivation of latent infection in the sensory ganglia after primary or secondary infection. Foci appear at the site of primary infection or in surrounding areas innervated by the same sensory nerve. The characteristic feature of HSV recurrence is that lesions are observed not only in immunocompromized patients with underlying diseases, but even in healthy people who have become fatigued or who are exposed to ultraviolet light. VZV also becomes latent in the sensory ganglia like HSV after varicella, and reactivation usually happens only once in healthy humans as in herpes zoster. Recurrence of VZV is seen only in immunocompromized patients. Rapid diagnosis and immediate treatment are essential as HSV can quickly be spread among healthy people, and there is no radical therapeutic method with the exception of some antiviral drugs.

FINDINGS AND DIAGNOSTIC SIGNIFICANCE

Immunofluorescence (IF) is an important method of rapid diagnosis for herpes viral infections. The method has been applied not only for vesicular content and dermal tissue, but also for the examination of internal organ lesions in connection with viruses[551]. HSV infections show various clinical symptoms, depending upon age or underlying diseases, so it is sometimes extremely difficult to establish a diagnosis of varicella- or zoster-like HAC lesions from the clinical signs alone. In these cases, IF is the most reliable and useful method for the detection of viral antigens and is the first choice for rapid diagnosis.

Usually smears from vesicular content or skin ulcers and mucosa are employed. Viral antigens are observed in the cytoplasm and nucleus, and sometimes correspond to the inclusion bodies of multinuclear giant or ballooned cells (1)[551]. Conventional Giemsa, Papanicolaou, haematoxylin and eosin staining do not clarify the differentiation of HSV or VZV. IF is the most useful method for definitive diagnosis, as the positive ratio of antigen detection in IF is much higher than in electron microscopy (negative staining) or virus isolation[551]. In addition, the histopathological findings of HSV and VZV muco-cutaneous tissue infections are too similar to differentiate by light microscopy.

Vesicular lesions are usually localized in the epidermis, and haemorrhages and intranuclear inclusion body-bearing endothelial cells are observed in the dermis or subcutaneous areas. In the epidermis, Cowdry's type A or full-type intranuclear inclusion bodies are frequently seen in the epithelial cells. The degenerated cells show ballooning and go into vesicles. Multinuclear giant cell formation, which occurs by fusion of infected cells, is also a common histological feature in HSV and VZV infection.

In mucosa, lesions appear by forming an ulcer, particularly on the tongue and genital organs. By immunofluorescence, the distribution of viral antigens of HSV is clear and relatively sharply demarcated. Specific fluorescence is detected in the nucleus, inclusion bodies and cytoplasm of infected epithelial cells (2)[551], giant cells, vascular endothelia, hair follicles, and sebaceous glands. In VZV lesions, in addition to the HSV findings, intranuclear inclusion bodies are revealed in the swollen fibroblasts of dermis or submucosa, and antigens are seen in these cells (3) and in the surrounding connective tissues (4)[551].

The use of anti-viral drugs sometimes makes it difficult to isolate the virus from lesions, but viral antigens are demonstrable in the foci, irrespective of treatment. For these reasons, antigen detection is recommended for all cases.

Viral antigens have been revealed in liver, lungs, adrenals, spleen, brain, pancreas, intestines, thymus, oesophagus, and kidneys in HSV infection. Further, VZV antigens and intranuclear inclusion bodies are observed in almost all organs including thyroid glands, thymus, lymph nodes, uterus, ovary, heart, and testes (5). It is not rare to find viral antigens in the vascular endothelia of dermis (6)[551]. In these cells, no deposition of immunoglobulin is shown, it seems, therefore, that vascular lesions in HSV or VZV are not caused by immune complex as in HB virus infection.

Erythema multiforme, clinically known as one of the allergic lesions (virusid) of HSV by detection of viral antigens[552], has been reported, but isolation of the agent has not yet been achieved.

TECHNICAL POINTS

Vesicular content and samples from the ulcer are smeared on spot slides (4 to 12 wells), fixed in acetone, and stored at −20 to −70°C until used. These antigens are stable for between two and three years.

In formalin-fixed materials (10% buffered formalin), viral antigens are easily detected by proteolytic enzyme treatment of 0.25% trypsin or 0.1% protease[553].

For direct and/or indirect IF methods, antibodies from the following four sources are used: (1) monoclonal antibody, (2) antibody from active virus infection, (3) hyperimmunized antibody from purified virus, and (4) human convalescent serum. The advantage of specific monoclonal antibodies to HSV or VZV is the differentiation of the type of the virus[554].

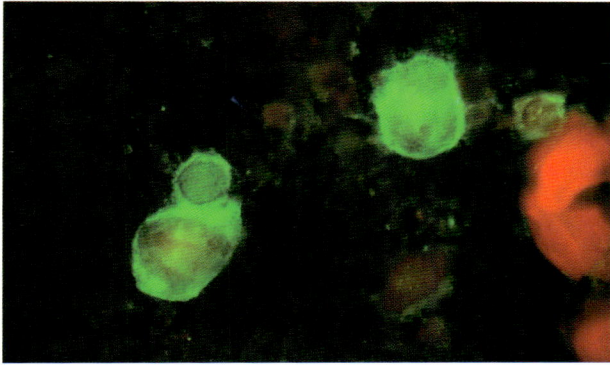

Fig. 1. Type 1 HSV: Viral antigens of smear from vaginal erosion (monoclonal antibody, acetone-fixed, indirect). (× 132)

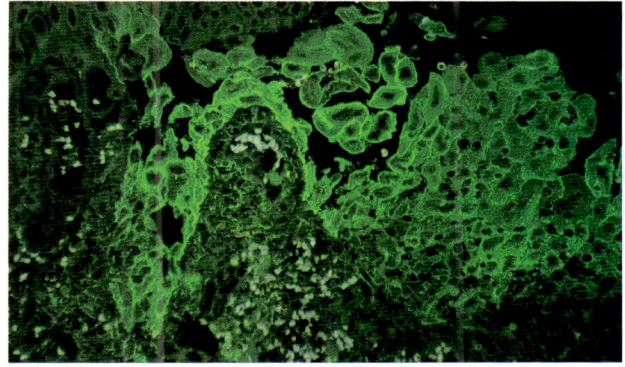

Fig. 2. Type 1 HSV: Viral antigens of oral herpes (rabbit antibody, formalin-fixed paraffin section, indirect). (× 66)

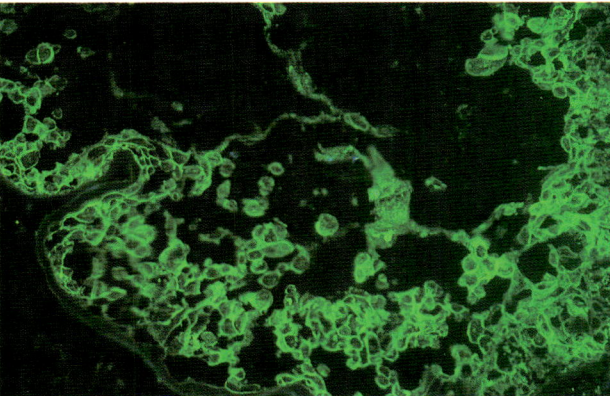

Fig. 3. VZV: Viral antigens found in the vesicle of epidermis (varicella) (human antibody, frozen section, direct). (× 66)

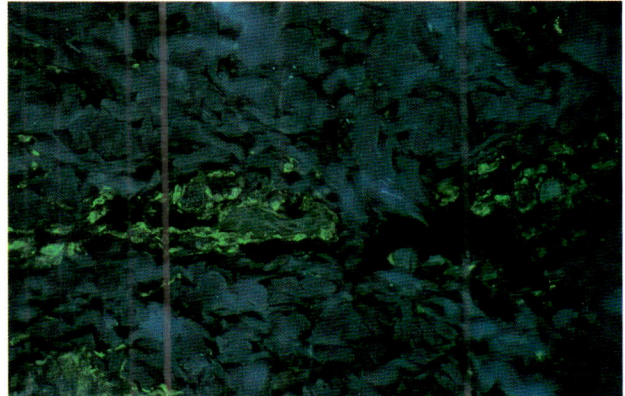

Fig. 4. VZV: Viral antigens in the connective tissue of dermis (monoclonal antibody, paraffin section, indirect). (× 66)

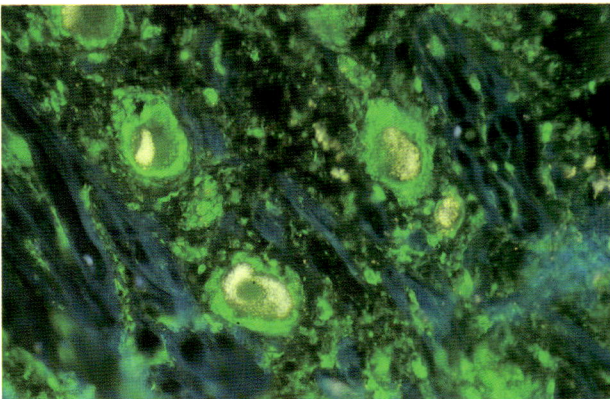

Fig. 5. VZV: Specific fluorescence in the neurons, satellite cells and neurofibres of spinal root ganglion (LTh7, zoster) (rabbit antibody, paraffin section, indirect). (× 132)

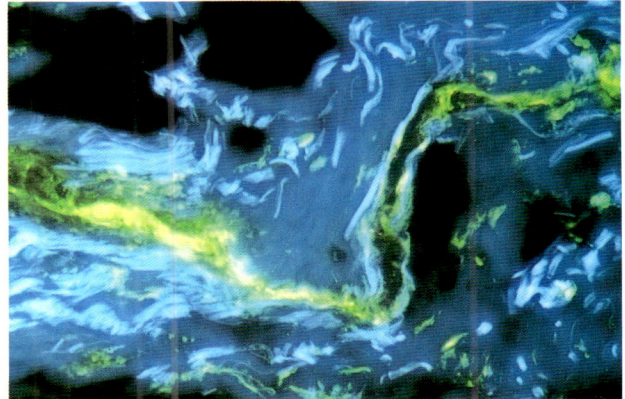

Fig. 6. VZV: Viral antigens in the dermal vascular wall of the purpuric vesicle (systemic varicella) (human antibody, frozen section, direct). (× 132)

Epithelial tumours

INTRODUCTION

Keratin intermediate filaments (keratin IFs) are one of the most important markers for diagnosis of epithelial tumours. They are also used in the studies on tumour differentiation and origin. Keratins are divided biochemically into two subgroups: acidic keratins and neutral-basic keratins. Additionally, keratins can be divided from the viewpoint of differentiation; $65-70 \times 10^3$ and 56.5×10^3 keratins are markers for keratinization, 48×10^3 and 56×10^3 are markers for proliferation, and 50×10^3 and 58×10^3 are markers for epidermal cells[555]. Monoclonal antibodies which react to each of these groups of keratins are now employed for pathological studies of tumours. Polyclonal keratins against total keratins can be used for the differentiation of epithelial cells and non-epithelial cells. Recently, many types of monoclonal antibodies against various keratins have been developed and utilized for the diagnosis of epithelial tumours[556-63]. Among these, monoclonal anti-keratin antibodies specific for sweat gland cells are included[559].

IMPORTANT FINDINGS

Normal epidermis. Polyclonal anti-keratin antibodies react with whole epidermis (**1a**). However, anti-keratin antibodies against marker keratins for keratinization bind to suprabasal cells (**1b**). No anti-keratin antibodies react with cells in the dermis[555], except for pilar apparatus and sweat glands.

Epithelial tumours. Antibodies against $65-70 \times 10^3$ keratins, markers for keratinization, react with tumour cells of seborrhoeic keratosis, keratoacanthoma, calcifying epithelioma, keratosis senilis, Bowen's disease and squamous cell carcinoma. However, the malignant cases of these tumours reveal a distinctive staining profile. They show focally positive cells with $65-70 \times 10^3$ keratins in an irregular arrangement. Figure 2 illustrates a case of squamous cell carcinoma, which contains both positive and negative cells for $65-70 \times 10^3$ keratins. Benign tumours have been shown to react with $65-70 \times 10^3$ keratins in the keratinized portions, but not in the basal layer.

Mouse monoclonal keratin antibody AE_1[564], reacts with 50×10 and 56.5×10^3 keratins and recognizes basal cell carcinoma, while the keratinization-marker antibody does not react with these. It is of interest that normal epidermal keratinocytes close to basal cell carcinoma cells turn to positive for their monoclonal antibody in the suprabasal layer[563]. In the so-called mixed tumour of the skin, individual tumour cells embedded in the mucous matrix are positive for keratinization marker and anti-total keratin antibodies, indicating that these free tumour cells are epithelial cells (**3**)[557]. The skin lesions of extramammary Paget's disease often consist of tumour cells scattered throughout the epidermis. These tumour cells are negative for $65-70 \times 10^3$ keratins and total epidermal keratins; when stained with these anti-keratin antibodies these cells appeared as black unstained cells in bright positive epidermis (**4**). However, Paget's cells are stained with anti-keratin antibodies against 40×10^3, 45×10^3, 52.5×10^3 and 54×10^3 keratins[556], which do not react with the normal epidermal cells surrounding the Paget's cells.

DIAGNOSTIC SIGNIFICANCE

Antibodies against $65-70 \times 10^3$ keratins react with tumour cells derived from epidermal cells but not with adenocarcinomas, and thus they are used for differential diagnosis of squamous cell carcinoma and adenocarcinomas. In this respect, monoclonal antibodies which react with 40×10^3, 45×10^3, 52.5×10^3 and 54×10^3 keratins, stain adenocarcinomas but not squamous cell carcinomas[556, 564]. These antibodies are useful tools for the determination of carcinoma cells scattered in mesenchymal tissues. Some of these polyclonal and monoclonal anti-keratin antibodies are now commercially available. In addition to the advantage of differential diagnosis of squamous cell carcinoma, adenocarcinoma and non-epithelial tumour cells, these antibodies can be used for the identification of epithelial cells in culture systems[565]. However, none of these differentiate malignant cells from benign cells.

TECHNICAL POINTS

Although formalin-fixed, paraffin-embedded tissue can be used, it is much better to use biopsy specimens embedded in OCT and snap-frozen in isopentane or n-hexane and cooled with liquid nitrogen after washing with phosphate-buffered saline. Formalin-fixed, paraffin-embedded tissue sections often produce false-negative results and reduce the reactivity. Digestion of the surface of the sections with trypsin (0.25%) for between five and thirty minutes may increase the reactivity to antibodies. A brief 8M urea treatment may also unmask the antigen and recover antibody reactivity. In negative reaction cases, the possibility of a false-negative should be taken into consideration.

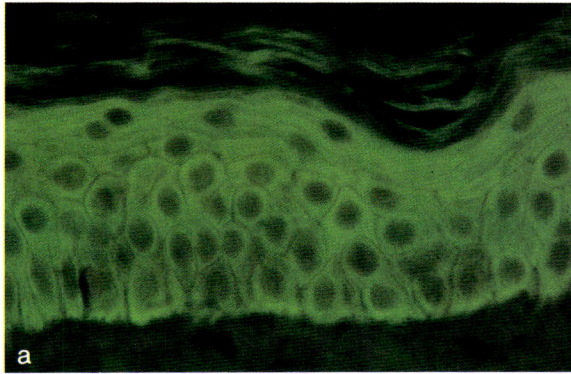

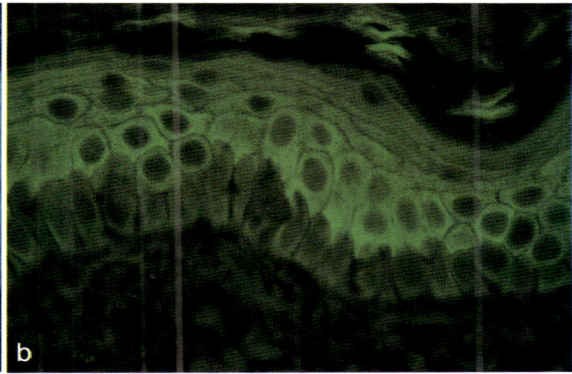

Fig. 1. a: Normal human epidermis stained with rabbit antibody against total epidermal keratins. (× 400)

b: Normal human epidermis stained with rabbit antibody against 67×10^3 keratins. (× 400)

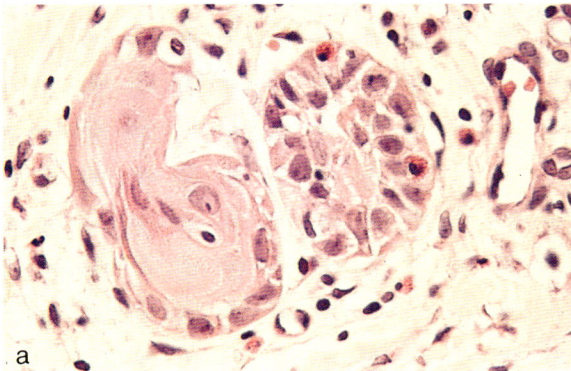

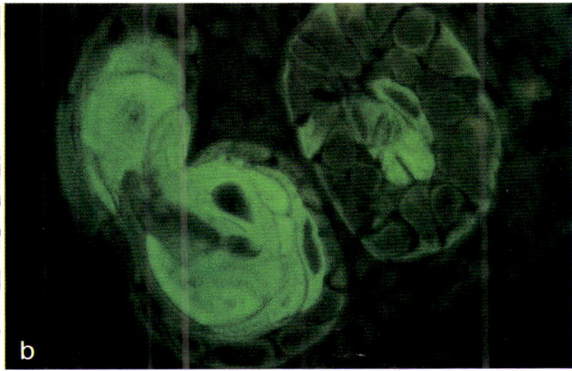

Fig. 2. a: Squamous cell carcinoma stained with haematoxylin and eosin. (× 400)

b: The same section stained with 67×10^3 keratins. (× 400)

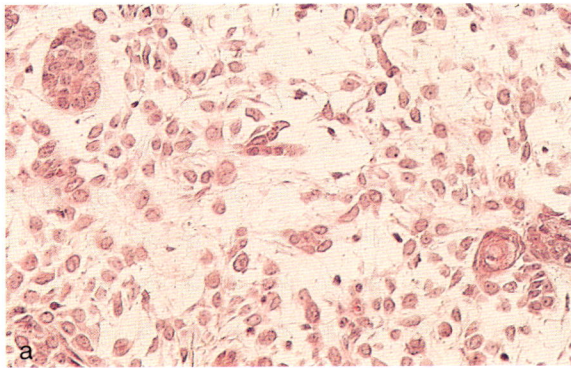

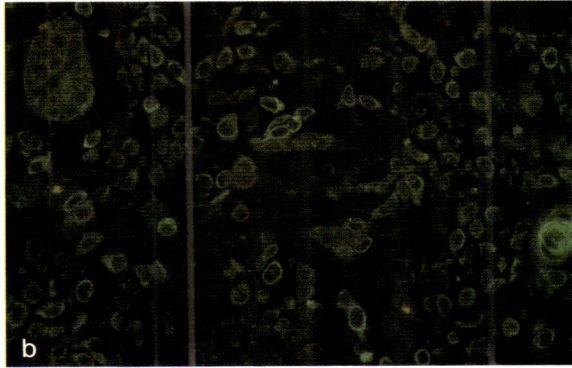

Fig. 3. a: Mixed tumour of the skin stained with haematoxylin and eosin. (× 400)

b: The same section stained with rabbit antibody against total epidermal keratins. Individual cells scattered throughout the matrix are stained with the antibody to show epithelial cells. (× 400)

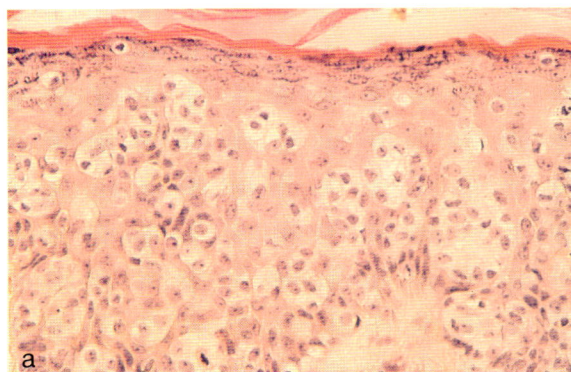

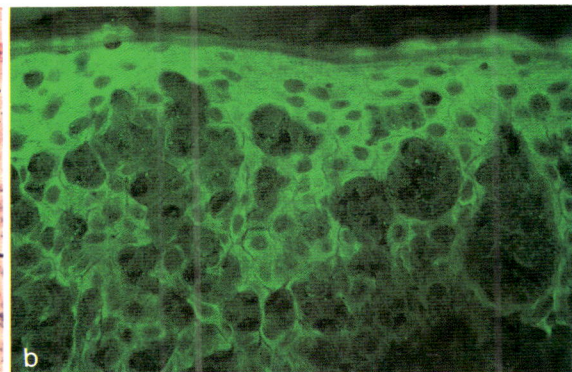

Fig. 4. a: Extramammary Paget's disease stained with haematoxylin and eosin. (× 400)

b: The same section stained with rabbit antibody against total epidermal keratins. This antibody does not react with Paget's cells but does react with normal keratinocytes. (× 400)

Paget's disease

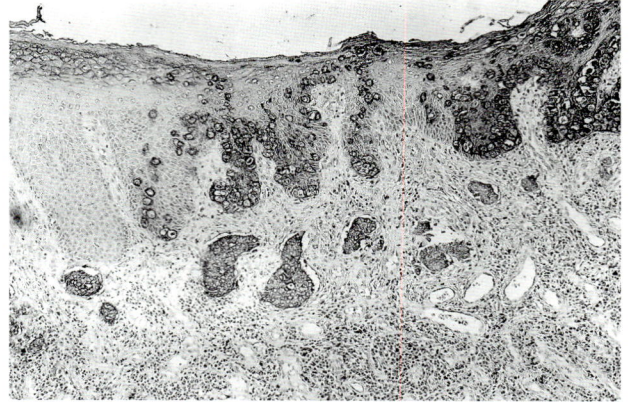

Fig. 1. Extramammary (genital) Paget's disease.
CEA was stained with PAP method. Tumour nests in the dermal invasion were also positive for CEA.

INTRODUCTION

Paget's disease is generally classified into two categories, mammary Paget's disease and extramammary Paget's disease[566]. The former was first reported by James Paget in 1874[567], and the latter by Crocker in 1889[568]. Although the nature and histogenesis of Paget cells are still controversial[566, 569-71], the recent progress in immunohistological methods may bring new clues to these particular points.

IMMUNOHISTOLOGIC FINDINGS

The detection of carcinoembryonic antigen (CEA) in Paget's disease. In 1981, Penneys et al. demonstrated the localization of CEA in normal sweat glands using a PAP method with anti-CEA antibody[572]. Subsequently, CEA was found in benign[573] and malignant sweat gland tumours[574]. Furthermore, it was suggested that Paget cells were of sweat gland origin since CEA was also positive in Paget cells but not in keratinocytes[575]. In our nine cases of extramammary Paget's disease, including three lymphnode metastasis, CEA was detected (1)[576]. The increased serum value of CEA in the patient with widespread metastasized Paget's disease suggested that the serum CEA level might serve as one of the tumour markers for Paget's disease[577].

Lectin binding sites in Paget's disease and double stain with CEA. It is well known that Paget cells contain a large amount of muco-polysaccharides using conventional histochemical stains (2)[566]. Lectins are proteins which specifically bind to various oligosaccharide residues[578]. We examined the lectin binding sites of normal sweat glands[579], mammary gland[579], sweat gland tumours[580, 81] and Paget's disease[579].

In contrast to the membrane staining pattern of eccrine glands, eccrine gland tumours and mammary glands, a cytoplasmic staining pattern was noted in apocrine glands and cells of Paget's disease, indicating apocrine differentiation of Paget cells[579].

Since CEA is a glycoprotein which possesses a considerable amount of oligosaccharides[582], double staining of lectin binding sites and CEA was performed. The double staining showed that (1) wheat germ agglutinin (WGA) binding sites always coincided with the location of CEA, (2) peanut agglutinin (PNA) binding sites seldom covered CEA-positive sites, and (3) Paget cells generally lacked PNA binding sites on cell membranes. Ogusa reported that dolichos biflorus agglutinin (DBA) was highly specific for the oligosaccharide residues of Paget cells.

The ongoing immunohistologic studies on sweat gland tumours and Paget's disease not only provide new insights into the nature and differentiation process of constitutive neoplastic cells, but may also serve to modify the conventional morphological classification of these tumours.

TECHNICAL POINTS

The above-mentioned immunohistologic method can be performed using paraffin sections. It is important to dilute the first antibody sufficiently, as is necessary in other PAP methods.

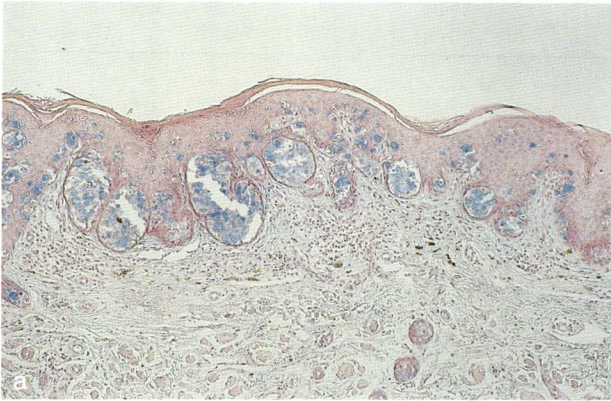

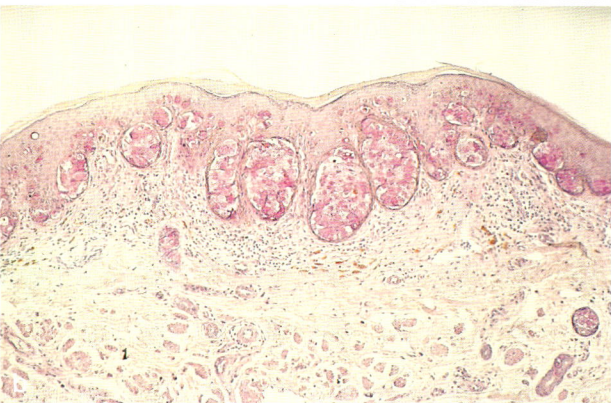

Fig. 2a. Alcian – blue stain.
Fig. 2b. PAS stain.
The deposition of muco-polysaccharides noted in the Paget cell cytoplasm.

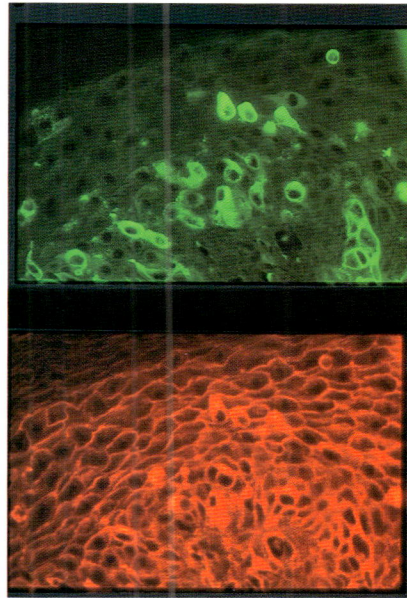

Fig. 3. Double stain of CEA (fluoroscein, green) and WGA binding sites (rhodamine, red).
WGA delineates the intercellular spaces of normal keratinocytes and cell membrane and cytoplasm of Paget cells. CEA-positive area is completely covered by WGA binding sites.

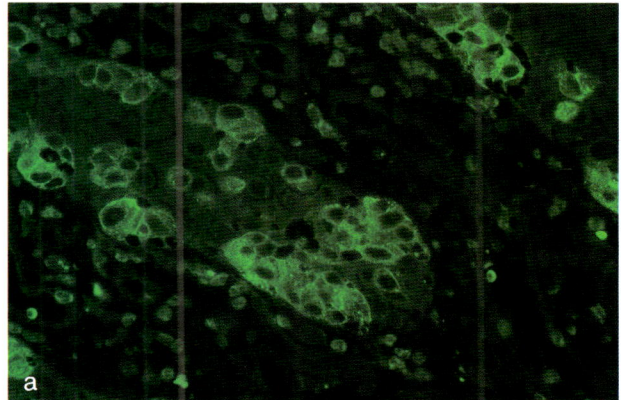

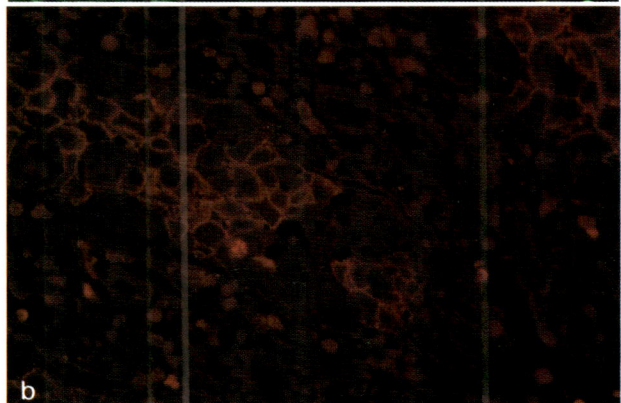

Fig. 4. Double stain of CEA (a: fluoroscein, green) and PNA binding sites (b: rhodamine, red).
PNA binding sites noted in the intercellular space of normal keratinocytes, but not on the Paget cell membrane.

Malignant melanoma

INTRODUCTION

S-100 protein[583] and neuron-specific enolase (NSE)[584] are markers for malignant melanoma for which antisera have been developed and utilized for the immunohistological diagnosis of melanoma. S-100 protein, of a family of acidic proteins with a molecular weight of 20K daltons, is composed of alpha and beta chains in three different combinations classified as S-100aO (alpha-chain, alpha-chain), S-100a (alpha-chain, beta-chain) and S-100b (beta-chain, beta-chain). Formerly S-100 protein was detected only in nervous tissues but recently it has been demonstrated in various cells of non-nervous tissues such as melanocytes, Langerhans cells, myoepithelial cells and fat cells and their related tumours. NSE is also an acidic protein with a molecular weight of 90K daltons and is termed gamma-enolase. S-100 protein acts as a hydrolase of the glycolytic pathway. NSE is demonstrated in neurons, para-neurons, neuroendocrine tumours and melanoma.

In 1978, Koprowski et al.[585] first reported the development of monoclonal antibodies against melanoma, since then many monoclonal antibodies to melanoma have been developed, some of which are now commercially available.

However, there are few monoclonal antibodies that react only with melanoma; most react with other tumours of neuroectodermal or epidermal origin and moreover these monoclonal antibodies react with some normal and foetal tissues. Therefore these antibodies define melanoma-associated antigens in that they recognize antigens expressed in melanoma cells but not in mature melanocytes. The antigens recognized by these antibodies are primarily glycoproteins present on the melanoma cell surface with molecular weight ranging from 28K to 550K daltons. Monoclonal antibodies have also been reported to recognize cytoplastic and glycolipid antigens whose expression is correlated with the malignant transformation of melanocytes. Moreover, melanoma cells express class I and class II histocompatibility antigens[586,587], and vimentin[588], one of the intermediate filaments

FINDINGS

S100 protein and NSE. S100 protein is present in the cytoplasm and nucleus of melanoma cells. Both primary and metastatic melanoma are highly positive for S100 (**1–3**). Primary lesions typically stain heterogeneously, while metastatic lesions stain more consistently. The intensity of the staining depends upon the amount of melanin, rather than the morphology of melanoma cells.

NSE is present in the cytoplasm of melanoma cells and also in pigmented nevi, Merkel cell tumours and normal melanocytes.

Monoclonal antibodies. Anti-human melanoma monoclonal antibody (225.28S)[589,590] reacts with a majority of melanomas, both primary and metastatic lesions such as amelanotic melanoma and atypical melanocytes of lentigo maligna (Table I). Specific staining for this monoclonal antibody is observed exclusively on the plasma membrane of the melanoma cells (**4**). The intensity of staining is heterogeneous depending on area but there seems to be no correlation between the clinical stage, the amount of melanin or cell morphology. This monoclonal antibody also shows cross-reactivity with pigmented nevi, basal cell carcinoma (**5**) and squamous cell carcinoma but the staining pattern is homogeneous compared to that of melanoma. Blue nevi, normal melanocytes and melanophages are negative for this antibody.

HLA-heavy chain and beta2-microglobulin[586] are expressed on the melanoma cell membrane. In particular, HLA-DR antigens[587] are expressed on the advancing portion of melanoma nest. On the other hand, expression of HLA-heavy chain and beta2-microglobulin is less on pigmented nevi and HLA-DR are completely negative.

Vimentin[588] is present in the cytoplasm of melanoma and pigmented nevi cells.

DERMATOLOGICAL SIGNIFICANCE

S-100 protein is known as a member of the group of calcium binding protein, but its exact function is still obscure. However, S-100 protein is very useful for immunohistological diagnosis of melanotic tumours due to its high reactivity to melanotic tumours.

Since most melanoma monoclonal antibodies show cross-reactivity to other tumours, particularly pigmented nevi, the

REACTIVITY OF ANTI-HUMAN MELANOMA MONOCLONAL ANTIBODY (225.28S) WITH MELANOMA, NEVI AND OTHER TISSUES

tissue	number of positive cases	total number of cases
malignant melanoma		
primary melanoma	6	8
metastatic melanoma	13	15
malignant blue nevus	1	1
pigmented nevi		
junctional nevi	2	2
compound nevi	1	3
intradermal nevi	6	20
blue nevi		
common blue nevi	0	6
cellular blue nevi	0	2
malignant tissues		
BCE	5	12
SCC	2	8
ML	0	3
tumors of nervous system		
meningioma	0	6
glioma	0	1
schwannoma	1	1
ependymoma	0	1
glioblastoma	0	3
fetal tissues		
skin (9–16 weeks)	8	10
brain (9–16 weeks)	0	5

No. of positive cases/ No. of total cases

immunohistological diagnosis of melanoma may be more effective by using several monoclonal antibodies. Recently, however, there has been a report of a monoclonal antibody which reacts only with melanoma and dysplastic nevus, and does not react with nevi[591]. This type of antibody would be very useful for clinical applications.

HLA-DR antigens are expressed on melanoma cells and not expressed on normal melanocytes or pigmented nevi, therefore expression of HLA-DR antigens on a melanocyte lineage might be a useful diagnostic marker for malignancy. But the significance of HLA-DR antigen expression is still unknown.

TECHNICAL POINTS

S-100 protein and NSE can be stained on formalin-fixed or paraffin-embedded sections. Unfortunately, most monoclonal antibodies do not react with formalin-fixed or paraffin-embedded sections. Thus, immunodiagnosis with monoclonal antibodies is limited to frozen tissue sections.

To reduce non-specific background staining in the indirect immunofluorescence assay, an FITC-labelled second antibody directed specifically to the subclass of the first antibody, such as FITC-labelled IgG_1 or FITC-labelled IgG_{2a}, is recommended.

In the avidin-biotin-peroxidase complex staining method, it is difficult to distinguish the peroxidase product from melanin granules. This can be overcome by lightly counterstaining with diluted Giemsa solution which causes a metachromatic colour change in the melanin granules, making the melanin granules and peroxidase product easily distinguishable (**1**).

Alkaline phosphatase[592] can be substituted for peroxidase to give a dark blue or dark red product which is clearly distinguishable from melanin granules (**2, 3**).

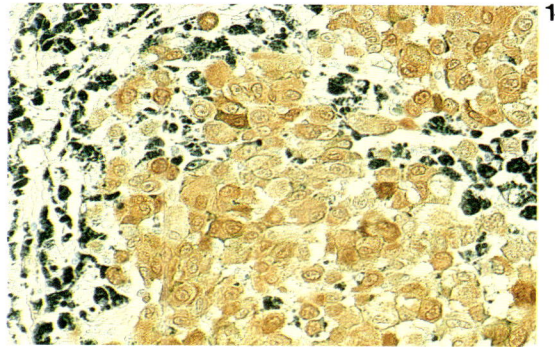

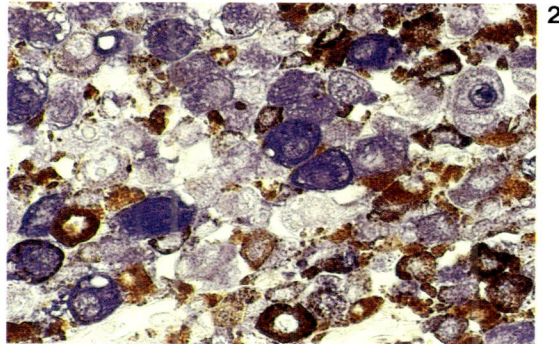

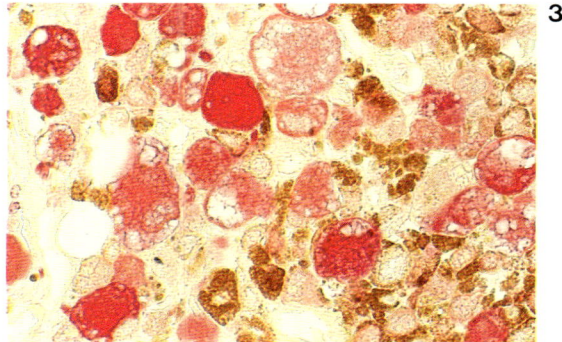

Fig. 1. Staining of melanoma for S100 protein by avidin-biotin-peroxidase method. Counter-stained with diluted Giemsa solution. Positive reaction is seen in the cytoplasm of melanoma cells. Melanin granules appear dark green. ($\times$ 200)

Fig. 2. Staining of melanoma for S-100 protein by avidin-biotin-alkaline phosphatase method. The enzyme label was reacted with naphthol AS-MX plus last Blue BB salt substrate which gives dark blue products, providing good contrast with the melanin granules. ($\times$ 400)

Fig. 3. Staining of melanoma for S-100 protein by avidin-biotin-alkaline phosphatase method. The enzyme label was reacted with naphthol AS-MX plus Fast Red Violet LB salt, thus giving dark red products. ($\times$ 400)

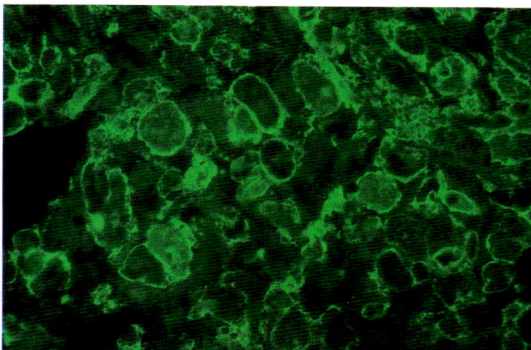

Fig. 4. Indirect immunofluorescence staining of primary melanoma using anti-human melanoma monoclonal antibody (225.28S). The heterogeneous staining pattern appears to be restricted to the melanoma cell plasma membrane. ($\times$ 200)

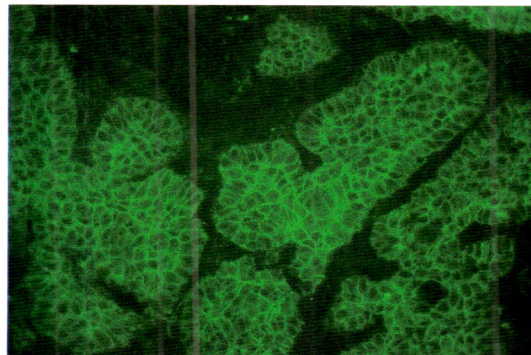

Fig. 5. Indirect immunofluorescence staining of basal cell carcinoma using anti-human melanoma monoclonal antibody (225.28S). The homogeneous staining pattern is specific for the tumour cell membrane. ($\times$ 200)

Nevus cell nevus

INTRODUCTION
There is no specific marker for pigmented nevi. But most markers for melanoma react with pigmented nevi, because pigmented nevi, like melanoma, originate from the neural crest. S-100 protein[593] and anti-human melanoma monoclonal antibody are described below.

FINDINGS
S-100 protein. S-100 protein is present in the cytoplasm of various types of pigmented nevus cells, with the exception of blue nevus cells[593]. In pigmented nevi, the degree of staining for intradermal components is stronger than that for junctional components (**1**).

Monoclonal antibodies. Anti-human melanoma antibody (225.28S)[594, 595], which recognizes cell surface glycoproteins with a molecular weight of 280K and 550K daltons, cross-reacts with pigmented nevus cells (**2**). The staining pattern is homogeneous. But this monoclonal antibody does not react with normal melanocytes or blue nevus.

HLA-heavy chain and beta$_2$-microglobulin[596] are weakly expressed on pigmented nevus cells but HLA-DR antigens are completely negative. In dysplastic nevus, HLA-heavy chain and beta$_2$-microglobulin are strongly expressed; however HLA-DR antigens are still negative.

DERMATOLOGICAL SIGNIFICANCE
Clinically, it is most important to distinguish melanoma from pigmented nevi, but the immunohistological diagnosis is difficult. The expression of HLA-DR antigens of a melanocytic lineage might be a useful marker for malignancy.

TECHNICAL POINTS
S100 protein can be stained on formalin-fixed and paraffin-embedded sections. Most monoclonal antibodies are limited to frozen-tissue sections.

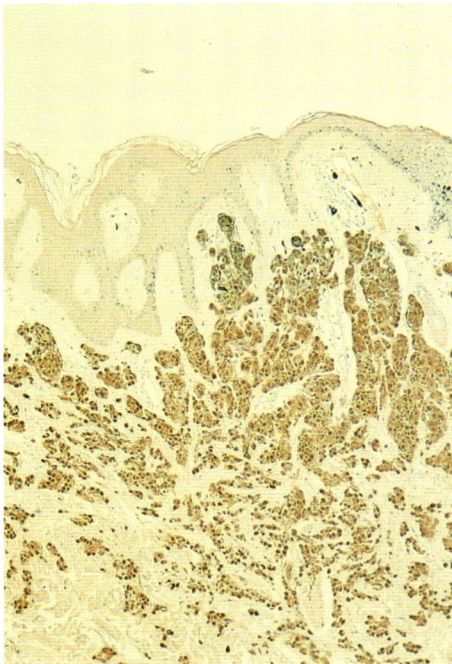

Fig. 1. Staining of pigmented nevus for S-100 protein by avidin-biotin-peroxidase complex method. Positive reactions are seen in the cytoplasm of nevus cells. ($\times$ 200)

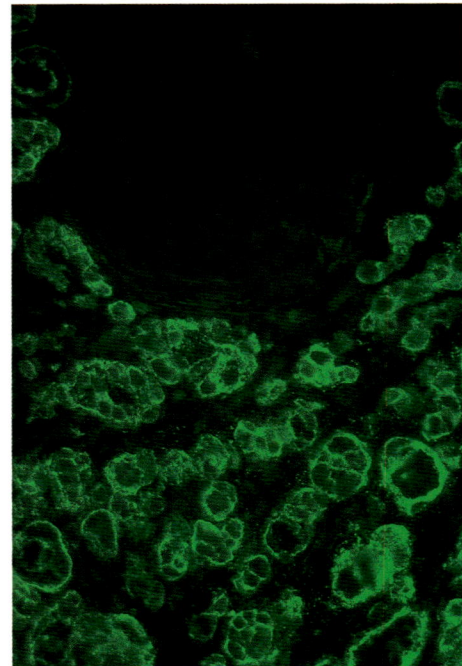

Fig. 2. Indirect immunofluorescence staining of pigmented nevus using anti-human melanoma monoclonal antibody (225.28S). The homogeneous staining pattern appears to be restricted to the nevus cell plasma membrane. ($\times$ 200)

Kimura's disease

CLINICAL ENTITY

Kimura's disease is characterized by unusual chronic granuloma accompanied by proliferation of lymphoid tissue and marked eosinophil infiltration[597]. Since it was first described by Kimura in 1948, over 350 cases have been reported in Japan. More males than females suffer from this disease, particularly those between the ages of 16 and 45 years. The lesion location is usually the face, neck, axilla, groin or elbow. These lesions may be single or multiple, dermal or subcutaneous, elastic soft or elastic hard in stiffness, and may range in size extending to the palm. Laboratory findings are marked peripheral blood eosinophilia and hyperimmunoglobulinaemia E. Immediate-type hypersensitivity reaction against *Candida albicans* is often strongly positive in the intracutaneous test, while the delayed-type hypersensitivity finding is proliferation of lymphfolliculoid structures of various sizes in dermis and subcutaneous tissues and nonspecific granulation tissue consisting mainly of eosinophils, and a varying number of plasma cells, lymphocytes and mast cells in the peripheral area and fibrosis of vessels among lymphfolliculoid structures (**1**).

IMMUNOFLUORESCENT FINDINGS

IgM, IgG and IgE can be detected in the germinal centre of the lymphfolliculoid structure by using the direct immunofluorescent technique[598]. In the present case, IgE was also detected in the germinal centre by using anti-sheep human IgE antibody purchased from Cappel Lab. Oc., (F/P ratio 2.69)[600, 601] (**2**). The deposition of IgE which was seen in the germinal centre of the lymphfolliculoid structure, was detected on the cell membrane and intracell by immunoelectron microscopical techniques[601]. But to confirm that the cells of the germinal centre produced IgE was impossible, as fixation was not complete and the micro-organelle, particularly the rough endoplasmic reticulum, was obscure in this case. We examined the lymphocyte subpopulation of the lymphfolliculoid structure by using anti-HLA-DR and Leu-4 antibody (Becton-Dickinson company). It appears that the B cells are mainly in the germinal centres of the lymphfolliculoid structure, while the T cells are mainly in the margin of the germinal centre. These findings were identical to the previously reported structure of the lymph node[601].

PATHOGENESIS

This disease was thought to be not a tumour but a reaction disease, but at present the aetiology is not fully understood. The immunological findings of this disease are summarized as follows: (1) IgE deposition is observable in the germinal centre[598, 599]. (2) IgE deposition is observable on the cell membrane and intracellularly in the germinal centres by the immunoelectron microscopic technique[601]. (3) The lymph cell subpopulation of the lymphfolliculoid structure is almost identical to that of lymph nodes[601]. (4) The level of serum IgE decreases according to the decrease in tumour size by irradiation. (5) A high level of IgE was detected in the lymph cell culture medium obtained from the lymph node[599]. (6) The sera from patients with this disease selectively enhances *in vitro* IgE plaque-forming cells' response more effectively than that from normal subjects[602]. (7) Immediate skin reaction to *Candida* allergen extract is positive[598, 599]. (8) 80% of serum IgE is absorbed by using the adsorption test of *Candida* mannan. But only 11% of serum IgE is adsorbed by Candida binding paper disc adsorption test[599].

As mentioned above, the IgE antibody against the soluble antigenic substance of *Candida albicans* or other antigens is produced in the germinal centres of the lymphfolliculoid structure and causes degradation of mast cells. The granules of mast cells are said to contain an eosinophilic chemotactic factor for anaphylaxis, and a relationship to infiltration of eosinophils has been suggested. There have been many objections to the relation to type 1 allergy. This hypothesis does not explain all of the mechanisms.

TECHNICAL POINTS

A tumour which contains lymphfolliculoid structure should be used as a specimen. The method is the same as that for a routine immunofluorescent technique. The autofluorescence of eosinophils must be noted.

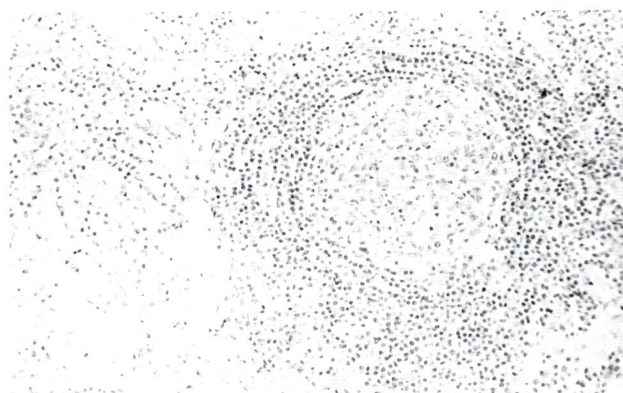

Fig. 1. Histological finding of lymphfolliculoid structure in the present case. ($\times$ 250)

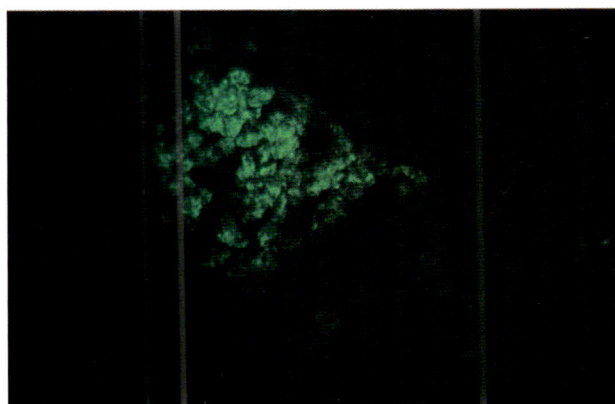

Fig. 2. IgE deposition in the lymphfolliculoid structure germinal centre in the present case. ($\times$ 250)

Lymphoma

INTRODUCTION

Currently, malignant lymphoma (ML) is investigated through the techniques of enzyme histochemistry, immunohisto-chemistry, and monoclonal antibodies. By these methods, it has been proved that tumour cells have some surface markers similar to those of normal lymphocytes that show various types of differentiation. Malignant lymphoma (cutaneous malignant lymphoma: C-ML) is mainly described here. The relationship between these types of lymphoma[603–5] and immunohistological features is being researched.

IMPORTANT FINDINGS

Most types of C-MLs are malignant proliferations of peripheral $T(T_2)$ lymphocytes. It has been shown in Western countries that more than half of MLs are B-cell malignant lymphomas (B-ML). Whereas in most patients in Japan, particularly those born in the southern prefectures of Kyushu, most MLs are shown to be T-ML in nature. Here in Kagoshima, we have observed 37 C-ML patients, and of these, 17 had mycosis fungoides (MF); 10 were adult T cell leukaemia (ATL); and 8 of the remaining 10 showed T cell leukaemia patterns. However 2 of the 37 patients were shown to have B-cell patterns. By using monoclonal antibodies that recognize the differentiated antigens of lymphocytes, subsets of tumour cells are easily identified. We can divide peripheral T-ML into 2 main groups. One group is the helper/inducer T cell type ($T_{H/I}$; ATL, MF Sézary syndrome) and the other is the suppressor/cytotoxic T cell type ($T_{S/C}$; IBL-like lymphoma, T zone lymphoma, Lennert lymphoma). Other T_2 lymphomas also show $T_{H/I}$ or $T_{S/C}$ patterns, but the relationship between the clinical and pathological features should be examined hereafter. It should be mentioned that of the $T_{H/I}$ and $T_{S/C}$ groups, $T_{H/I}$ is the most common. To date, we have not experienced any cases of transformation from $T_{H/I}$ to $T_{S/C}$ or vice versa; therefore, it is necessary to reorganize the study of ML immunological research. Both MF and ATL show $T_{H/I}$ cell surface markers. Tumour cells of MF show helper functions and those of ATL show suppressor functions and have $T_{S/C}$ antigen.

In the immunohistological diagnosis of C-ML, like MFD, it is necessary to study surface markers of proliferative tumour cells. However, cell markers of tumour cells sometimes disappear, and we occasionally find $T_{S/C}$ lymphocytes, histiocytes, eosinophils, and plasma cells in the $T_{H/I}$ pro-liferating lesion. In recent reports it has been noted that the helper/suppressor ratio is helpful for the diagnosis and understanding of the prognosis of C-ML such as MF, and this is suggested as very useful for the analysis of inflammatory stage to tumour stage alterations. But, some recent reports have mentioned that in early stages of cutaneous T cell lymphoma (CTCL), such analysis is not so useful[606]. The existence and proliferation of Langerhans cells (LC) in skin tissue and lymph node biopsy specimens is considered to be a casual relation to the pathogenesis of ML[607] (5); and it is thought LC may be co-operating with $T_{H/I}$ cells in C-ML. The characterization of human lymphoid neoplastic cells using cell surface markers of T and B cells will give us a better understanding of the origin and nature of neoplastic cells and deeper insight into the concept, classification, prognosis and even the pathogenesis of ML[608].

BIOPSY PROCEDURE

For the skin biopsy of C-ML, an excision biopsy is preferable to the punch biopsy. In immunological research there are two biopsy methods, one using a tumour cell suspension and the other using a tissue specimen. The former method is used for studying T and B cell surface markers (E Rosettes (1), EAC Rosettes, surface immunoglobulins), and for determining chromosomes and for functions of the subsets of tumour cells (2) by using monoclonal antibodies. The latter is useful for making stump specimens, freeze sections, PLP-fixed specimens, and for examining surface markers by monoclonal antibodies (OKT, Leu, B series) by means of fluorescein, PAP, ABC staining methods and immunoelectron microscopy (3, 4, 6). The technique of free suspension preparation from the skin tissues is very complicated. Additionally, cell suspensions include tumour cells and inflammatory cells, thus tissue specimens are recommended.

TECHNICAL POINTS

For classifying lymphoid neoplastic diseases based on cell surface marker analysis, it is necessary to use several kinds of antibodies, due to cross-reactions.

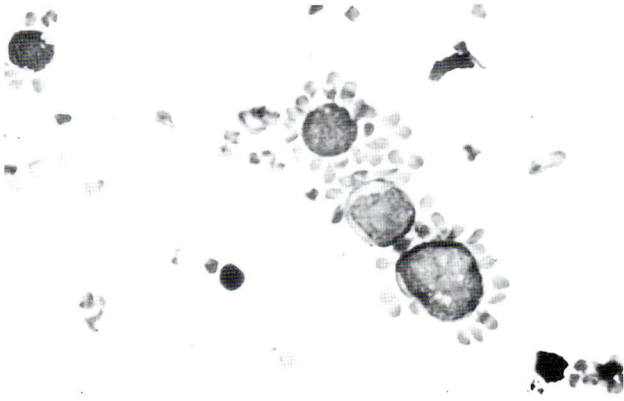

Fig. 1. Tumour cells in MF
E Rossette formation, positive lymphocyte (T cell) in cell
suspension method. (× 400)

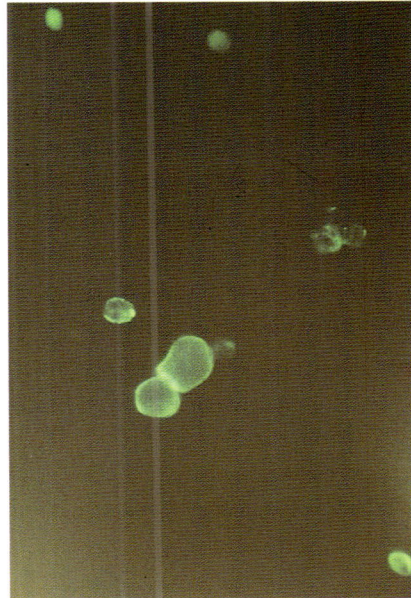

Fig. 2. Cutaneous B-cell lymphoma
B lymphocytes in tumour cell suspensions show fluorescent IgG-
Fc-receptor by the immunofluorescent direct method.

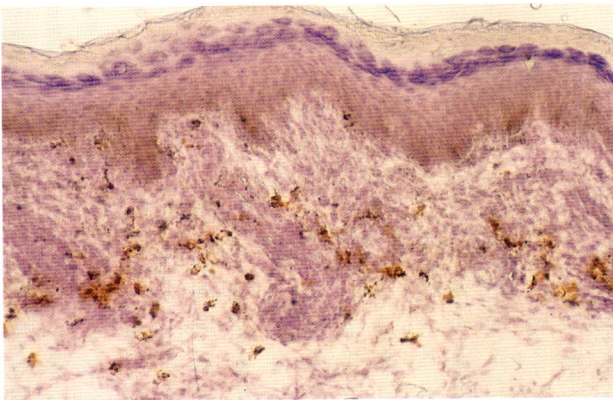

Fig. 3. Leu-2a antigen-positive cells in MF lesion. (PAP
method: × 400)

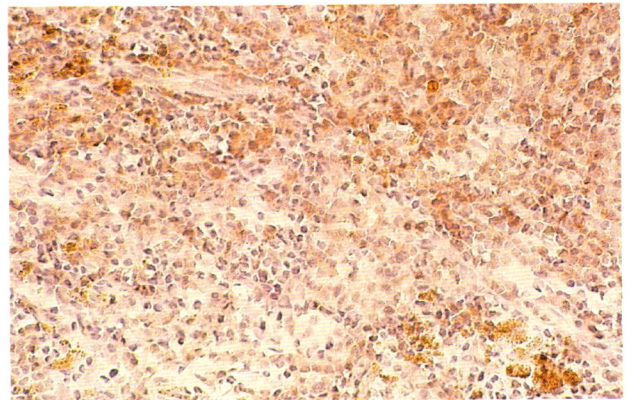

Fig. 4. Leu-4 antigen-positive cells in MF lesion. (PAP method:
× 100)

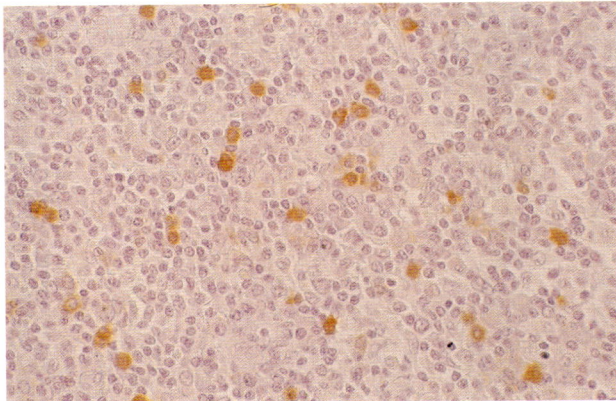

Fig. 5. S-100 protein antigen-positive cells in MF lesion. (PAP
method: × 100)

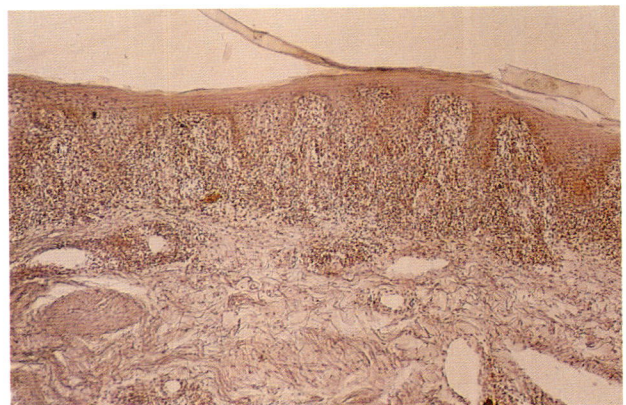

Fig. 6. Pautrier's microabscess at the epidermis and Leu-3a
antigen-positive cells at the upper dermis in MF. (PAP method:
× 100)

Histiocytosis-X

INTRODUCTION
Histiocytosis-X (HX)[609] is an unusual disorder which refers to the histiocytosis syndrome that includes Letterer-Siwe disease, Hand-Schüller-Christian disease, and eosinophilic granuloma. The histopathological features are characterized by the proliferation of distinctive histiocytic cells. These histiocytic cells are generally considered to be abnormal Langerhans cells (LC).

FINDINGS
Light microscopically, HX cells appear as large, (15–25 μm diameter) ovoid cells with pink, granular cytoplasm. The nucleus is often folded and lobulated, and has an irregular granular chromatin pattern.

Electron microscopically, HX cells have Langerhans granules (Birbeck granules) similar to those of LC in the cytoplasm.

Immunohistochemical profiles of the HX cell, LC, and macrophage are shown in Table I. HX cells and LC share many surface markers and morphological features and both cells show positive staining for S100 protein and monoclonal antibody (OKT6). However, the presence of T_4 antigen may be useful in differentiating HX cells from normal LC[610].

AETIOLOGY
Although the aetiology of this disease is unclarified yet, HX is regarded as a proliferative disorder of cells of Langerhans lineage. Recently, it has been suggested that histiocytosis syndromes may represent a reactive immunological disorder[611].

TECHNICAL POINTS
Frozen tissue is required for the method using monoclonal antibody. Formalin-fixed and paraffin-embedded tissue specimens are used for the study of S100 protein.

TABLE I   COMPARATIVE FEATURES OF HX CELLS, LC, AND MACROPHAGES

CHARACTERISTIC	HISTIOCYTOSIS-X CELL	LANGERHANS CELL	MACROPHAGE
ATPase	+	+	0
acid phosphatase	+/−	+/−	+ to ++++
esterase	+/−	+/−	+ to ++++
Fc receptor IgG	+	+	+
Ia-like antigenicity	++++	++++	0 to ++++
T-6 antigenicity	+	+	0
T-4 antigenicity	+	0	0
S-100 antigenicity	+	+	0
ultrastructure	Birbeck granules	Birbeck granules	non-specific

(Favara, B.E., McCarthy, R.C., Mierau, G.W.: Human Pathology **14**:663, 1983)

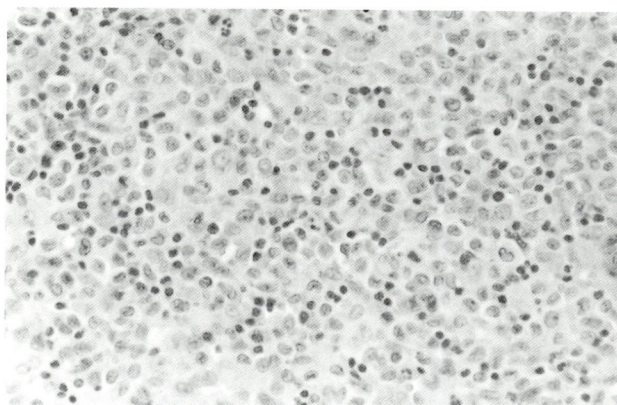

Fig. 1. Infiltration of ovoid histiocytic cells.
(HE staining, × 100)
(Courtesy of Dr. Mori, Dept. of Pathology, Tsukuba Univ.)

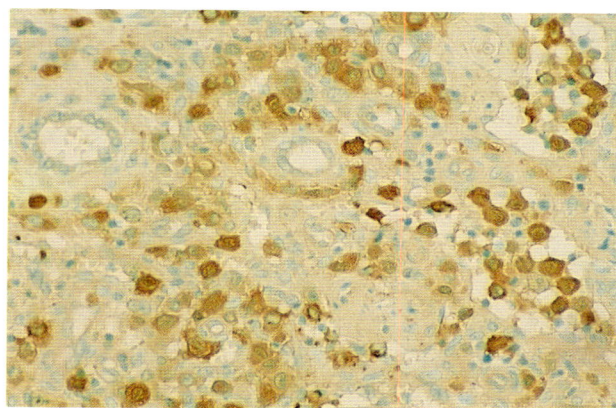

Fig. 2. Staining for S100 protein
(PAP, × 200)
HX cells are positive.
(Courtesy of Dr. Mori, Dept. of Pathology, Tsukuba Univ.)

Plasmacytoma cutis

INTRODUCTION

In plasmacytoma it is commonly believed that plasma cells grow in the bone marrow[612]. However, there are cases in which plasmacytoma appears in other extramedullary sites. Although rare, extramedullary plasmacytoma has been found to occur in various organs; the upper respiratory tract being the most common site[613–20], and the skin the least commonly involved[614,621]. Clinicopathologically, plasmacytoma is divided into three groups: (1) multiple myeloma (MM), (2) solitary plasmacytoma of the bone (SPB) and (3) extramedullary plasmacytoma (EMP). MM are highly malignant generalized bone diseases with a characteristic roentgenogram, and bone marrow findings of frequently abnormal proteins and Bence-Jones proteinuria. SPB is a solitary lesion arising in the bone marrow and often develops to MM. EMP, however, does not seem to be such a malignant tumour, because it rarely develops into MM as SPB.

FINDINGS

Clinically, we must consider other diseases such as malignant lymphoma, some sarcomas and metastatic carcinoma in the differential diagnosis. The present case, of a 76-year-old Japanese man, is a very interesting one, in which the first tumour appeared on the right upper extremity and, one year later, another tumour appeared in the left maxillary sinus. Histologically, both tumour cells were distinctly plasmacytoid and showed cell size variation and abnormal figures. Every laboratory investigation was normal except for serum IgA, which was slightly elevated. This case was examined immunologically and electron microscopically to determine the proper diagnosis[613]. An intracytoplasmic monoclonal immunoglobulin (IgA, gamma-type) was demonstrated by the immunofluorescence method and the peroxidase anti-peroxidase method (**1, 2**). By electron microscopy, the tumour cells were plasmacytoid and showed a mature, well-organized cytoplasm with a markedly dilated, rough endoplasmic reticulum.

TECHNICAL POINTS

The immunofluorescence method and peroxidase anti-peroxidase method are very useful in the diagnosis of this disease.

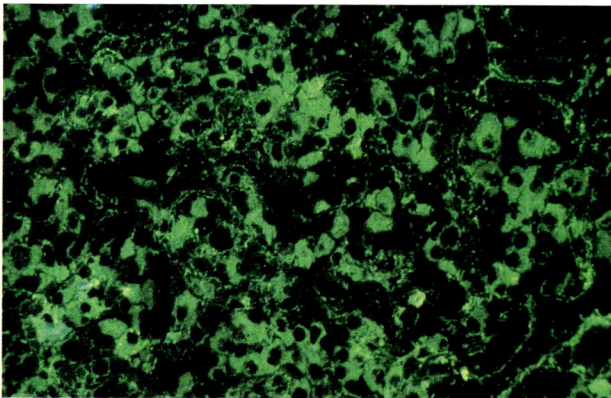

Fig. 1. Direct immunofluorescence method.

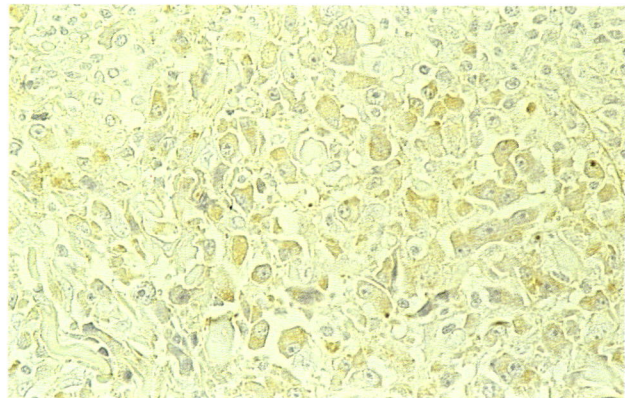

Fig. 2. An intracytoplasmic monoclonal immunoglobulin (IgA, gamma-type) was demonstrated by peroxidase anti-peroxidase method.

Overview

Progress in dermato-immunohistology has contributed significantly both to basic research and also to clinical diagnosis. Especially noteworthy has been the leadership of dermatologists in the clinical application of immunoelectron microscopy (IEM). Since the inception of IEM, it has been applied clinically in dermatology. However, many dermato-immunohistopathological techniques are still in the development stages due to the unique character (specificity) of skin. Each researcher has had to develop new techniques or modify existing ones for each specific research purpose. Despite this ever-increasing technical complexity, clinical application dictates that the simpler the technique, the better. How to rationalize this situation is the current question.

We anticipate the advent of techniques for observing immune reactions in live subjects without the use of biopsy or fixative. It is our hope that this book may serve to inform the rising generation of dermatologists about developments in the field of dermato-immunohistology, and that in so doing this book may be a contribution to future progress in dermatology.

References

Introduction

1. Coons, A.H., Creech, H.J., Jones, R.N.: Immunological properties of an antibody containing a fluorescent group. *Proc. Soc. Exp. Biol. Med. (NY).* **47**:200, 1941.
2. Coons, A.H., Creech, H.J., Jones, R.N., Berliner, E.: The demonstration of pneumococcal antigen in tissues by the use of fluorescent antibody. *J. Immunol.* **45**:159, 1942.
3. Riggs, J.L., Seiwald, R.J., Burckhalter, J., Downs, C.M., Metcalf, T.G.: Isothiocyanate compounds as fluorescent labelling agents for immune serum. *Am. J. Pathol.* **34**:1081, 1958.
4. Felton, L.C., McMillion, C.R.: Chromatographically pure fluorescein and tetramethylrhodamine isothiocyanates. *Anal. Biochem.* **2**:178, 1961.
5. Oi, V.J., Glaser, A.N., Stryer, L.: Fluorescent phycobiliprotein conjugates for analysis of cells and molecules. *J. Cell. Biol.* **93**:981, 1982.
6. Plem, J.S.: The use of a vertical illuminator with interchangeable dichroic mirrors for fluorescent microscopy with incident light. *Z. Wiss. Mikr.* **68**:129, 1967.
7. Kawamura, A-Jr., Aoyama, Y.: *Immunofluorescence in Medical Science.* University of Tokyo Press, Tokyo, pp. 75–91, 1982.
8. Nakane, P.K., Pierce, G.B.: Enzyme-labelled antibodies: Preparation and application for the localization of antigens. *J. Histochem. Cytochem.* **14**:929, 1966.
9. Avrameas, S.: Coupling of enzymes to proteins with glutar-aldehyde: Use of the conjugates for the detection of antigens and antibodies. *Immunochemistry.* **6**:43, 1969.
10. Roth, J., Bendayan, M., Orci, L.: Ultrastructural localization of intracellular antigens by the use of protein A-gold complex. *J. Histochem. Cytochem.* **26**:1074, 1978.
11. Holgate, C.S., Jackson, P., Cowen, P.N. et al: Immunogold-silver staining: New method of immuno-staining with enhanced sensitivity. *J. Histochem. Cytochem.* **31**:938, 1983.
12. Talmage, D.W., Baker, H.R., Akeson, W.: The separation and analysis of labelled antibodies. *J. Infec. Dis.* **94**:199, 1954.
13. Kumon, H.: Morphologically recognizable markers for scanning immunoelectron microscopy II: An indirect method using T and TMV. *Virology.* **74**:93, 1976.
14. Sternberger, L.A., Hardy, P.H. Jr., Cuculis, J.J., Meyer, H.G.: The unlabelled antibody enzyme method of immunohistochemistry: Preparation and properties of soluble antigen-antibody complex (horseradish peroxidase-antihorseradish peroxidase) and its use in identification of spirochetes. *J. Histochem. Cytochem.* **18**:315, 1970.
15. Hsu, S-M., Raine, L., Fanger, H.: Use of avidin-biotin peroxidase complex (ABC) in immunoperoxidase techniques: A comparison between ABC and unlabelled antibody (PAP) procedures. *J. Histochem. Cytochem.* **29**:577, 1981.
16. Kaplan, M.H.: Localization of streptococcal antigens in tissues. I. Histological distribution and persistence of M protein, types 1, 5, 12 and 19 in the tissues of the mouse. *J. Exp. Med.* **107**:341, 1958.
17. Parish, W.E., Rhodes, E.L.: Bacterial antigens and aggregated gamma globulin in the lesions of nodular vasculitis. *Brit. J. Derm.* **79**:131, 1967.
18. Epstein, W.L., Senecal, I., Kranobrod, H.: Viral antigens in human epidermal tumours: Localization of an antigen to molluscum contagiosum. *J. Invest. Dermatol.* **40**:51, 1963.
19. Weller, T.H., Coons, A.H.: Fluorescent antibody studies with agents of varicella and herpes zoster propagated in vitro. *Proc. Soc. Exp. Biol. Med.* **80**:789, 1954.
20. Aoyama, Y., Kurata, T., Kurata, K., Hondo, R., Ogiwara, H.: Demonstration of viral antigens in herpes simplex and varicella-zoster infections. *Recent advances in RES. Res.* **14**:60, 1974.
21. Mahony, J.D.H., Harris, J.R.W., Sydney, M.J., Kennedy, J., Doughan, H.: Evaluation of the C.S.F.F.T.A.ABS test in latent and tertiary treated syphilis. *Acta Dermatovenereol.* **52**:71, 1972.
22. Friou, G.J.: Identification of the nuclear component of the interaction of lupus erythematosus globulin and nuclei. *J. Immunol.* **80**:476, 1958.
23. Beck, J.S.: Variations in the morphological patterns of 'autoimmune' nuclear fluorescence. *Lancet.* **1**:1203, 1961.
24. Beutner, E.H., Tordon, R.E.: Demonstration of skin antibodies in sera of pemphigus vulgaris patients by indirect immunofluorescent staining. *Proc. Soc. Exp. Biol. Med.* **117**:505, 1964.
25. Jordan, R.E., Beitner, E.H., Witebsky, E.: Basement zone antibodies in bullous pemphigoid. *JAMA.* **100**:751, 1967.
26. Burnham, T.K., Neblett, T.R., Fine, G.: The application of the fluorescent antibody technique to the investigation of lupus erythematosus and various dermatoses. *J. Invest. Dermatol.* **41**:451, 1963.
27. Ueki, H., Wolff, H.H., Brown-Falco, O.: Cutaneous localization of human γ-globulins in lupus erythematosus. An electron microscopical study using the peroxidase labelled antibody technique. *Arch. Derm. Res.* **248**:297, 1974.
28. Sams, W.M. Jr., Thorne, E.C., Small, P., Mass, M.F., McIntosh, R.M.: Leucocytoclastic vasculitis. *Arch. Dermatol.* **112**:219, 1976.
29. Ueki, H. et al: Transient immune deposits in the papillary dermis and in the epidermis. *Arch. Dermatol. Res.* **269**:51, 1980.
30. Ueki, H., Meurer, M.: Immunkomplexe in der dermatologie heute (Eine kritische Bestandsaufnahme). *Der Hautarzt.* **34**:371–376, 1983.
31. Ruiter, D.J., Dingjan, G.M., Steijlen, P.M. et al: Monoclonal antibodies selected to discriminate between malignant melanomas and nevocellular nevi. *J. Invest. Dermatol.* **85**:4, 1985.
32. Kitajima, Y., Inoue, S., Yoneda, K. et al: Alteration in the arrangement of the keratin-type intermediate filaments during mitosis in cultured human keratinocytes. *Eur. J. Cell. Biol.* **38**:219, 1985.
33. Foidart, J.M., Bere, E.W., Yaar, M. et al: Distribution and immunoelectron microscopic localization of laminin, a noncollagenous basement membrane glycoprotein. *Lab. Invest.* **42**:336, 1980.

34. Nagata, H., Ueki, H. *et al*: The localization of fibronectin in normal human skin, granulation tissue, hypertrophic scar, mature scar, PSS skin and other fibrosing dermatoses. *Arch. Dermatol.* **121**:995, 1985.

35. Konomi, H., Hayashi, T., Nakayasu, K. *et al*: Localization of type V collagen and type IV collagen in human cornea, lungs and skin. *Am. J. Pathol.* **116**:417, 1984.

36. Davison, P.M., Bensch, K., Karasek, M.A.: Isolation and growth of endothelial cells from the microvessels of the newborn human foreskin in cell culture. *J. Invest. Dermatol.* **75**:316, 1980.

37. Cocchia, D., Michetti, F.: S-200 protein in satellite cells of the adrenal medulla and the superior cervical ganglion of the rat. An immunochemical and immunocytochemical study. *Cell Tissue Res.* **215**:103, 1981.

38. Kohler, G., Milstein, C.: Continuous cultures of fused cells secreting antibody of predefined specificity. *Nature.* **256**:495, 1975.

39. Bjerke, J.R.: Subpopulations of mononuclear cells in lesions of psoriasis, lichen planus and discoid lupus erythematosus studied using monoclonal antibodies. *Acta Dermatovenereol.* **62**:477, 1982.

40. Kohchiyama, A., Oka, D., Ueki, H.: Immunohistologic studies of squamous cell carcinoma: Possible participation of Leu-7 (natural killer) cells as anti-tumour effector cells. *J. Invest. Dermatol.* **87**:515–518, 1986.

Technical Procedures in Immunohistocytology

A Immunofluorescence technique

41. Coons, A.H., Creech, H.J., Jones, R.N.: Immunological properties of an antibody containing a fluorescent group. *Proc. Soc. Exp. Biol. Med. (NY).* **47**:200, 1941.

42. Kawamura, A. Jr., Aoyama, Y.: Synopsis of immunofluorescence and labelled antibody preparation. *Immunofluorescence in Medical Science.* Univ. Tokyo Press, Tokyo, pp. 9–30, 1982.

43. Beutner, E.H., Chorzelski, T.P., Bean, S.F.: *Part 1. Indications, methods, and concepts for immunopathologic studies Immunopathology of the skin.* 2nd edition. A Wiley Medical Publication, N.Y., pp. 1–182, 1979.

44. Riggs, J.L., Seimald, R.J., Burckhalter, J., Downs, C.M., Metcalf, T.G.: Isothiocyanate compound as fluorescent labelling agents for immune serum. *Am. J. Pathol.* **34**:1081, 1958.

45. Bergquist, N.R., Nilsson, P.: The conjugation of immunoglobulins with tetramethylrhodamine isothiocyanate by utilzation of dimethylsulphoxide (DMSO) as a solvent. *J. Immunol. Methods.* **5**:189, 1974.

46. Oi, V.J., Glazer, A.N., Stryer, L.: Fluorescent phycobiliprotein conjugates for analysis of cells and molecules. *J. Cell Biol.* **93**:981, 1982.

47. Ploem, J.S.: The use of a vertical illuminator with interchangeable dichroic mirrors for fluorescent microscopy with incident light. *Z. Wiss. Mikr.* **68**:129, 1967.

48. Ueki, H.: The application of the fluorescent antibody technic in dermatology. 1. Localization of tissue-bound globulin in the skin lesions. *Jpn. J. Dermatol. Ser. B.* **77**:32, 1967.

49. Ueki, H., Wolff, H.H.: Immunohistochemie in der Dermatologie. *Hautarzt.* **24**:323, 1973.

B Enzyme-labelled antibody method

50. Ram, J.S., Nakane, P.K., Rawlinson, E.G., Pierce, G.B.: Enzyme-labelled antibody for ultrastructural studies. *Fed. Proc.* **25**:732, 1966.

51. Mclean, I.W., Nakane, P.K.: Periodate-lysin-paraformaldehyde fixative: A new fixative for immunoelectron microscopy. *J. Histochem. Cytochem.* **22**:1077, 1974.

52. Boorsma, D.M.: *Immunoperoxidase: Technical Aspects and Some Applications in Dermatology.* Amsterdam, Academische Press. 1977.

53. Sternberger, L.A.: Electron microscopic immunocytochemistry. *J. Histochem. Cytochem.* **15**:139, 1967.

54. Yaoita, H., Gullino, M., Katz, S.I.: Herpes gestationis. Ultrastructural localization of *in vivo*-bound complement. *J. Invest. Dermatol.* **66**:383, 1976.

55. Guesdon, J.L., Ternyck, T., Avrameas, S.: The use of avidin-biotin interaction in immunoenzymatic techniques. *J. Histochem. Cytochem.* **27**:1131, 1979.

56. Hsu, S.M., Raine, I., Franger, H.: Use of avidin-biotin-peroxidase complex (ABC) in immunoperoxidase techniques: A comparison between ABC and unlabelled antibody (PAP) procedure. *J. Histochem. Cytochem.* **29**:577, 1981.

57. Holuber, K., Wolfee, K., Konrad, K., Beutner, E.G.: Ultrastructural localization of immunoglobulins in bullous pemphigoid skin. Employment of a new peroxidase-antiperoxidase method. *J. Invest. Dermatol.* **74**:220, 1975.

58. Roth, J., Bendayan, M., Carlemalm, E., Villiger, W., Garavito, M.: Enhancement of structural preservation and immunocytochemical staining in low temperature embedded pancreatic tissue. *J. Histochem. Cytochem.* **29**:663, 1981.

C Immunoelectron microscopy
1 Horseradish peroxidase-labelled method

59. Yaoita, H., Gullino, M., Katz, S.I.: Herpes gestationis. Ultrastructure and ultrastructural localization of *in vivo*-complement. *J. Invest. Dermatol.* **66**:383–388, 1976.

60. Boorsma, D.M.: *Immunoperoxidase: Technical Aspects and Some Applications in Dermatology.* Amsterdam, Academisch Press. 1977.

2 Immunoferritin electron microscopic method

61. Tanaka, H.: Detection of unique proteins by ferritin-antibody method. *Protein, Nucleic Aid and Enzyme.* **13**:954, 1968.

62. Kishida, Y. Olson, B.K. *et al*: Two improved methods for preparing ferritin-protein conjugates for electron microscopy. *J. Cell Biol.* **64**:331, 1975.

63. Takigawa, M., Imamura, S. *et al*: Distribution and mobility of specific antigen on isolated guinea pig epidermal cells. *J. Ultrastruct. Res.* **65**:246, 1978.

64. Takigawa M., Iwatsuki, K. *et al*: The Langerhans cell granules is an absorptive endocytic organelle. *J. Invest. Dermatol.* **85**:12, 1985.

3 Colloidal gold-labelled antibody method

65. Faulk, W.P., Taylor, G.M.: An immunocolloidal method for electron microscopy. *Immunochemistry* **8**:1081, 1971.

66. Larsson, L.I.: Simultaneous ultrastructural demonstration of multiple peptides in endocrine cells by a novel immunocytochemical method. *Nature.* **282**:743, 1979.

67. Pinto da Silva, P., Kan, F.W.K.: Label-fracture – A method for high resolution labelling of cell surfaces. *J. Cell Bio.* **99**:1156, 1984.

68. Hiramoto, T., Kitajima, Y., Yaoita, H.: Ultrastructural localization of pemphigus foliaceus antibody binding sites on the plasma membrane of keratinocytes. *3rd Immunodermatological Symposium, Oct. Milano*, pp. 68–69, 1986.

69. Slot, J.W., Geuze, H.J.: A new method of preparing gold probe for multiple-labelling cytochemistry. *Eur. J. Cell Bio.* **38**:87, 1985.

4 Scanning immunoelectron microscopy

70. Kumon, H.: T4-bacteriophage as a surface marker for scanning electron microscopy. *Biomedical Res 2 (suppl)*: 41, 1981.
71. Molday, R.S.: Labelling of cell surface antigens for SEM. In *Techniques in Immunocytochemistry*, 1983, II ed. Bullock G.R. and Petrusz P., Academic Press, p. 117, 1983.
72. Kumon, H.: Morphologically recognizable markers for scanning immunoelectron microscopy. II. An indirect method using T4 and TMV. *Virology.* **74**:93, 1976.
73. Nakaye, M., Nakagawa, S., Mimura, S., Ueki, H., Kumon, H., Ohmori, H.: Demonstration of DNP groups on *in vitro* dinitrophenylated lymph node cells of the guinea pig by a scanning immunoelectron microscopic method. *J. Dermatol.* (Tokyo) **7**:148, 1980.
74. Nakaye, M., Nakagawa, S., Ueki, H., Kumon, H., Ohmori, H.: Ultrastructural localization of 2, 4-dinitrophenyl groups on draining lymph node cells of guinea pigs following skin painting with 2, 4-dinitrochlorobenzene: I. Scanning immunoelectron microscopic studies. *J. Dermatol.* (Tokyo) **10**:251, 1983.
75. Oka, D., Nakagawa, S., Ueki, H., Kumon, H., Ohmori, H.: Antigen in contact sensitivity: II. Scanning immunoelectron microscopic studies of the distribution of DNP groups on the epidermal cells of guinea pigs following skin painting with DNCB. *J. Dermatol.* (Tokyo) **11**:15, 1984.
76. Kumon, H., Kaneshige, T., Ohmori, H.: T4-labelling technique and its applications with particular reference to blood group antigens in bladder tumours. In *Scanning Electron Microscopy*, 1983, II ed. Om Johari, SEM Inc., Chicago, p. 939, 1983.

D Application of monoclonal antibodies

77. Kehler, G., Milatein, C.: Continuous cultures of fused cells secreting antibody of predefined specificity. *Nature.* **256**:495, 1975.
78. Brown, J.P., Hewick, R.M., Hellström, K.E., Doolittle, R.F., Dreyer, W.J.: Human melanoma-associated antigen p97 is structurally and functionally related to transferrin. *Nature.* **296**:171, 1982.
79. Nakane, P.K., Pierce, G.B.: Enzyme-labelled antibodies: Preparation and application for the localization of antigens. *J. Histochem. Cytochem.* **14**:929, 1966.
80. Sternberger, L.A.: *Immunocytochemistry*, 2nd ed. New York, John Wiley & Sons, 1979.
81. Nohara, M.: Monoclonal antibodies raised against human malignant trichilemmoma cell line. *Kitasato Medicine.* **15**(5):345, 1985 (English in preparation).

Cellular and Extracellular Components in Normal Skin

A Cells
1 Keratinocytes
1.1 Cytoskeleton

82. Lazarides, E.: Intermediate filaments as mechanical integrators of cellular shape. *Nature.* **283**:249, 1980.
83. Kitajima, Y., Inoue, S., Yaoita, H.: Reorganization of keratin intermediate filaments by the drug-induced disruption of microfilaments in cultured human keratinocytes. *J. Invest. Dermatol.* **87**:565–569, 1986.
84. Kitajima, Y., Inoue, S., Yoneda, K., *et al*: Alteration in the arrangement of the keratin-type intermediate filaments during mitosis in cultured human keratinocytes. *Eur. J. Cell Biol.* **38**:219, 1985.
85. Woodcock-Mitchell, J., Eichner, R., Nelson, W.G. *et al*:

Immunolocalization of keratin polypeptides in human epidermis using monoclonal antibodies. *J. Cell Biol.* **95**:580, 1982.
86. Sun, T.T., Eichner, R., Nelson, W.G. *et al*: Keratin classes: Molecular markers for different types of epithelial differentiation. *J. Invest. Dermatol.* **81**:109, 1983.
87. Yoneda, K., Kitajima, Y., Furuta, H. *et al*: The distribution of keratin-type intermediate-sized filaments in so-called mixed tumour of the skin. *Br. J. Dermatol.* **109**:393, 1983.
88. Weiss, R.A., Guillet, G.Y.A., Freedberg, I.M. *et al*: The use of monoclonal antibody to keratin in human epidermal disease: Alterations in immunohistochemical staining pattern. *J. Invest. Dermatol.* **81**:224, 1983.
89. Hashimoto, K., Eto, H., Matsumoto, M. *et al*: Anti-keratin monoclonal antibodies: Production, specificities and application. *J. Cutan. Patho.* **10**:529, 1983.
90. Kitajima, Y., Inoue, S., Yaoita, H.: Effects of pemphigus antibody on organization of microtubules and keratin-intermediate filaments in cultured human keratinocytes. *Br. J. Dermatol.* **114**:171, 1986.

1.2 Hair keratin

91. Gillespie, J.M.: The structural proteins of hair: Isolation, characterization, and regulation of biosynthesis: *Biochemistry and Physiology of the Skin*, Vol.1, ed. Goldsmith, L.A, New York, Oxford University Press, pp. 475·510, 1983.
92. Baden, H.P., McGilvray, N., Lee, L.D. *et al*: Comparison of stratum corneum and hair fibrous proteins. *J. Invest. Dermatol.* **75**:311, 1980.
93. Marshall, R.C.: Characterization of the proteins of human hair and nail by electrophoresis. *J. Invest. Dermatol.* **80**:519, 1983.
94. Ito, M., Tazawa, T., Ito, K. *et al*: Immunological characteristics and histological distribution of human hair fibrous proteins studied with anti-hair keratin monoclonal antibodies, HKN-2, HKN-4 and HKN-6. *J. Histochem. Cytochem.* **34**:269, 1986.
95. Ito, M., Tazawa, T., Shimizu, N. *et al*: Cell differentiation in human anagen hair and hair follicle studied with anti-hair keratin monoclonal antibodies. *J. Invest. Dermatol.* **86**:563, 1986.
96. Ito, M.: The innermost cell layer of the outer root sheath in anagen hair follicle: Light and electron microscopic study. *Arch. Dermatol. Res.* **279**:112–119, 1986.

1.3 Desmosome

97. Kitajima, Y., Mori, S.: Plasma membrane ultrastructure of the human skin keratinocyte as observed by freeze-fracture electron microscopy. *J. Dermatol.* (Tokyo) **6**:153, 1979.
98. Hennings, H., Michael, D., Cheng, C. *et al*: Calcium regulation of growth and differentiation of mouse epidermal cells in culture. *Cell.* **19**:245, 1980.
99. Franke, W.W., Moll, R., Schiller, D.L. *et al*: Desmoplakins of epithelial and myocardial desmosomes are immunologically and biochemically related. *Differentiation.* **23**:115, 1982.
100. Cowin, P., Mattey, D., Garrod, D.: Identification of desmosomal surface components (desmocollins) and inhibition of desmosome formation by specific Fab. *J. Cell Sci.* **70**:41, 1984.
101. Eto, H., Matsumoto, M., Tazawa, T. *et al*: A monoclonal anti-hair keratin monoclonal antibody recognizes keratinocyte membrane substance. *J. Invest. Dermatol.* **80**:337, 1982.
102. Eto, H., Matsumoto, M., Hashimoto, K. *et al*: Immunohistochemical studies of acantholytic cells in pemphigus

141

vulgaris, Darier's disease and Hailey-Hailey's disease using monoclonal anti-desmosome antibody HK-1. *Proc. Jpn. Soc. Invest. Dermatol.* **9**:73, 1985.

1.4 Lysozyme

103. Jollès, J., Jollès, P.: Human tear and milk enzyme. *Biochemistry.* **6**:411, 1967.
104. Charlemagne, D., Jollès, P.: Les lysozyme des leucocytes et du plasma d'origine humaine. *Nouvelle Revue Français d'Haematologie.* **6**:355, 1966.
105. Ogawa, H., Miyazaki, H., Kimura, M.: Isolation and characterization of human skin lysozyme. *J. Invest. Dermatol.* **57**:111, 1971.
106. Ogawa, H., Miyazaki, H.: Immunochemical studies on the human skin lysozyme. *J. Invest. Dermatol.* **58**:59, 1972.
107. Ogawa, H.: Immunoenzymatic studies on human skin lysozyme. *J. Dermatol.* (Tokyo) **2**:45, 1975.
108. Kubagawa, H., Hamajima, Y., Ogawa, H.: Blood cell differentiation and lysozyme. *Igaku-no-Ayumi.* **94**:56, 1975 (in Japanese).
109. Takahashi, H., Negi, M., Ogawa, H.: A case of leukaemia cutis (myelomonocytic leukaemia). *J. Clin. Dermatol.* **35**:1075, 1981.

1.5 Cyclic AMP

110. Mizumoto, T., Ohkawara, A.: The localization of cyclic nucleotides in the human epidermis: An immunohisto-chemical study. In: *Biochemistry of Normal and Abnormal Epidermal Differentiation,* ed. Bernstein, I.A., Seiji, M., Univ. Tokyo Press, Tokyo, pp. 67–81, 1980.
111. Wedner, H.J., Hoffer, B.J., Battenberd, E. *et al*: A method for detecting intracellular cyclic adenosine monophosphate by immunofluorescence. *J. Histochem. Cytochem.* **20**:293–295, 1972.
112. Miyachi, Y., Imamura, S., Tanaka, C. *et al*: Immuno-histochemical localization of cyclic nucleotides in guinea pig lip. *Arch. Dermatol. Res.* **269**:233–237, 1980.
113. Adachi, K., Iizuka, H., Halprin, K.M. *et al*: Epidermal cyclic AMP is not decreased in psoriasis lesions. *J. Invest. Dermatol.* **74**:74–76, 1980.
114. Yoshikawa, K., Adachi, K., Halprin, K.M. *et al*: Cyclic AMP in skin: Effects of acute ischaemia. *Br. J. Dermatol.* **94**:611–614, 1976.

1.6 DNase and RNase A

115. Nohara, T.: Immunohistochemical study of the localiz-ation of deoxyribonuclease I and ribonuclease A in epidermal keratinocytes. *Jpn. J. Dermatol.* **94**:137, 1984 (in Japanese).
116. Nohara, T., Suzuki, H., Morioka, S., Kawaoi, A.: Immunohistochemical study of the localization of deoxyribonuclease in cornified cells of epidermis. *Jpn. J. Dermatol.* **93**:871, 1985 (in Japanese).
117. Yasui, Y.: Immuno-light and electron microscopy deoxyribonuclease localization in the nuclei of keratino-cytes and changes following UVB irradiation. *Jpn. J. Dermatol.* **96**:997, 1986 (in Japanese).
118. Suzuki, H., Fukuyama, K., Epstein, W.L.: Changes in nuclear DNA and RNA during epidermal keratinization. *Cell and Tissue Res.* **184**:871, 1977.
119. Usuba, S.: Distribution of DNase and RNase in psoriasis and their changes following PUVA. A study using immunohistochemical methods. *Jpn. J. Dermatol.* **97**:729–736, 1987 (in Japanese).
120. Suzuki, H., Fukuyama, K., Epstein, J.H., Epstein, W.L.: Ultrastructural study of the nuclei in premitotic

and repair DNA synthesis following UVB injury. *J. Invest. Derm.* **71**:334, 1978.

2 Thy-1 positive d-EC

121. Cantor, H., Weissman, I.: Development and function of subpopulations of thymocytes and T lymphocytes. *Prog. Allergy.* **20**:1, 1976.
122. Tamaki, K.: Heterogeneity of epidermal Thy-1-positive cells defined by lectin-binding sites. *J. Invest. Dermatol.* **86**:222, 1986.
123. Bergstresser, P.R., Tigelaar, R.E., Dees, J.H. *et al*: Thy-1 antigen-bearing dendritic cells populate murine epi-dermis. *J. Invest. Dermatol.* **81**:286, 1983.
124. Sheid, M., Boyse, E.A., Carswell, E.A. *et al*: Serologically demonstrable alloantigens of mouse epidermal cells. *J. Exp. Med.* **135**:938, 1972.
125. Tschachler, E., Schuler, G., Hutterer, J. *et al*: Expression of Thy-1 antigen by murine epidermal cells. *J. Invest. Dermatol.* **81**:282, 1983.
126. Breathnach, S.M., Katz, S.I.: Thy-1$^+$ dendritic cells in murine epidermis are bone-marrow derived. *J. Invest. Dermatol.* **83**:74, 1984.
127. Bergstresser, P.R., Tigelaar, R.E., Streilein, J.W.: Thy-1 antigen-bearing dendritic cells in murine epidermis are derived from bone marrow precursors. *J. Invest. Dermatol.* **83**:83, 1984.
128. Romani, N., Stingl, G., Tschachler, E. *et al*: The Thy-1-bearing cell of murine epidermis: A distinctive leucocyte perhaps related to natural killer cells. *J. Exp. Med.* **161**:1368, 1985.
129. Cooper, K.D., Breathnach, S.M., Caughman, S.W. *et al*: Fluorescence microscopic and flow cytometric analysis of bone marrow-derived cells in human epi-dermis. A search for the human analogue of murine dendritic Thy-1$^+$ epidermal cells. *J. Invest. Dermatol.* **85**:546, 1985.

3 Langerhans cells

130. Langerhans, P.: Über die Nerven der menschlichen Haut. *Virchow Arch. Path. Anat.* **44**:325, 1968.
131. Stingl, G., Tamaki, K., Katz, S.I.: Origin and function of Langerhans cells. *Immunol. Rev.* **53**:149, 1980.
132. Toews, G.B., Bergstresser, P.R., Streilein, J.W.: Epi-dermal Langerhans cell density determines whether contact sensitivity or unresponsiveness follows skin painting with DNFB. *J. Immunol.* **124**:445, 1980.
133. Chen, H.D., Silvers, W.K.: Influence of Langerhans cells on the survival of H-Y incompatible skin grafts in rats. *J. Invest. Dermatol.* **81**:20, 1983.
134. Fithian, E., Kung, P., Goldstein, G. *et al*: Reactivity of Langerhans cells with hybridoma antibody. *Proc. Natl. Acad. Sci.* **78**:2541, 1981.
135. Cocchia, D., Michetti, F., Donato, R.: Immunochemical and immunohistochemical localization of S-100 antigen in normal human skin. *Nature.* **294**:85, 1981.
136. Tamaki, K., Katz, S.I., Stingl, G.: Collection and isolation of epidermal Langerhans cells. In: *Manual of Macrophage Methodology.* ed. Herocowitz, H.B., Holden, H.T., Hellanti, J.A., Ghaffar, A. Marcell Dekker Inc., New York, 1981.

4 Melanocytes
4.1 Tyrosinase in melanocytes

137. Hearing, V.J. *et al*: Mammalian tyrosinase: isozymic forms of the enzyme. *Int. J. Biochem.* **13**:99, 1981.
138. Tomita, Y. *et al*: Transfer of tyrosinase to melanosomes in Harding-Passey mouse melanoma. *Arch. Biochem.*

Biophys. **225**:75, 1983.

139. Tomita, Y. *et al*: Inactivation of tyrosinase by dopa. *J. Invest. Dermatol.* **75**:379, 1980.

140. Tomita, Y., *et al*: Anti-(T$_4$) tyrosinase monoclonal antibodies-specific markers for pigmented melanocytes. *J. Invest. Dermatol.* **85**:426, 1985.

141. Tomita, Y. *et al*: Monoclonal antibodies to mouse T4-tyrosinase identify human melanocytes. *J. Invest. Dermatol.* **84**:294, 1985.

142. Tomita, Y., Hearing, V.J.: Monoclonal antibodies produced against murine tyrosinase identify pigmented human melanocytes. *Diagnostic Immunol.* **4**:149, 1986.

4.2 Cell membrane and organelle (melanosome) in melanocytes and melanoma

143. Jimbow, K., Fitzpatrick, T.B., Quevedo, W.C. Jr.: Formation, chemical compositions and functions of melanin pigments in mammals. In: *Biology of the Integument, Vol. 2*, ed. Matoltsy, A.G., Springer Verlag, Berlin, pp. 278–292, 1986.

144. Jimbow, M., Kanoh, H., Jimbow, K.: Characterization of biochemical properties of melanosomes for structural and functional differentiation: Analysis of the compositions of lipids and proteins in melanosomes and their subfractions. *J. Invest. Dermatol.* **79**:97–102, 1982.

145. Jimbow, K., Jimbow, M., Chiba, M.: Characterization of structural properties for morphological differentiation of melanosomes: II. Electron microscopic and SDS-PAGE comparison of melanosomal matrix proteins in B16 and Harding-Passey melanomas. *J. Invest. Dermatol.* **78**:76–81, 1982.

146. Takahashi, H., Horikoshi, T., Jimbow, K.: Fine structural characterization of melanosomes in dysplastic nevi. *Cancer.* **56**:111–123, 1985.

147. Jimbow, K., Szabo, G., Fitzpatrick, T.B.: Ultrastructure of giant pigment granules (macromelanosomes) in the cutaneous pigmented macules of neurofibromatosis. *J. Invest. Dermatol.* **61**:300–309, 1973.

148. Hunter, J.A.A., Zaynoun, S., Paterson, W.D., Bleehen, S.S., Mackie, R., Cochran, A.J.: Cellular fine structure in the invasion nodules of different histogenetic types of malignant melanoma. *Br. J. Dermatol.* **98**:255–272, 1978.

149. Akutsu, Y., Jimbow, K.: Development and characterization of a mouse monoclonal antibody, MoAb HMSA-1, against melanosomal fraction of human malignant melanoma. *Cancer Res.* **46**:2904–2911, 1986.

150. Maeda, K., Jimbow, K.: Development of MoAb HMSA-2 for melanosomes of human melanoma and its application to immunohistopathologic diagnosis of neoplastic melanocytes. *Cancer.* **59**:415–423, 1987.

151. Akutsu, Y., Jimbow, K.: Characterization of biological and biochemical properties of melanosomal protein in human malignant melanoma by development of monoclonal antibody, MoAb HMSA-1. *J. Invest. Dermatol.* **87**:442a, 1986.

152. Yamana, K., Maeda, K., Jimbow, K.: Application of MoAb HMSA-2 for immunohistopathological diagnosis of amelanotic and/or regressed lesions of human melanoma on routine paraffin sections. *J. Invest. Dermatol.* **87**:429a, 1986.

153. Maeda, K., Yamana, K., Jimbow, K., Akutsu, Y., Takahashi, H.: MoAb HMSA-2 as a differentiation marker for dysplastic melanocytic nevi from common melanocytic nevi on routine histology section. *J. Invest. Dermatol.* **87**:438a, 1986.

5 Sweat gland cells

154. Leidal, R., Rapini, R., Sato, K. *et al*: Evolution and development of human axillary sweat glands. *J. Invest. Dermatol.* **78**:352, 1982.

155. Penneys, N.S., Nadji, M., Mckinney, E.C.: Carcinoembryonic antigen present in human eccrine sweat. *J. Am. Acad. Dermatol.* **40**:401, 1981.

156. Nakama, T.: Carcinoembryonic antigen in several skin tumours. *Jpn. J. Dermatol.* **93**:1271, 1983 (in Japanese).

157. Nakajima, T., Watanabe, S., Sato, Y. *et al*: Immunohistochemical demonstration of S-100 in malignant melanoma and pigmented nevus, and its diagnostic application. *Cancer.* **50**:912, 1982.

158. Tamada, S., Hirose, T., Sano, T. *et al*: Immunohistochemical localization of S-100 protein in sweat gland neoplasms. *Jpn. J. Dermatol.* **94**:937, 1984 (in Japanese).

159. Eto, H., Hashimoto, K., Kobayashi, H. *et al*: Eccrine gland associated antigens. A demonstration by monoclonal antibodies. *J. Invest. Dermatol.* **80**:339, 1983.

160. Kanitakis, J., Schmitt, D., Bernard, A. *et al*: Anti-D47: A monoclonal antibody reacting with the secretory cells of human eccrine sweat glands. *Br. J. Dermatol.* **109**:509, 1983.

161. Tourville, D.R., Adler, R.H., Bienenstock, J. *et al*: The human secretory immunoglobulin system: Immunohistochemical localization of gamma-A, secretory piece and lactoferrin in normal human tissues. *J. Exp. Med.* **129**:411, 1969.

162. Heyderman, E., Steele, K., Ormerod, M.G.: A new antigen on the epithelial membrane: Its immunoperoxidase localization in normal and neoplastic tissue. *J. Clin. Pathol.* **32**:35, 1979.

163. Mazoujian, G., Pinkus, G.S., Davis, S. *et al*: Immunohistochemistry of a gross cystic disease fluid protein (GCDFP-15) of the breast. *Am. J. Pathol.* **110**:105, 1983.

164. Ookusa, Y., Takata, K., Nagashima, M., Hirano, H.: Lectin-binding pattern in extramammary Paget's disease by horseradish (HRP)-labelling method – specific staining with Dolichos biflorus agglutinin (DBA). *Arch. Dermatol. Res.* **277**:65, 1985.

165. Hori, K., Hashimoto, K., Eto, H., Dekio, S.: Keratin-type intermediate filament in sweat gland myoepithelial cells. *J. Invest Dermatol.* **85**:453, 1985.

166. Eto, H., Hashimoto, K., Kobayashi, H. *et al*: Monoclonal antikeratin antibody: Production, characterization and immunohistochemical application. *J. Invest. Dermatol.* **84**:404, 1985.

167. Hashimoto, K., Eto, H., Matsumoto, M. *et al*: Anti-keratin monoclonal antibodies: Production, specificities and application. *J. Cutan. Pathol.* **10**:529, 1983.

6 Pilosebaceous cells

168. Lever, W.F., Schaumburg-Lever, G.: Embryology of the skin. In: *Histopathology of the Skin*, ed. Lever, W.F., Schaumburg-Lever, G., Lippincott, Philadelphia, pp. 3–7, 1983.

169. Eto, H. *et al*: Eccrine gland-associated antigens. A demonstration by monoclonal antibodies. *J. Invest. Dermatol.* **80**:339, 1983.

170. Hashimoto, K., Eto, H. *et al*: Anti-keratin monoclonal antibodies: Production, specificities and applications. *J. Invest. Dermatol.* **10**:429, 1983.

171. Eto, K., Hashimoto, K., Matsumoto, M., Kanzaki, T. *et al*: Monoclonal antikeratin antibody: Production, characterization and immunohistochemical application. *J. Invest. Dermatol.* **84**:404, 1985.

172. Ito, M. *et al*: Immunological specificity of hair fibrous proteins studied by antihair keratin monoclonal antibodies (HKN-2, 3, 4 and 6). *Proc. Jpn. Soc. Invest. Dermatol.* **9**:1, 1985.

173. Lever, W.F., Schaumburg-Lever, G.: Tumours of epidermal appendages. In: *Histopathology of the Skin*, ed. Lever, W.F., Schaumburg-Lever, G., Lippincott, Philadelphia, p. 551, 1983.
174. Kanzaki, T., Eto, H., Umezawa, *et al*: Morphological, biological, and biochemical characteristics of a benign human trichilemmoma cell line *in vivo* and *in vitro*. *Cancer Res.* **41**:2468, 1981.
175. Kanzaki, T., Kanamaru, T., Nishiyama, S., Eto, H. *et al*: Three-dimensional hair differentiation of a trichilemmoma cell line *in vitro*. *Dev. Biol.* **99**:324, 1983.
176. Kanzaki, T., Eto, H., Tsukamoto, K. *et al*: Differentiation of trichilemmoma cells toward eccrine gland and syringoma *in vitro*. *Proc. Jpn. Soc. Invest. Dermatol.* **8**:186, 1984.

7 Fibroblasts
7.1 Cytoskeleton

177. Lazarides, E., Weber, K.: Actin antibody: The specific visualization of actin filaments in non-muscle cells. *Proc. Natl. Acad. Sci. USA.* **71**:2268, 1974.
178. Hynes, R.O., Destree, A.T.: Relationships between fibronectin (LETS protein) and actin. *Cell.* **16**:875, 1978.
179. Brinkley, B.R., Fistel, S.H., Marcum, J.M. *et al*: Microtubules in cultured cells: Indirect immunofluorescence staining with tubulin antibody. *Int. Rev. Cytol.* **63**:59, 1980.
180. Steinert, P.M., Jones, J.C.R., Goldman, R.D.: Intermediate filaments. *J. Cell Biol.* **99**:22, 1984.
181. Wulf, E., Deboben, A., Bautz, F.A. *et al*: Fluorescent phallotoxin, a tool for the visualization of cellular actin. *Proc. Natl. Acad. Sci. USA.* **76**:4498, 1979.

7.2 Immunological phenomena

182. Ueki, A. *et al*: The receptor sites for complement (C3) on human diploid fibroblasts. *Virchows Arch. B.* **18**:101, 1975.
183. Al-Adnani, M.S. *et al*: Clq production and secretion by fibroblasts. *Nature.* **263**:145, 1976.
184. Reid, K.B.M. *et al*: Biosynthesis of the first component of complement by human fibroblasts. *Biochem. J.* **167**:647, 1977.
185. Bianco, C. *et al*: Complement receptors. *Contemp. Top. Mol. Immunol.* **6**:145, 1977.

8 Vascular endothelial cells

186. Jaffe, E.A., Holer, L.W., Nachman, R.L.: Synthesis of anti-haemophilic factor antigen by cultured human endothelial cells. *J. Clin. Invest.* **52**:2757, 1973.
187. Hoyer, L.M., de los Santos, R.P., Hoyer, J.R.: Anti-haemophilic factor antigen: Localization in endothelial cells by immunofluorescence microscopy. *J. Clin. Invest.* **52**:2737, 1973.
188. Holthofer, H. *et al*: Ulex europaeus I lectin as a marker for vascular endothelial cells in human tissues. *Lab. Invest.* **47**:60, 1982.
189. Suzuki, Y., Masuzawa, M., Kanzaki, T., Nishiyama, S.: The biological nature of vascular endothelial cells in cutaneous tissues – the second report: by the immunoperoxidase method of UEA-I lectin-. *Jpn. J. Dermatol.* **93**:1289, 1983 (in Japanese).
190. Todd, A.S.: The histological localization of plasminogen activator. *J. Pathol. Bacteriol.* **78**:281, 1959.
191. Larsson, A., Asteat, B.: Immunohistochemical localization of tissue plasminogen activator and urokinase in the vessel wall. *J. Clin. Pathol.* **38**:140, 1985.
192. Linder, E.: Binding of Clq and complement activation by vascular endothelium. *J. Immunol.* **126**:648, 1981.

193. Ryan, T.J.: Dermal vasculature. In: *Methods in Skin Research*, ed. Skerrow, D., Skerrow, C.J., John Wiley & Sons Ltd, London pp. 527–558, 1985.
194. Davison, P.M., Bensch, K., Karasek, M.A.: Isolation and growth of endothelial cells from the microvessels of the newborn human foreskin in cell culture. *J. Invest. Dermatol.* **75**:316, 1980.
195. Caldwell, P.R. *et al*: Angiotensin-converting enzyme: Vascular endothelial localization. *Science.* **191**:1050, 1976.

9 Nerve cells

196. Lillie, R.D., Fullmer, H.M.: Glia and nerve cells and fibres. In: *Histopathologic Technic and Practical Histochemistry*. 4th ed., McGraw-Hill, New York, pp. 765–786, 1976.
197. Roman, N.A., Ford, D., Montagna, W.: The demonstration of cutaneous nerves. *J. Invest. Dermatol.* **53**:328, 1969.
198. Falck, B.: Observations of the possibilities of the cellular localization of monoamines by fluorescence method. *Acta. Physiol. Scand. 56: Suppl.* **197**:1, 1962.
199. Moore, B.W.: A soluble protein characteristic of the nervous system. *Biochem. Biophys. Res. Commun.* **19**:739, 1965.
200. Cocchia, D., Michetti, F.: S-100 protein in satellite cells of the adrenal medulla and the superior cervical ganglion of the rat: An immunochemical and immunocytochemical study. *Cell Tissue Res.* **215**:103, 1981.
201. Marangos, P.J., Zimzely-Neurath, C., Luk, D.C.M., York, C.: Isolation and characterization of the nervous system-specific protein 14-3-2 from rat brain: Purification, subunit composition, and comparison to the beef brain protein. *J. Biol. Chem.* **250**:1884, 1975.
202. Schmechel, D., Marangos, P.J., Brightman, M., Goodwin, F.K.: Brain enolases as specific markers of neuronal and glial cells. *Science.* **199**:313, 1978.
203. Hachisuka, H., Mori, O., Sakamoto, F., Sasai, Y., Nomura, F.: Immunohistological demonstration of S-100 protein in the cutaneous nervous system. *Anatomical Record.* **210**:639, 1984.
204. Hachisuka, H., Sakamoto, F., Mori, O., Nomura, F., Sasai, Y., Nakamura, Y., Uno, H.: Immunohistochemical demonstration of neuron specific enolase (NSE) on cutaneous nerves: Comparative study using NSE and S-100 protein antibodies on denervated skin. *Acta Histochem.* **81**:227–235, 1987.
205. Sakamoto, F., Hachisuka, H., Mori, O., Nomura, F., Sasai, Y.: Immunohistochemical investigation of S-100 protein and neuron specific enolase in skin tumours. *J. Dermatol.* (Tokyo) **95**:969, 1985.
206. Hachisuka, H., Sakamoto, F., Nomura, F., Mori, O., Sasai, Y.: Immunohistochemical study of S-100 protein and neuron specific enolase (NSE) in melanocytes and the related tumours. *Acta Histochem.* **80**:215, 1986.
207. Bjerke, J.R.: Subpopulations of mononuclear cells in lesions of psoriasis, lichen planus and discoid lupus erythematosus studied using monoclonal antibodies. *Acta Derm. Venereol.* **62**:477, 1982.
208. Gomes, M.A., Schmitt, D.S. *et al*: Lichen planus and chronic graft-versus-host reaction. *In situ* identification of immunocompetent cell phenotypes. *J. Cutan. Pathol.* **9**:249, 1982.
209. Buechner, S.A., Winkelmann, R.K. *et al*: T cell and T cell subsets in mycosis fungoides and parapsoriasis: A study of 18 cases with anti-human T cell monoclonal antibodies and histochemical techniques. *Arch. Dermatol.* **120**:897, 1984.
210. Willemze, R., Graaff-Reitsma, C.B. *et al*: Characterization of T cell subpopulations in skin and peripheral

blood of patients with cutaneous T cell lymphomas and benign inflammatory dermatoses. *J. Invest. Dermatol.* **80**:60, 1983.

211. Buechner, S.A., Winkelmann, R.K. *et al*: Identification of T cell subpopulations in granuloma annulare. *Arch. Dermatol.* **119**:125, 1983.

212. Narayanan, R.B., Bhutani, L.K. *et al*: T cell subsets in leprosy lesions: *In situ* characterization using monoclonal antibodies. *Clin. Exp. Immunol.* **51**:421, 1983.

213. Poulter, L.W., Seymour, G.J. *et al*: Immunohistological analysis of delayed-type hypersensitivity in man. *Cell. Immunol.* **74**:358, 1982.

214. Margolis, R.J., Tonnesen, M.G. *et al*: Lymphocyte subsets and Langerhans cells/indeterminate cells in erythema multiforme. *J. Invest. Dermatol.* **81**:403, 1983.

215. Kohchiyama, A., Hatamochi, A., Ueki, H.: Increased number of OKT 6-positive dendritic cells in the hair follicles of patients with alopecia areata. *Dermatologica.* **171**:327, 1985.

216. Kohchiyama, A., Oka, D., Ueki, H.: T cell subsets in lesions of systemic and discoid lupus erythematosus. *J. Cutan. Pathol.* **12**:497, 1985.

217. Kohchiyama, A., Oka, D., Ueki, H.: Immunohistologic studies of squamous cell carcinoma: Possible participation of Leu7+ (natural killer) cells as anti-tumour effector cells. *J. Invest. Dermatol.* **87**:515, 1986.

218. Kohchiyama, A., Oka, D., Ueki, H.: Expression of HLA-DR antigen on tumour cells in basal cell carcinoma. *J. Am. Acad. Dermatol.* **16**:833–838, 1987.

10 Subsets of infiltrated lymphocytes in the skin

219. Cerio, R., Dupuy, P.F. *et al*: Monoclonal antibody labelling of mononuclear cell surface antigens in formaldehyde-fixed paraffin-embedded cutaneous tissue. *J. Invest. Dermatol.* **87**:499, 1986.

B Ground substance
1 Synopsis

220. Fawcett, D.W.: Connective tissue proper. In: *A Textbook of Histology, Eleventh Edition*, ed. Bloom, W., Fawcett, D.W., W.B. Saunders Co., Philadelphia, pp. 136–173, 1986.

221. Bornstein, P., Byers, P.H.: Disorders of collagen metabolism. In: *Metabolic Control and Disease, 8th Edition*, ed. Bondy, P.K., Rosenberg, L.E., W.B. Saunders Co., Philadelphia, pp. 1089–1153, 1980.

222. Timpl, R.: Components of basement membranes. In: *Immunochemistry of the Extracellular Matrix, Vol. II, Applications*, ed. Furthmayr H., CRC Press, Inc., Boca Raton, FL, pp. 119–150, 1982.

223. Martinez-Hernandez, A., Amenta, P.S.: The basement membrane in pathology. *Lab. Invest.* **48**:656, 1983.

224. Sano, J., Fujiwara S., Sato, S. *et al*: AB (type V) and basement membrane (type IV) collagens in the bovine lung parenchyma: Electron microscopic localization by the peroxidase-labelled antibody method. *Biomedical Res.* **2**:20, 1981.

225. Odermatt, E., Risteli, J., Van Delden, V. *et al*: Structural diversity and domain composition of a unique collagenous fragment (intima collagen) obtained from human placenta. *Biochem. J.* **211**:295, 1983.

226. Bentz, H., Morris, N.P., Murray, L.W. *et al*: Isolation and partial characterization of a new human collagen with an extended triple-helical structural domain. *Proc. Natl. Acad. Sci. USA.* **80**:3168, 1983.

227. Sage, H., Balian, G., Vogel, A.M. *et al*: Type VIII collagen: Synthesis by normal and malignant cells in culture. *Lab. Invest.* **50**:219, 1984.

228. Yasui, N., Benya, P.D., Nimni, M.E.: Identification of a large interrupted helical domain of disulfide-bonded cartilege collagen. *J. Biol. Chem.* **259**:14175, 1984.

229. Schmid, T.M., Linsenmayer, T.F.: A short chain (pro)-collagen from aged endochondral chondrocytes. *J. Biol. Chem.* **258**:9504, 1983.

230. Kivirikko, K.I., Myllyla, R.: Biosynthesis of the collagens. In: *Extracellular Matrix Biochemistry*, ed. Piez, K.A., Reddi, A.H., Elsevier·Science Publishing Co Inc, New York, pp. 83–118, 1984.

231. Burgeson, R.E., El Adli, F.A., Kaitila, I.I. *et al*: Fetal membrane collagens: Identification of two new collagen alpha chains. *Proc. Natl. Acad. Sci. USA.* **73**:2579, 1976.

232. Gosline, J.M., Rosenbloom, J.: Elastin. In: *Extracellular Matrix Biochemistry*, ed. Piez, K.A., Reddi, A.H., Elsevier Science Publishing Co. Inc., New York, pp. 191–227, 1984.

233. Tajima, S., Nishikawa, T., Hatano, I.I. *et al*: Distribution of macromolecular components in human dermal connective tissue. *Arch. Dermatol. Res.* **273**:115, 1982.

234. Fujii, N., Nagai, Y.: Isolation and characterization of a proteodermatan sulfate from calf skin. *J. Biochem.* **90**:1249, 1981.

235. Onodera, S., Nagai, Y.: Isolation and characterization of cartilage proteoglycans immunoreactive with an antibody to skin proteodermatan sulfate core protein. *Biochem. Biophys. Res. Commun.* **129**:95, 1985.

236. Hakomori, S., Fukuda, M., Sekiguchi, K., Carter, W.G.: *In Extracellular Matrix Biochemistry*, ed. Piez, K.A., Reddi, A.H., Elsevier Science Publishing Co. Inc., New York, pp. 229–275, 1984.

237. Hewitt, A.T., Varner, H.H., Silver, M.H. *et al*: The role of chondronectin and cartilage proteoglycan in the attachment of chondrocytes to collagen. *Limb Development and Regeneration Part B*, Alan R. Liss, Inc, New York, pp. 25–33, 1983.

238. Terranova, V.P., Rao, C.N., Kalebic, T. *et al*: Laminin receptor on human breast carcinoma cells. *Proc. Natl. Acad. Sci. USA.* **80**:444, 1983.

239. Carlin, B., Jaffe, R., Bender, B. *et al*: Entactin, a novel basal lamina-associated sulfated glycoprotein. *J. Biol. Chem.* **256**:5209, 1981.

2 Laminin

240. Timple, R., Rohde, H., Robey, P.G. *et al*: Laminin – a glycoprotein from basement membranes. *J. Biol. Chem.* **254**:9933, 1979.

241. Chung, A.E., Freeman, I.L., Braginski, J.E.: A novel extracellular membrane elaborated by a mouse embryonal carcinoma-derived cell line. *Biochem. Biophys. Res. Commun.* **79**:859, 1977.

242. Sakashita, S., Ruoslahti, E.: Laminin-like glycoproteins in extracellular matrix of endodermal cells. *Arch. Biochem. Biophys.* **205**:283, 1980.

243. Wewer, U., Albrechtsen, R., Ruoslahti, E.: Laminin, a noncollagenous component of epithelial basement membranes synthesized by a rat yolk sac tumour. *Cancer Res.* **41**:1518, 1981.

244. Foidart, J.M., Bere, E.W., Yaar, M. *et al*: Distribution and immunoelectron microscopic localization of laminin, a noncollagenous basement membrane glycoprotein. *Lab. Invest.* **42**:336, 1980.

245. Howe, C., Dietzschhold, B.: Structural analysis of three subunits of laminin from tetracarcinoma-derived parietal endodermal cells. *Devel. Biol.* **98**:385, 1983.

246. Engel, J., Odermatt, E., Engel, A. *et al*: Shapes, domain organizations and flexibility of laminin and fibronectin, two multifunctional proteins of the extracellular matrix. *J. Mol. Biol.* **150**:97, 1981.

247. Maekawa, Y., Nogita, T., Arao, T.: Two cases of so-called mixed tumour of the skin – distribution of fibronectin and laminin in the stroma. *Nishinihon J. Dermatol.* **47**:220, 1985 (in Japanese).

248. Nelson, D.L., Little, C.D., Balian, G.: Distribution of fibronectin and laminin in basal cell epitheliomas. *J. Invest. Dermatol.* **80**:446, 1983.

249. Nogita, T., Nogami, R., Maekawa, Y.: Distribution of fibronectin and laminin in basal cell carcinoma and squamous cell carcinoma. *Jpn. J. Dermatol.* **95**:1547, 1985 (in Japanese).

250. Hashimoto, H., Kuroda, K., Sakashita, S.: Laminin basement membrane-specific glycoprotein in bladder carcinoma. *Jpn. J. Urol.* **75**:580, 1984 (in Japanese).

3 Fibronectin

251. Yamada, K.M., Olden, K.: Fibronectin-adhesive glycoproteins of cell surface and blood. *Nature.* **275**:179, 1978.

252. Yamada, K.M., Kennedy, D.W.: Fibroblast cellular and plasma fibronectins are similar but not identical. *J. Cell Biol.* **80**:492, 1980.

253. Stenman, S., Vaheri, A.: Distribution of a major connective tissue protein, fibronectin, in normal human tissues. *J. Exp. Med.* **147**:1054, 1978.

254. Fyrand, O.: Studies on fibronectin in the skin. 1. Indirect immunofluorescence studies in normal skin. *Br. J. Dermatol.* **101**:263, 1979.

255. Fleischmajor, R., Dessau, W. *et al*: Immunofluorescent analysis of collagen, fibronectin and basement membrane protein in scleroderma skin. *J. Invest. Dermatol.* **75**:270, 1980.

256. Briggaman, R.A.: Biochemical composition of the epidermal-dermal junction and other basement membranes. *J. Invest. Dermatol.* **78**:1, 1982.

257. Kubo, M., Norris, D.A. *et al*: Human keratinocytes synthesize, secrete and deposit fibronectin in the pericellular matrix. *J. Invest. Dermatol.* **82**:580, 1984.

258. Nagata, H., Ueki, H. *et al*: The localization of fibronectin in normal skin, granulation tissue, hypertrophic scar, mature scar, PSS skin and other fibrosing dermatoses. *Arch. Dermatol.* **121**:995, 1985.

4 Type I, III, V collagens

259. Ooshima, A.: Immunohistochemical localization of prolyl hydroxylase in rat tissues. *J. Histochem. Cytochem.* **25**:1294, 1977.

260. Uitto, J., Eisen, A.Z.: Collagen. In: *Dermatology in General Medicine*, Eds. Fitzpatrick, T.B. *et al*, 3rd ed. McGraw-Hill, 1987.

261. Meigel, W.N., Gay, S., Weber, L.: Dermal architecture and collagen distribution. *Arch. Dermatol. Res.* **259**:1, 1977.

262. Epstein, E.H., Münderloh, N.H.: Human skin collagen, presence of type I and III at all levels of the dermis. *J. Biol. Chem.* **253**:1336, 1978.

263. Konomi, H., Hayashi, T., Nakayasu, K. *et al*: Localization of type V collagen and type IV collagen in human cornea, lungs and skin. *Am. J. Pathol.* **116**:417, 1984.

264. Cauwenberge, D.E., Pierard, G.E., Foidert, J.M. *et al*: Immunohistochemical localization of laminin, type IV and type V collagen in basal cell carcinoma. *Br. J. Dermatol.* **108**:163, 1983.

265. Peltonen, J., Aho, H., Halme, T. *et al*: Distribution of different collagen types and fibronectin in neurofibromatosis tumours. *Acta. Path. Microbiol. Immunol. Scand.* (Sect A). **92**:345, 1984.

266. Gay, S.: Immunological studies on collagen-type distribution in tissues. *Thrombosis and Haemostasis suppl.* **63**:171, 1978.

5 Type IV collagen

267. Brinker, J.M. *et al*: Immunochemical characterization of type IV procollagen from anterior lens capsule. *Collagen Relat. Res.* **5**:233, 1985.

268. Timple, R. *et al*: Laminin-A glycoprotein from basement membranes. *J. Biol. Chem.* **254**:9933, 1979.

269. Kobayashi, T. *et al*: Degradation of dermal fibrils: Effect of collagenase, elastase, dithiothreitol and citrate buffer (abst.). *J. Ultrastruct. Res.* **57**:229, 1976.

270. Uitto, V. *et al*: Degradation of basement-membrane collagen by neutral protease from human leucocytes. *Eur. J. Biochem.* **105**:409, 1980.

271. Yaoita, H. *et al*: Localization of the collagenous component in skin basement membrane. *J. Invest. Dermatol.* **70**:191, 1978.

6 Bullous pemphigoid antigen

272. Woodley, D., Didierjean, L., Regnier, M. *et al*: Bullous pemphigoid antigen synthesized *in vitro* by human epidermal cells. *J. Invest. Dermatol.* **75**:148, 1980.

273. Stanley, J.R., Hawley-Nelson, P., Yuspa, S.H. *et al*: Characterization of bullous pemphigoid antigen: a unique basement membrane protein of stratified squamous epithelia. *Cell.* **24**:897, 1981.

274. Beutner, E.H., Jordan, R.E., Chorzelski, T.P.: The immunopathology of pemphigus and bullous pemphigoid. *J. Invest. Dermatol.* **51**:63, 1968.

275. Holubar, K., Wolff, K., Konrad, K. *et al*: Ultrastructural localization of immunoglobulins in bullous pemphigoid skin. *J. Invest. Dermatol.* **64**:220, 1975.

276. Stanley, J.A., Alvarez, O.M., Bere, E.W. *et al*: Detection of basement membrane zone antigens during epidermal wound healing in pigs. *J. Invest. Dermatol.* **77**:240, 1981.

277. Stanley, J.R., Foidert, J.M., Murray, J.C. *et al*: The epidermal cell which selectively adheres to a collagen substrate is the basal cell. *J. Invest. Dermatol.* **74**:54, 1980.

278. Stanley, J.R., Yuspa, S.H.: Specific epidermal protein markers are modulated during calcium-induced differentiation. *J. Cell Biol.* **96**:1809, 1983.

279. Okada, N., Kitano, Y., Miyagawa, S., *et al*: Expression of pemphigoid antigen by SV40-transformed human keratinocytes. *J. Invest. Dermatol.* **86**:399, 1986.

7 Glycosaminoglycan

280. Maeda, H.: Observations on the fine structure of glycoseaminoglycans in normal and abnormal skin. *Jpn. J. Dermatol.* **90**:411, 1980 (in Japanese).

281. Ishikawa, H., Maeda, H.: Macromolecular structure of proteoglycans in the skin. *Nishinihon Hifuka.* **43**:1024, 1981 (in Japanese).

282. Wieslander, J., Heinegård, D.: Immunochemical analysis of cartilage proteoglycans. Antigenic determinants of substructures. *Biochemical J.* **179**:35, 1979.

283. Kitabatake, M., Ishikawa, H., Maeda, H.: Immuno-histochemical demonstration of proteoglycans in the skin of patients with sytemic scleroderma. *Br. J. Dermatol.* **108**:257, 1983.

284. Maeda, H., Ishikawa, H., Ohta, S.: Circumscribed myxoedema of lichen myxoedematosus as a sign of faulty formation of the proteoglycan macromolecule. *Br. J. Dermatol.* **105**:239, 1981.

Findings in Various Dermatoses

A Bullous dermatoses

1 Pemphigus

285. Beutner, E.H., Jordan, R.E.: Demonstration of skin antibodies in sera of pemphigus vulgaris patients by indirect immunofluorescence staining. *Proc. Soc. Exp. Biol. Med.* **117**:505, 1964.

286. Beutner, E.H., Lever, W.F., Witebsky, E. *et al*: Auto-antibodies in pemphigus vulgaris. *J. Am. Med. Assoc.* **192**:682, 1965.

287. Jordon, R.E., Triftshanser, C.T., Schroeter, A.L.: Direct immunofluorescence studies of pemphigus and bullous pemphigoid. *Arch. Dermatol.* **103**:486, 1971.

288. Jordon, R.E., Schroeter, A.L., Rogers, R.S. *et al*: Classical and alternate pathway activation of complement in pemphigus vularis lesions. *J. Invest. Dermatol.* **63**:256, 1974.

289. Jordon, R.E., Sams, W.M. Jr., Diaz, G. *et al*: Negative complement immunofluorescence in pemphigus. *J. Invest. Dermatol.* **57**:407, 1971.

290. Nishikawa, T., Kurihara, S., Harada, T. *et al*: Capability of complement fixation of pemphigus antibodies *in vitro*. *Arch. Dermatol. Res.* **260**:1, 1977.

291. Schliz, J.R., Michel, B.: Production of epidermal acantholysis in normal skin *in vitro* by the IgG fraction from pemphigus serum. *J. Invest. Dermatol.* **67**:254, 1976.

292. Uehara, Y.: *In vitro* leucocyte attachment to skin via autoantibodies of pemphigus and pemphigoid and the complement system. *Keigo Igaku.* **60**:731, 1983 (in Japanese).

293. Hashimoto, K., Shafran, K.M., Webber, P.S. *et al*: Anti-cell surface pemphigus autoantibody stimulates plasminogen activator activity of human epidermal cells. A mechanism for the loss of epidermal cohesion and blister formation. *J. Exp. Med.* **157**:259, 1983.

294. Katz, S.I., Halprin, K.M., Inderbitzin, T.M.: The use of human skin for the detection of antiepithelial auto-antibodies. *J. Invest. Dermatol.* **53**:390, 1969.

2 Pemphigoid

295. Lever, W.F., Schaumburg-Lever, G.: In: *Histopathology of the skin*, 6th Ed., ed. Lever, W.G., Schaumburg-Lever, G., Lippincott, Philadelphia, pp. 92–135, 1983.

296. Horiguchi, Y., Danno, K., Ikai, K. *et al*: Colloid body formation in bullous pemphigoid. *Arch. Dermatol. Res.* **277**:167, 1985.

297. Gammon, W.R., Briggaman, R.A., Inman, A.O. *et al*: Differentiating anti-lamina lucida and anti-sublamina densal anti-BMZ antibodies by indirect immunofluorescence on 1.0 M sodium chloride-separated skin. *J. Invest. Dermatol.* **82**:139, 1984.

298. Masutani, M., Ogawa, H., Taneda, A. *et al*: Ultrastructural localization of immunoglobulins in the dermo-epidermal junction of a patient with bullous pemphigoid. *J. Dermatol.* (Tokyo) **5**:107, 1978.

299. Horiguchi, Y., Imamura, S.: Discrepancy between the localization of *in vivo*-bound immunoglobulins in the skin and *in vitro*-binding sites of circulating anti-BMZ antibodies in bullous pemphigoid: Immunoelectron microscopic studies. *J. Invest. Dermatol.* **87**:715–719, 1986.

300. Pehamberger, H., Gschnait, F., Konrad, K. *et al*: Bullous pemphigoid, herpes gestationis and linear dermatitis herpetiformis. Circulating anti-basement membrane zone antibodies: *in vitro* studies. *J. Invest. Dermatol.* **74**:105, 1980.

301. Mutasim, D.F., Takahashi, Y., Labib, R.S. *et al*: A pool of bullous pemphigoid antigen(s) is intracellular and associated with the basal cell cytoskeleton-hemidesmosome complex. *J. Invest. Dermatol.* **84**:47, 1985.

302. Stanley, J.R., Hawley-Nelson, P., Yuspa, S.H. *et al*: Characterization of bullous pemphigoid antigen: A unique basement membrane protein of stratified squamous epithelia. *Cell.* **24**:897, 1981.

303. Gammon, W.R., Lewis, D.M., Carlo, J.R. *et al*: Pemphigoid antibody mediated attachment of peripheral blood leucocytes at the dermal-epidermal junction of human skin. *J. Invest. Dermatol.* **75**:334, 1980.

304. Naito, K., Morioka, S., Ogawa, H.: The pathogenic mechanism of blister formation in bullous pemphigoid. *J. Invest. Dermatol.* **79**:303, 1982.

3 Herpes gestationis

305. Schaumburg-Lever, G., Saffold, O.E., Orfanos, C.E. *et al*: Herpes gestationis; Histopathology and ultrastructure. *Arch. Dermatol.* **107**:888, 1973.

306. Yaoita, H., Gullino, M., Katz, S.I.: Herpes gestationis: Ultrastructure and ultrastructural localization of *in vivo*-bound complement. *J. Invest. Dermatol.* **66**:383, 1976.

307. Jordon, R.E.: Cutaneous immunopathology: Investigative and clinical applications. In: *Recent Advances in Dermatology*, ed. Rook, A., Savin J., Churchill Livingstone, New York, p. 15, 1980.

308. Provost, T.T., Tomasi, T.B. Jr.: Evidence for complement activations via the alternative pathway in skin diseases. I Herpes gestationis, SLE and bullous pemphigoid. *J. Clin. Invest.* **52**:1779, 1973.

309. Hönigsman, H., Stingl, G., Holubar, K. *et al*: Herpes gestationis: Fine structural pattern of immunoglobulin deposits in the skin *in vivo*. *J. Invest. Dermatol.* **66**:389, 1976.

310. Jordon, R.E., Heine, K.C., Tappeiner, G. *et al*: The immunopathology of herpes gestationis: Immunofluorescence studies and characterization of 'HG factor'. *J. Clin. Invest.* **57**:1426, 1976.

311. Katz, S.I., Hertz, K.C., Yaoita, H.: Herpes gestationis: Immunopathology and characterization of the HG factor. *J. Clin. Invest.* **57**:1434, 1976.

312. Cholzelski, T.P., Jablonska, S., Beutner, E.H. *et al*: Herpes gestationis with identical lesions in the newborn. *Arch. Dermatol.* **112**:1129, 1976.

313. Katz, A., Minta, J.O., Toole, J.W.P., *et al*: Immunopathologic study of herpes gestationis in mother and infant. *Arch. Dermatol.* **113**:1069, 1977.

314. Holmes, R.C., Black, M.M., Williamsen, D.M. *et al*: Herpes gestationis and bullous pemphigoid: A disease spectrum. *Br. J. Dermatol.* **103**:535, 1980.

315. Roscoe, J.T., Mutasim, D., Labib, R.S. *et al*: Autoantibodies from a patient with herpes gestationis identify bullous pemphigoid antigens by immunoblotting. (Abstr). *J. Invest. Dermatol.* **86**:503, 1986.

316. Miyagawa, S., Yoshioka, J., Morita, M. *et al*: Herpes gestationis associated with ectopic pregnancy. *J. Dermatol.* (Tokyo) **9**:203, 1982.

4 Epidermolysis bullosa acquisita

317. Kablitz, R.: Ein Beitrag zur frage der epidermolysis bullosa traumatica (hereditaria et acquisita). *Rostock Med. Diss, Rostock*, April 20, 1904.

318. Elliot, G.T.: Two cases of epidermolysis bullosa. *J. Cutan. Genitourin. Dis.* **13**:10, 1895.

319. Fox, T.C.: Pemphigus in a woman of nine years duration. *Br. J. Dermatol.* **9**:341, 1897.

320. Roenigk, H.H. Jr., Ryan, J.G., Bergfeld, W.F.: Epidermolysis bullosa acquisita: Report of three cases and review of all published cases. *Arch. Dermatol.* **103**:1, 1971.

321. Kushniruk, W.: The immunopathology of epidermolysis bullosa acquisita. *Can. Med. Assoc. J.* **108**:1143, 1973.

322. Nieboer, C., Boorsman, D.M., Woertdeman, M.J.,

Kalsbeek, G.L.: Epidermolysis bullosa acquisita: Immunofluorescence, electron microscopic and immunoelectron microscopic studies in four patients. *Br. J. Dermatol.* **102**:383, 1980.

323. Yaoita, H., Briggaman, R.A., Lawley, T.J., Provost, T.T., Katz, S.I.: Epidermolysis bullosa acquisita: Ultrastructural and immunologic studies. *J. Invest. Dermatol.* **76**:288, 1981.

324. Woodley, D.T., Briggaman, R.A., O'Keefe, E.J., Inman, A.O., Queen, L.L., Gammon, W.R.: Identification of the skin basement-membrane autoantigen in epidermolysis bullosa acquisita. *N. Engl. J. Med.* **310**:1007, 1984.

325. Wilson, B.D., Birnkrant, A.F., Beutner, E.H., Maige, J.C.: Epidermolysis bullosa acquisita: A clinical disorder of varied etiologies. *J. Am. Acad. Dermatol.* **3**:280, 1980.

326. Holubar, K., Wolff, K., Konrad, K., Beutner, E.H.: Ultrastructural localization of immunoglobulins in bullous pemphigoid skin. *J. Invest. Dermatol.* **64**:220, 1975.

327. Fine, J.D., Neiss, G.R., Katz, S.I.: Immunofluorescence and immunoelectron microscopic studies in cicatricial pemphigoid. *J. Invest. Dermatol.* **82**:39, 1984.

328. Woodley, D., Sauder, D., Talley, M.J., Silver, M., Grotendorst, G., Qwarnstrom, E.: Localization of basement membrane components after dermal-epidermal junction separation. *J. Invest. Dermatol.* **81**:149, 1983.

329. Furue, M., Iwata, M., Tamaki, K., Ishibashi, Y.: Anatomical distribution and immunological characteristics of epidermolysis bullosa acquisita and bullous pemphigoid antigen. *Brit. J. Dermatol.* **114**:651–659, 1986.

5 Linear IgA bullous dermatosis

330. Katz, S.I., Strober, W.: The pathogenesis of dermatitis herpetiformis. *J. Invest. Dermatol.* **70**:63, 1978.

331. Honeyman, J.F., Honeyman, A.R., Dela Parra, M.A. *et al*: Polymorphic pemphigoid. *Arch. Dermatol.* **115**:423, 1979.

332. Chorzelski, T.P., Jablonska, S.J., Beutner, E.H. *et al*: Linear IgA bullous dermatosis. In: *Immunopathology of the Skin*, ed. Beutner, E.H., Chorzelski, T.P., Bean, S.F., 2nd Ed., John Wiley and Sons. New York, pp. 315–323, 1979.

333. Pehamberger, H., Konrad, K., Holubar, K.: Circulating IgA anti-basement membrane antibodies in linear dermatitis herpetiformis Duhring. IF and immunoelectron microscopic studies. *J. Invest. Dermatol.* **59**:490, 1977.

334. Yaoita, H., Katz, S.I.: Circulating IgA anti-basement membrane zone antibodies in dermatitis herpetiformis. *J. Invest. Dermatol.* **69**:558, 1977.

335. McLean, I.E., Nakane, P.K.: Periodate-lysine-paraformaldehyde fixative. A new fixative for immunoelectron microscopy. *J. Histochem. Cytochem.* **22**:1077, 1974.

336. Yaoita, H., Katz, S.I.: Immunoelectron microscopic localization of IgA in skin of patients with dermatitis herpetiformis. *J. Invest. Dermatol.* **67**:502, 1976.

337. Yamasaki, Y., Hashimoto, T., Nishikawa, T.: Dermatitis herpetiformis with linear IgA deposition: Ultrastructural localization of *in vivo*-bound IgA. *Acta Derm. Venereol.* (Stockholm) **62**:401, 1982.

6 Dermatitis herpetiformis

338. Duhring, L.: Dermatitis herpetiformis. *JAMA.* **3**:225, 1884.

339. Yaoita, H., Katz, S.I.: Immunoelectron microscopic

localization of IgA in skin of patients with dermatitis herpetiformis. *J. Invest. Dermatol.* **67**:502, 1976.

340. Katz, S.I., Strober, W.: The pathogenesis of dermatitis herpetiformis. *J. Invest. Dermatol.* **70**:63, 1978.

341. Beutner, E.H., Chorzelski, T.P., Jordan, R.E.: *Autosensitization in Pemphigus and Bullous Pemphigoid.* Charles C. Thomas Pub. 1970.

342. Fry, L., Seah, P.P.: *Dermatitis Herpetiformis.* John Wiley and Sons, New York, 1974.

343. Yaoita, H.: Identification of IgA binding structures in skin of patients with dermatitis herpetiformis. *J. Invest. Dermatol.* **71**:213, 1978.

B Collagen diseases and related disorders
1 Lupus erythematosus

344. Moleden, D.P. *et al*: Standardization of the immunofluorescence test for autoantibody to nuclear antigens (ANA): Use of reference sera of defined antibody specificity. *Am. J. Clin. Pathol.* **82**:57, 1984.

345. Burnham, T.K. *et al*: The application of fluorescent antibody technique to the investigation of lupus erythematosus and various dermatoses. *J. Invest. Dermatol.* **41**:451, 1963.

346. Cormane, R.H.: 'Bound' globulin in the skin of patient with chronic discoid lupus erythematosus. *Lancet.* **1**:534, 1964.

347. Tuffanelli, D.L., Epstein, J.H.: Discoid lupus erythematosus. In: *Lupus Erythematosus*, 2nd Ed., ed. Dubois, E.L., Los Angeles, University of Southern California Press. p. 225. 1974.

348. Carlo, J.R. *et al*: Demonstration of B1H globulin together with C3 in the dermal-epidermal junction of patients with systemic lupus erythematosus. *Arthritis Rheum.* **22**:13, 1979.

349. Ueki, H., Wolff, H.H., Braw-Falco, O.: Cutaneous localization of human -globulins in lupus erythamatosus. An electron microscopical study using the peroxidase-labelled antibody technique. *Arch. Dermatol. Res.* **248**:297–314, 1974.

350. Winkelman, R.K., *et al*: Direct immunofluorescence in the diagnosis of scleroderma syndromes. *Br. J. Dermatol.* **96**:231, 1972.

351. Kay, D.M., Tuffanelli, D.L.: Immunofluorescent techniques in clinical diagnosis of cutaneous disease. *Ann. Intern. Med.* **71**:753, 1969.

352. Grossman, J., Callerame, M.L., Condemi, J.J.: Skin immunofluorescent studies in lupus erythematosus and other antinuclear antibody positive diseases. *Ann. Intern. Med.* **80**:496, 1974.

353. Ullman, S., Spielvogel, R.L., Kersey, J.H. *et al*: Immunoglobulins and complement in skin in graft-versus-host disease. *Ann. Intern. Med.* **85**:205, 1976.

354. Davis, B.M., Gilliam, A.N.: Prognostic significance of subepidermal immune deposits in uninvolved skin of patients with systemic lupus erythematosus: 10-year longitudinal study. *J. Invest. Dermatol.* **83**:242, 1984.

355. Kohchiyama, A., Oka, D., Ueki, H.: T cell subsets in lesions of systemic and discoid lupus erythematosus. *J. Cutan. Pathol.* **12**:493–499, 1985.

356. Bos, J.D., Emsbroek, J.A., Krieg, S.R.: T cell subsets and Langerhans cells in cutaneous lupus erythematosus. In: *Immuno-dermatopathology*, ed. Macdonald, D.M., Butterworth, London, p. 261. 1984.

2 Scleroderma

357. Hatano, H.: Classification of scleroderma. *Jpn. J. Dermatol.* **90**:1200, 1980 (in Japanese).

358. Winkelman, R.K.: Classification and pathogenesis of

scleroderma. *Mayo Clin. Proc.* **46**:83, 1971.

359. Sharp, G.C., Irwin, W.S., Tan, E.M. *et al*: Mixed connective tissue disease – an apparently distinct rheumatic disease syndrome associated with a specific antibody to an extractable nuclear antigen (ENA). *Am. J. Med.* **52**:148, 1972.

360. Nishikawa, T., Tajima, S., Kurihara, S. *et al*: *In vivo*-bound immunoglobulins and antinuclear antibodies in scleroderma and the scleroderma-like disorders. *Rinsho Hifuka.* **32**:973, 1978 (in Japanese).

361. Galoppin, L., Saurat, J-H.: *In vitro* study of the binding of anti-ribonucleoprotein antibodies to the nuclei of isolated living keratinocytes. *J. Invest. Dermatol.* **76**:264, 1981.

362. Iwatsuki, K., Tagami, H., Imaizumi, S. *et al*: The speckled epidermal nuclear immunofluorescence of epidermis seems to develop as an *in vitro* phenomenon. *Br. J. Dermatol.* **107**:653, 1982.

363. Takehara, K., Nakabayashi, Y., Ishibashi, Y. *et al*: Anti-nuclear antibodies in localized scleroderma. *Jpn. J. Dermatol.* **92**:883, 1982 (in Japanese).

364. Yamasaki, Y., Hashimoto, T., Kato, H. *et al*: Ultrastructural localization of immunoglobulin deposition in the dermo-epidermal junction seen in a few cutaneous disorders. *Jpn. J. Dermatol.* **93**:570, 1983 (in Japanese).

3 Behçet's disease

365. Behçet, H.: Uber rezidivierende, aphthose, durch Virus verursachte Geschwure am Mund, am Auge und an den Genitalien. *Dermatol. Wochenschr.* **105**:1152, 1937.

366. Mortada, A., Imam, I.Z.E.: Virus aetiology of Behçet's syndrome. *Br. J. Ophthalmol.* **48**:250, 1964.

367. Matsumura, N.: Aetiological experimental studies on Behçet's syndrome. *J. Jpn. Allergol.* **17**:62, 1968 (in Japanese).

368. Barile, M.F., Graykowsky, E.A. *et al*: L form of bacteria isolated from recurrent aphthous stomatitis lesions. *Oral Surg.* **16**:1395, 1963.

369. Kaneko, F., Kaneda, T. *et al*: Bacterial infectious allergy in Behçet's disease. (1) Chronic infectious foci and immunological responses to bacterial antigens *in vivo* and *in vitro*. *J. Jpn. Allergol.* **27**:440, 1978 (in Japanese).

370. Shimizu, T., Katsuta, Y., Oshima, Y.: Immunological studies on Behçet's syndrome. *Ann. Rheum. Dis.* **24**:494, 1965.

371. Lehner, T.: Behçet's syndrome and autoimmunity. *Lancet.* **1**:465, 1967.

372. Nishiyama, S., Hori, Y. *et al*: Behçet's disease and heavy metals. *Nishi Nihon Hifu.* **37**:7, 1975 (in Japanese).

373. Ohno, S., Asanuma, T. *et al*: HLA-BW51 and Behçet's disease. *JAMA.* **240**:529, 1978.

374. Shimizu, T., Ehrlich, G.E. *et al*: Behçet's disease (Behçet's syndrome). *Semin. Arthritis Rheum.* **8**:223, 1979.

375. Aoki, K., Ohno, S.: Behçet's disease in Japan. *J. Ophthalmol.* **14**:797, 1972.

376. Adachi, K., Kaneko, F. *et al*: Behçet's disease in Hokkaido Prefecture. *J. Jpn. Dermatol.* **93**:585, 1983 (in Japanese).

377. Kaneko, F., Kubota, K. *et al*: Immunocytological studies on aphthous lesions in Behçet's disease. In: *Behçet's Disease.* ed. Inaba, G., Univ. Tokyo Press, pp. 421–428, 1982.

378. Reimer, G., Steinkohl, S. *et al*: Lytic effect of cytotoxic lymphocytes on oral epithelial cells in Behçet's disease. *Br. J. Dermatol.* **107**:529, 1982.

379. Nishiyama, S.: Cutaneous histology of Behçet's disease. *Saishin Igaku.* **26**:445, 1971 (in Japanese).

380. Kaneko, F., Sido, M. *et al*: Infectious allergy in Behçet's disease. (2) On Serum immunological reactions and immunopathology. *J. Jpn. Allergol.* **29**:217, 1980 (in Japanese).

381. Kaneko, F., Takahashi, Y. *et al*: Immunological studies on aphthous ulcer and erythema nodosum-like eruptions in Behçet's disease. *Br. J. Dermatol.* **113**:303, 1985.

382. Kaneko, F., Takahashi, Y. *et al*: Natural killer cell numbers and function in peripheral lymphoid cells in Behçet's disease. *Br. J. Dermatol.* **113**:313, 1985.

4 Graft-versus-host (GvH) reaction

383. James, W.D., Odom, R.B.: Graft-versus-host disease. *Arch. Dermatol.* **119**:683, 1983.

384. Rolink, A.G., Gleichmann, E.: Allosuppressor- and allohelper-T cells in acute and chronic graft-versus-host diseases. III. Different Lyt subsets of donor T cells induce different pathological syndromes. *J. Exp. Med.* **158**:546, 1983.

385. Glazier, A., Tutschka, P.J., Farmer, E.R. *et al*: Graft-versus-host disease in cyclosporin A-treated rats after syngeneic and autologous bone marrow reconstitution. *J. Exp. Med.* **158**:1, 1983.

386. Shiohara, T., Narimatsu, H., Nagashima, M.: Induction of cutaneous graft-versus-host disease by allo- or self-Ia reactive helper T cells in mice. *Transplantation.* **43**: 692–698, 1987.

387. Shiohara, T., Ruddle, N.H., Horowitz, M. *et al*: Antitumour activity of class II MHC antigen-restricted cloned autoreactive T cells. I. Destruction of B16 melanoma cells mediated by by-stander cytolysis *in vitro*. *J. Immunol.* **138**:1971–1978, 1987.

5 Human GvH reaction

388. Rolink, A.G., Gleichmann, E.: Allosuppressor- and allohelper-T cells in acute and chronic graft-versus-host (GvH) disease. *J. Exp. Med.* **158**:546, 1983.

389. Thomas, E.D., Storb, R., Clift, R.A. *et al*: Bone-marrow transplantation. *N. Engl. J. Med.* **292**:895, 1975.

390. Saurat, J.H., Gluckman, E.: Lichen-planus-like eruption: A marker for chronic graft-versus-host reaction. *Br. Med. J.* **2**:1480, 1977b.

391. Saurat, J.H., Gluckman, E., Bussel, A. *et al*: The lichen planus-like eruption after bone marrow transplantation. *Br. J. Dermatol.* **92**:675, 1975.

392. Lampert, I.A., Janossy, G., Suitters, A.J. *et al*: Immunological analysis of the skin in graft-versus-host disease. *Clin. Exp. Immunol.* **2**:42s, 1982.

393. Janossy, G., Montano, L., Selby, W.S. *et al*: T cell subset abnormalities in tissue lesions developing during autoimmune disorders, viral infection and graft-versus-host disease. *J. Clin. Immunol.* **2**:42S, 1982.

394. Fujii, H., Ohashi, M., Nagura, H.: Immunohistochemical analysis of oral lichen-planus-like eruption in graft-versus-host disease after allogeneic bone marrow transplantation. *Am. J. Clin. Pathol.* **89**:177, 1988.

395. Uchiyama, T., Broder, S., Waldman, T.A.: A monoclonal antibody (anti-Tac) reactive with activated and functionally mature human T cells: 1. Production of anti-Tac monoclonal antibody and distribution of Tac (+) cells. *J. Immunol.* **126**:1393, 1981.

396. Sloane, J.P., Thomas, J.A., Imrie, S.F. *et al*: Morphological and immunohistological changes in the skin in allogenic bone marrow recipients. *J. Clin. Pathol.* **37**:919, 1984.

397. Basham, T., Nickoloff, B.J., Merigan, T.C. *et al*: Recombinant gamma interferon induces HLA-DR expression on cultured human keratinocytes. *J. Invest. Dermatol.* **83**:88, 1984.

149

C Erythematous diseases and vasculitis
1 Pityriasis rosea (Gibert)

398. Panisson, R., Bloch, P.H.: Histopathology of pityriasis rosea Gibert: Quantitative and qualitative light microscopic study of 62 biopsies of 40 patients. *Dermatologica.* **165**:551–558, 1982.
399. Aiba, S., Tagami, H.: Immunohistological studies in pityriasis rosea. Evidence for cellular immune reaction in the lesional epidermis. *Arch. Dermatol.* **121**:861–765, 1985.
400. Okamoto, H., Imamuro, S., Aoshima, T. *et al*: Dyskeratotic degeneration of epidermal cells in pityriasis rosea: Light and electron microscope studies. *Br. J. Dermatol.* **107**:189–1984, 1982.
401. Takaki, Y., Miyazaki, H.: Cytolytic degeneration of keratinocytes adjacent to Langerhans cells in pityriasis rosea Gibert. *Acta Dermatovenereol.* **56**:99–103, 1976.
402. Mobacken, H., Bjursten, L.M., Lowhagen, G.B. *et al*: Failure to detect immune complexes in the secondary stage of pityriasis rosea. *Arch. Dermatol. Res.* **275**:92–94, 1983.
403. Aiba, S., Tagami, H.: HLA-DR antigen expression on the keratinocyte surface in dermatoses characterized by lymphocytic exocytosis (e.g. pityriasis rosea). *Br. J. Dermatol.* **111**:285–294, 1984.

2 Erythema exudativum multiforme

404. Orfanos, C.E., Schaumberg-Lever, G., Lever, W.F.: Dermal and epidermal types of erythema multiforme. *Arch. Dermatol.* **109**:682, 1974.
405. Imamura, S., Yanase, K., Taniguchi, S., Ofuji, S, Mamgaoil, L.: Erythema multiforme: Demonstration of immune complexes in the sera and skin lesions. *Br. J. Dermatol.* **102**:161, 1980.
406. Kazmierowski, J.A., Wuepper, K.D.: Erythema multiforme: Immune complex vasculitis of the superficial cutaneous microvasculature. *J. Invest. Dermatol.* **71**:366, 1978.
407. Bushkell, L.L., Mackel, S.E., Jordon, R.E.: Erythema multiforme: Direct immunofluorescence studies and detection of circulating immune complexes. *J. Invest. Dermatol.* **74**:372, 1980.
408. Orton, P.W., Huff, J.C., Tonnensen, M.G., Weston, W.L.: Detection of a herpes simplex viral antigen in skin lesions of erythema multiforme. *Ann. Intern. Med.* **101**:48, 1984.

3 Urticarial vasculitis

409. McDuffie, F.C., Sams, M. Jr. *et al*: Hypocomplementemia with cutaneous vasculitis and arthritis. Possible immune complex disease. *Mayo Clin. Proc.* **48**:340, 1973.
410. Gammon, W.R., Wheeler, C.E.: Urticarial vasculitis. *Arch. Dermatol.* **115**:76, 1973.
411. Monroe, E.W.: Urticarial vasculitis, an up date review. *J. Am. Acad. Dermatol.* **5**:88, 1981.
412. Callen, J.P., Kalbfleisch, S.: Urticarial vasculitis, a report of nine cases and review of the literature. *Br. J. Dermatol.* **107**:87, 1982.
413. Sanchez, N.P., Winkelmann, P.K. *et al*: The clinical and histological spectra of urticarial vasculitis: Study of forty cases. *J. Am. Acad. Dermatol.* **7**:599, 1982.

4 Schönlein-Henoch purpura

414. Trygstad, C.W., Steim, E.R.: Elevated serum IgA globulin in anaphylactoid purpura. *Paediatrics.* **47**:1023, 1971.

415. Garcia-Fuentes, M., Chantler, C., Williams, D.G.: Cryoglobulinaemia in Schönlein-Henoch purpura. *Br. Med. J.* **16**:163, 1977.
416. Coppo, R., Basolo, B., Piccoli, G. *et al*: IgA 1 and IgA 2 immune complexes in primary IgA nephropathy and Schönlein-Henoch nephritis. *Clin. Exp. Immunol.* **57**:583, 1984.
417. Casanueva, B., Rodriquez-Valverde, V., Merino J. *et al*: Increased IgA-producing cells in the blood of patients with active Schönlein/Henoch purpura. *Arthritis Rheum.* **26**:854, 1983.
418. Bannister, K.M., Drew, R.A., Clarkson, A.R. *et al*: Immunoregulation in glomerulonephritis, Schönlein-Henoch purpura. *Arthritis Rhem.* **26**:854, 1983.

5 Vasculitis allergica cutis (Ruiter)

419. Ruiter, M.: Arteriolitis (vasculitis) allergica cutis (superficialis): A new dermatological concept. *Dermatologica.* **129**:217, 1964.
420. Stinga, S.G. *et al*: Allergic vasculitis Gougerot-Ruiter syndrome, immunofluorescent study. *Arch. Dermatol.* **95**:23, 1967.
421. Hermann, W.A. *et al*: Allergic vasculitis. *Arch. Dermatol. Res.* **269**:179, 1980.
422. Dambuyant, C. *et al*: Antigenic similarities within circulating immune complexes in patients suffering from cutaneous vasculitis. *Dermatologica.* **162**:429, 1981.

6 Erythema elevatum diutinum

423. Imamura, S. *et al*: Demonstration of circulating and tissue-fixed immune complexes in cutaneous necrotizing vasculitis. *Acta Derm. Venereol.* (Stockholm) **60**:389, 1980.
424. Katz, S.I. *et al*: Erythema elevatum diutinum: Skin and systemic manifestations, immunologic studies, and successful treatment with dapsone. *Medicine.* **56**:443, 1977.
425. Wolff, H.H. *et al*: Erythema elevatum diutinum. *Arch. Dermatol. Res.* **261**:17, 1978.

7 HB vasculitis

426. Gocke, D.J., Hsu, K., Morgan, C. *et al*: Association between polyarteritis and Australia antigen. *Lancet.* **II**:1149, 1970.
427. Shumacher, H.F., Gall, E.P.: Arthritis in acute hepatitis and chronic active hepatitis. Pathology of the synovial membrane with evidence for the presence of Australia antigen in synovial membranes. *Am. J. Med.* **57**:655, 1974.
428. Takekoshi, Y., Yanada, M., Miyakawa, Y.: Free 'small' and IgG-associated 'large' hepatitis Be antigen in the serum and glomerular capillary walls of two patients with membranous glomerulonephritis. *N. Engl. J. Med.* **300**:814, 1979.
429. Dienstag, J.L., Rhodes, A.R., Bhan, A.K. *et al*: Urticaria associated with acute viral hepatitis type B. *Ann. Intern. Med.* **89**:34, 1978.
430. Endoh, C., Katayama, H., Watanabe, C. *et al*: Leucocytoclastic vasculitis in a patient with so-called asymptomatic carrier of HB antigen: Demonstration of immune complex in the serum and the blood vessel walls in urticarial lesion. *Jpn. J. Dermatol.* **94**:781, 1984 (in Japanese).
431. Takahashi, T., Nakagawa, S., Hashimoto, T. *et al*: Large-scale isolation of Dane particles from plasma containing hepatitis B antigen and demonstration of a circular double-stranded DNA molecule extruding directly from their cores. *J. Immunol.* **117**:1392, 1976.

432. Kohler, G., Milstein, C.: Continuous cultures of fused cells secreting antibody of predefined specificity. *Nature*. **258**:485, 1975.

433. Tsuda, F., Miyakawa, Y., Mayumi, M.: Application of human erythrocytes to a radioimmuno-assay of immune complexes in serum. *Immunology*. **37**:681, 1979.

434. Gocke, D.J.: Extrahepatic manifestations of viral hepatitis. *Am. J. Med. Sci.* **270**:49, 1975.

435. Neumann, H.A.M., Berretty, P.J.M., Reinders Folmer, S.C.C. *et al*: Hepatitis B surface antigen deposition in the blood vessel walls of urticarial lesions in acute hepatitis B. *Br. J. Dermatol.* **104**:388, 1981.

8 Livedo vasculitis

436. Bard, J.W., Winkelmann, R.K.: Livedo vasculitis. *Arch. Dermatol.* **96**:489, 1967.

437. Winkelmann, R.K.: Livedoid vasculitis. *Jpn. J. Dermatol.* **82**:84, 1972 (in Japanese).

438. Schroeter, A.R. *et al*: Immunofluorescence of cutaneous vasculitis with systemic disease. *Arch. Dermatol.* **104**:254, 1971.

439. Gomes, M.A. *et al*: Semilogic value of Clq and C4 cutaneous deposits. An immunofluorescent study. *J. Cutan. Pathol.* **9**:169, 1982.

9 Wegener's granuloma tosis

440. Fauci, A.S., Wolff, S.M.: Wegener's granulomatosis: Studies in eighteen patients and a review of the literature. *Medicine*. **52**:535, 1973.

441. Horn, R.G. *et al*: Renal biopsy pathology in Wegener's granulomatosis. *Am. J. Pathol.* **74**:423, 1974.

442. Spector, W.G., Heesorm, N.: The production of granuloma by antigen-antibody complexes. *J. Pathol.* **98**:31, 1969.

10 Experimental cutaneous vasculitis

443. Uriuhara, T., Movat, H.Z.: The role of PMN-leucocyte lysosomes in tissue injury, inflammation and hypersensitivity. I. The vascular changes and the role of PMN-leucocytes in the reversed passive Arthus reaction. *Exp. Mol. Pathol.* **5**:539, 1966.

444. Venkatachalam, M.A., Cotran, R.S.: Ultrastructure of the local Arthus phenomenon using horseradish peroxidase as antigen. *Lab. Invest.* **23**:129, 1970.

445. Kniker, W.T., Cochrane, C.G.: The localization of circulating immune complexes in experimental serum sickness. *J. Exp. Med.* **127**:119, 1968.

446. Cream, J.J. *et al*: Disappearance of immunoglobulin and complement from the Arthus reaction and its relevance to studies of vasculitis in man. *Br. J. Dermatol.* **84**:107, 1971.

447. Cochrane, C.G., Janoff, A.: The Arthus reaction: a model of neutrophil and complement-mediated injury. In: *The Inflammatory Process*, 2nd ed., Vol. III, Academic Press, New York: 85, 1974.

448. Ueki, H. *et al*: Reversed passive Arthus reaction using horseradish peroxidase as antigen. *Arch. Dermatol. Forsch.* **250**:1, 1974.

449. Weber, K. *et al*: Ultrastructural evidence for lack of tissue damage in a local immune complex reaction. *Virchows Arch. Abt. B. Cell. Path.* **18**:213, 1975.

450. Ueki, H. *et al*: Transient immune deposits in the papillary dermis and in the epidermis. *Arch. Dermatol. Res.* **269**:51, 1980.

451. Kohda, M., Ueki, H.: The localization of immune complexes in epidermis and upper dermis, electron microscopic studies on reversed passive Arthus reaction. *J. Cutan. Pathol.* **8**:411, 1981.

D Eczematous diseases
1 Atopic dermatitis

452. Braathen, L.R., Føorre, Ø., Natvic, J.B., Eeg-Larsen, T.: Predominance of T lymphocytes in the dermal infiltrate of atopic dermatitis. *Br. J. Dermatol.* **100**:511–519, 1979.

453. Uno, H., Hanifin, J.M.: Langerhans cells in acute and chronic epidermal lesions of atopic dermatitis, observed by L-dopa histofluorescence, glycol methacrylate thin section, and electron microscopy. *J. Invest. Dermatol.* **75**:52–60, 1980.

454. Leung, D.Y.M., Bhan, A.K., Schneeberger, E.E., Geha, R.S.: Characterization of the mononuclear cell infiltrate in atopic dermatitis using monoclonal antibodies. *J. Allergy. Clin. Immunol.* **71**:47–56, 1983.

455. Zachary, C.B., Allen, M.H., Macdonald, D.M.: In situ quantification of T lymphocyte subsets and Langerhans cells in the inflammatory infiltrate of atopic eczema. *Br. J. Dermatol.* **112**:149–156, 1985.

456. Uehara, M.: Clinical and histological features of dry skin in atopic dermatitis. *Acta Dermatovenereol. Suppl.* **114**:82–86, 1985.

2 Contact dermatitis

457. McMillan, E.M., Stoneking, L., Burdick, S. *et al*: Immunophenotype of lymphoid cells in positive patch tests of allergic contact dermatitis. *J. Invest. Dermatol.* **84**:229–233, 1985.

458. Scheynius, A., Fischer, T., Forsum, U. *et al*: Immunohistochemical analysis of the cellular immune response in contact and irritant dermatitis in man. *J. Invest. Dermatol.* **80**:229, 1983.

459. Aiba, S., Tagami, H.: HLA-DR antigen expression on the keratinocyte surface in dermatoses characterized by lymphocytic exocytosis (e.g. pityriasis rosea). *Br. J. Dermatol.* **111**:285–294, 1984.

460. Aiba, S., Tagami, H.: Immunohistologic studies in pityriasis rosea. Evidence for cellular immune reaction in the lesional epidermis. *Arch. Dermatol.* **121**:761–765, 1985.

3 Distribution of antigen in allergic contact dermatitis

461. Eisen, H.N., Tabachnick, M.: Elicitation of allergic contact dermatitis in the guinea pig. The distribution of bound dinitrobenzene groups within the skin and quantitative determination of the extent of combination of 2,4-dinitrochlorobenzene with epidermal protein *in vivo*. *J. Exp. Med.* **108**:773, 1958.

462. Nakagawa, S., Ueki, H., Tanioku, K.: The distribution of 2,4-dinitrophenyl groups in guinea pig skin following surface application of 2,4-dinitrochlorobenzene: An immunofluorescent study. *J. Invest. Dermatol.* **57**:269, 1971.

463. Oka, D., Nakagawa, S., Ueki, H.: Antigen in contact sensitivity: I. Immunofluorescent studies on the distribution of bound DNCB within the epidermis of guinea pigs following skin painting with the sensitizer. *Kawasaki Med. J.* **9**:21, 1983.

464. Oka, D., Nakagawa, S. *et al*: Antigen in contact sensitivity; 11. Scanning immunoelectron microscopic studies of the distribution of DNP groups on the epidermal cells of guinea pigs following skin painting with DNCB. *J. Dermatol.* **11**:15–19, 1984.

465. Nishioka, K. *et al*: Induction of hapten-specific lymphoid cell proliferation by liposome-carrying molecules from haptenated epidermal cells in contact sensitivity. *J. Invest. Dermatol.* **83**:96, 1984.

466. Oka, D. *et al*: Distribution of 2,4-dinitrophenyl groups

on the epidermal Langerhans cells of guinea pigs following skin painting with 2,4-dinitrochlorobenzene. *Dermatologica*. **172**:12, 1986.

467. Nakagawa, S., Fujita, S., Tanioku, K.: The distribution of DNP groups in lymph nodes following application of DNCB to guinea pig skin. *Kawasaki Med. J.* **3**:67, 1977.

468. Nakagawa, S. *et al*: The distribution of 2,4-dinitrophenyl groups in lymphoid tissue of guinea pigs following skin painting with 2,4-dinitrochlorobenzene. *Immunology*. **36**:851, 1979.

469. Aoshima, T. *et al*: Studies on the dinitrophenylated lymphocytes in guinea pig painted with DNCB. *J. Dermatol*. (Tokyo) **4**:251, 1977.

470. Nakaye, M. *et al*: Ultrastructural localization of 2,4-dinitrophenyl groups on draining lymph node cells of guinea pigs following skin painting with 2,4-dinitrochlorobenzene: I. Scanning immunoelectron microscopic studies. *J. Dermatol*. (Tokyo) **10**:251, 1983.

471. Nakagawa, S. *et al*: Ultrastructural localization of DNP groups on draining lymph node cells of guinea pigs following skin painting with DNCB. II. Immunoferritin electron microscopic study. *Kawasaki Med. J.* **9**:181, 1983.

472. Forman, J. *et al*: Relationship between trinitrophenyl and H-2 antigens on trinitrophenyl-modified spleen cells. I. H-2 antigens on cells treated with trinitrobenzene sulfonic acid derivatized. *J. Immunol*. **118**:797, 1977.

473. Clement, L.T., Shevach, E.M.: Characterization of major histocompatibility antigens on trinitrophenyl-modified cells. *Mol. Immunol*. **16**:67, 1979.

474. Battisto, J.R., Bloom, B.R.: Dual immunological unresponsiveness induced by cell membrane coupled hapten or antigen. *Nature*. **212**:156, 1966.

475. Miller, S.D. *et al*: Nature of hapten-modified determinants involved in induction of T cell tolerance and suppressor T cells to DNCB contact sensitivity. *J. Immunol*. **124**:1187, 1980.

476. Ueki, H.: Hyaline bodies in subepidermal papillae. Immunohistochemical studies in several dermatoses. *Arch. Dermatol*. **100**:608, 1969.

E Inflammatory keratosis
1 Psoriasis

477. Gelsthorpe, K., Doughty, R.W.: A new HLA antigen. *TY Tissue Antigens*. **3**:316, 1973.

478. Ozawa, A., Ohkido, M., Tsuji, K.: Some recent advances in HLA and skin diseases. *J. Am. Acad. Dermatol*. **4**:205, 1981.

479. Weinstein, G.D., Van Scott, E.J.: Autoradiographic analysis of turnover times of normal and psoriatic epidermis. *J. Invest. Dermatol*. **45**:257, 1965.

480. Weinstein, G.D., McCullough, J.L., Ross, P.: Cell proliferation in normal epidermis. *J. Invest. Dermatol*. **82**:623, 1984.

481. Voorhees, J.J., Duell, E.A., Bass, L.J. *et al*: Decreased cyclic AMP in the epidermis of lesions of psoriasis. *Arch. Dermatol*. **105**:695, 1972.

482. Iizuka, H., Adachi, K., Halprin, K.M. *et al*: Cyclic AMP accumulation of psoriatic skin: Differential responses to histamine, AMP and epinephrine by the uninvolved and involved epidermis. *J. Invest. Dermatol*. **70**:250, 1978.

483. Greaves, M.W.: Neutrophil polymorphonuclears, mediators and the pathogenesis of psoriasis. *Brit. J. Dermatol*. **109**:115, 1983.

484. Langhof, H., Müller, H.: Leukotaktische Eigenschaften von Psoriasisschuppen. *Hautarzt*. **17**:101, 1966.

485. Krogh, H.K., Tönder, O.: Antibodies in psoriatic scales. *Scand. J. Immunol*. **2**:45, 1973.

486. Beutner, E.H., Chorzelski, T.P., Jablonska, S.: Autoimmunity in psoriasis. I: Studies on the possible significance of the universal stratum corneum antibodies in the pathogenesis of psoriasis. Psoriasis. Proceedings of the 2nd international symposium, ed. Faber, E.M., Cox, A.J., New York Medical Books, pp. 63–72, 1977.

487. Jablonska, S., Chorzelski, T.P., Beutner, E.H. *et al*: Autoimmunity in psoriasis. II. Immunohistologic studies on various forms of psoriasis and Köbner's phenomenon. ditto, pp. 73–80, 1977.

488. Tagami, H., Ofuji, S.: Characterization of a leukotactic factor derived from psoriatic scale. *Br. J. Dermatol*. **97**:509, 1977.

489. Kaneko, F., Gushiken, H., Kawagishi, I. *et al*: Analysis of immunological responses in psoriatic lesions. (1) Immunopathological studies on psoriatic lesions. *J. Invest. Dermatol*. **75**:436, 1980.

490. Kaneko, F.: Immunological analysis of psoriatic lesion. Current concepts on pathogenesis of psoriasis. *Hokkaido University Medical Library Series*. **18**:101, 1985.

491. Braun-Falco, O., Mannel, C., Scherer, R.: Nachweis von zirkulierenden loeslichen Immunokomplexen im Serum von Psoriatispatienten mit dem ^{125}J-Clq-Ablenkungstest. *Hautgarzt*. **28**:658, 1977.

492. Guilhou, J.J., Clot, J., Guillot, B. *et al*: Immunological aspects of psoriasis. *Br. J. Dermatol*. **102**:173, 1980.

2 Pustulosis palmaris et plantaris

493. Miyachi, Y., Danno, K., Yanase, K. *et al*: Acute generalized pustular bacterid and immune complexes. *Acta Dermatovenereol*. (Stockholm) **60**:66, 1980.

494. Miyachi, Y.: Pustular vasculitis. *J. Am. Acad. Dermatol*. **9**:774, 1983.

495. Uehara, M., Ofuji, S.: The morphogenesis of pustulosis palmaris et plantaris. *Arch. Dermatol*. **109**:518, 1974.

496. Uehara, M., Fujigaki, T., Hayashi, S.: Glucose tolerance in pustulosis palmaris et plantars. *Arch. Dermatol*. **116**:1275, 1980.

497. Tagami, H., Ofuji, S.: A leukotactic factor in the stratum corneum of pustulosis palmaris et plantaris: A possible mechanism for the formation of intraepidermal sterile pustules. *Acta Dermatovenereol*. (Stockholm) **58**:401, 1978.

498. Danno, K., Okamoto, H., Imamura, S. *et al*: Assessment of anti-stratum corneum antibody titres in pustulosis palmaris et plantaris. *Br. J. Dermatol*. **107**:183, 1982.

499. Takigawa, M., Miyachi, Y, Uehara, M. *et al*: Treatment of pustulosis palmaris et plantaris with oral doses of colchicine. *Arch. Dermatol*. **118**:458, 1982.

3 Lichen planus

500. Lever, W.F., Schaumburg-Lever, G.: Lichen planus. In: *Histopathology of the Skin*, 6th ed. Lippincott, Philadelphia, pp. 151–156, 1983.

501. Ueki, H.: Hyaline bodies in subepidermal papillae. Immunohistochemical studies in several dermatoses. *Arch. Dermatol*. **100**:610, 1969.

502. Abell, E., Presbury, D.G., Marks, R. *et al*: The diagnostic significance of immunoglobulin and fibrin deposition in lichen planus. *Br. J. Dermatol*. **93**:17, 1975.

503. Baart de la Faille-Kuyper, E.H., Baart de la Faille, H.: An immunofluorescence study of lichen planus. *Br. J. Dermatol*. **90**:365, 1974.

504. Konrad, K., Pehamberger, H., Holubar, K.: Ultrastructural localization of immunoglobulin and fibrin in lichen planus. *J. Am. Acad. Derm*. **1**:233, 1979.

505. Black, M.M.: What is going on in lichen planus? *Clin. Exp. Dermatol*. **2**:303, 1977.

F Metabolic diseases
1 Amyloidosis

506. Wright, J.R., Calkins, E., Humphrey, R.L.: Potassium permanganate reaction in amyloidosis: A histological method to assist in differentiating forms of this disease. *Lab. Invest.* **36**:274, 1977.
507. Fujihara, S., Balow, J.E., Costa, J.C., Glenner, G.G.: Identification and classification of amyloid in formalin-fixed, paraffin-embedded tissue sections by the unlabelled immunoperoxidase method. *Lab. Invest.* **43**:358, 1980.
508. Masu, S., Hosokawa, M. Seiji, M.: Amyloid in localized cutaneous amyloidosis: Immunofluorescent studies with anti-keratin antiserum especially concerning the difference between systemic and localized cutaneous amyloidosis. *Acta Derm. Venereol.* (Stockholm) **61**:381, 1981.
509. Maeda, H., Ohta, S., Saito, Y. *et al*: Epidermal origin of the amyloid in localized cutaneous amyloidosis. *Br. J. Dermatol.* **106**:345, 1982.
510. Kobayashi, H., Hashimoto, K.: Amyloidogenesis in organ-limited cutaneous amyloidosis: Antigenic identity between epidermal keratin and skin amyloid. *J. Invest. Dermatol.* **80**:66, 1983.
511. Eto, H., Hashimoto, K., Kobayashi, K. *et al*: Differential staining of cytoid and skin-limited amyloidosis with monoclonal anti-keratin antibodies. *Am. J. Pathol.* **116**:473, 1984.
512. Noren, P., Westermark, P., Cornwell, G.G. *et al*: Immunofluorescence and histochemical studies of localized cutaneous amyloidosis. *Br. J. Dermatol.* **108**: 277, 1983.
513. Ishii, M., Asai, Y., Hamada, T.: Evaluation of cutaneous amyloid employing anti-keratin antibodies and the immunoperoxidase technique (PAP method). *Acta Derm. Venereol.* (Stockholm) **64**:281, 1981.
514. Yoneda, K., Kitajima, Y., Yanagihara, M. *et al*: Immunofluorescent staining properties of amyloid substance in primary localized cutaneous amyloidosis using anti-keratin antibody. *Jpn. J. Dermatol.* **93**:151, 1984 (in Japanese).
515. Masuda, C., Hayashi, M., Kameda, Y. *et al*: Study on amyloid deposited in the skin of a patient with amyloidosis cutis nodularis atrophicans. *Rinsho Hifuka.* **38**:545, 1984 (in Japanese).
516. Breathnack, S.M., Melrose, S.M., Bhogal, B. *et al*: Ultrastructural localization of amyloid P component in primary localized cutaneous amyloidosis. *Clin. Exp. Dermatol.* **8**:355, 1983.
517. Kaneko, F., Kumakiri, M.: Immunopathological studies on cutaneous amyloidoses: Observations on interaction of amyloid substances, the dermo-epidermal junction and infiltrates in the dermis. *Jpn. J. Dermatol.* **94**:701, 1984 (in Japanese).

2 Porphyria cutanea tarda

518. Cormane, R.H., Szabo, E., Hoo, T.T.: Histopathology of the skin in acquired and hereditary porphyria cutanea tarda. *Br. J. Dermatol.* **85**:531, 1971.
519. Epstein, J.H., Tuffanelli, D.T., Epstein, W.L.: Cutaneous changes in the porphyrias. *Arch. Dermatol.* **107**:689, 1973.
520. Honigsmann, H., Gschnait, F., Konrad, K. *et al*: Mouse model for protoporphyria. III. Experimental production of chronic erythropoietic protoporphyria-like lesions. *J. Invest. Dermatol.* **66**:188, 1976.
521. Nonaka, S., Hirowatari, T., Honda, T. *et al*: Erythropoietic protoporphyria. *Jpn. J. Dermatol.* **87**:7, 1977 (in Japanese).

522. Wick, G., Honigsmann, H., Timpl, R.: Immunofluorescent demonstration of type IV collagen and non-collagenous glycoprotein in thickened vascular basal membranes in protoporphyria. *J. Invest. Dermatol.* **73**:335, 1979.
523. Honda, T., Nonaka, S., Murayama, F. *et al*: Introduction of chronic skin changes in intraperitonally haematoporphyrin-injected with metal halide lamp irradiation. *J. Dermatol.* (Tokyo) **13**:426, 1986.

G Alopecia

524. Igarashi, R. *et al*: Immunofluorescent studies of complement C3 in the hair follicle of normal scalp and of scalp affected by alopecia areata. *Acta Derm. Venereol.* (Stockholm) **60**:33, 1980.
525. Igarashi, R. *et al*: Immunofluorescent studies on complement components in the hair follicles of normal scalp and of scalp affected by alopecia areata. *Acta Derm. Venereol* (Stockholm) **63**:131, 1981.
526. Bystryn, J.C. *et al*: Direct immunofluorescence studies in alopecia areata and male pattern alopecia. *J. Invest. Dermatol.* **73**:317, 1979.
527. Nakajima, S.: Immunohistological study of alopecia areata. *Journal of Tokyo Women's Medical College.* **50**:592, 1980 (in Japanese).

H Infectious diseases
1 Mycoses

528. Coons, A.H., Creech, H.J., Jones, R.N., Berliner, E.: The demonstration of pneumococcal antigens in tissues by the use of fluorescent antibody. *J. Immunol.* **45**:157–170, 1942.
529. Kaplan, W., Ivens, M.S.: Fluorescent antibody staining of *Sporotrichum schenckii* in cultures and clinical materials. *J. Invest. Dermatol.* **35**:151–159, 1960.
530. Kaplan, W., Kraft, D.E.: Demonstration of pathogenic fungi in formalin-fixed tissues by immunofluorescence. *Am. J. Clin. Pathol.* **54**:420–437, 1969.
531. Chandler, F.W., Kaplan, W., Ajello, L.: *Color Atlas and Text of the Histopathology of Mycotic Diseases.* Year Book Medical, Chicago, pp. 1–333, 1980.
532. Palmer, D.F., Kaufman, L., Kaplan, W., Cavallaro, J.J.: *Serodiagnosis of Mycotic Diseases.* Charles C. Thomas, Springfield, pp. 1–191, 1977.

2 Spirochaetal diseases

533. Lomholt, G.: Syphilis, Yaws and Pinta. In: *Textbook of Dermatology.* eds. Rook, A., Wilkinson, D.S., Ebling, F.J.G. 3rd Ed., Blackwell Scientific, Oxford, pp. 701–736, 1979.
534. Kataniwa, Y., Sato, T., Nakazawa, M. *et al*: Three rare cases of symptomatic syphilis. *V D* **60**:56–63, 1979.
535. Warthin, A.S., Starry, A.C.: A more rapid and improved method of demonstrating spirochaetes in tissues. *Am. J. Syph.* **4**:97–103, 1920.
536. Ito, K., Ohtani, M., Haba, T.: Über ein zeitsparende Methode zur Anfärbung von *Treponema pallidum* in Geweben. *Der Hautarzt* **20**:85–88, 1969.
537. Tateshita, T., Asakuma, Y., Saito, T., Masumura, T., Fukushima, N.: A method of demonstrating spirochaetes in tissues embedded in paraffin. *Medical Technology* **8**:647–655, 1980 (in Japanese).

3 Bacterial infections – impetigo and staphylococcal scalded skin syndrome

538. Lillibridge, C.B., Melish, M.E., Glasgow, L.A.: Site of

action of exfoliative toxin in the staphylococcal scalded skin syndrome. *Paediatrics.* **50**:728–738, 1972.

539. Melish, M.E., Glasgow, L.A.: The staphylococcal scalded skin syndrome – development of an experimental model. *N. Engl. J. Med.* **282**:1114–1119, 1970.

540. Sakurai, S.: Studies of staphylococcal exfoliatin A and B. *Jikei Med. J.* **93**:1–15, 1978 (in Japanese).

541. Melish, M.E., Chen, F.S.: Demonstration of specific receptors for staphylococcal epidermolytic toxin in human and murine skin. *Clin. Res.* **29**:284A, 1981.

542. Fritsch, P., Elias, P., Varga, J.: The fate of staphylococcal exfoliatin in newborn and adult mice. *Br. J. Dermatol.* **95**::275–284, 1976.

4 Tsutsugamushi disease (Scrub typhus)

543. Suzuki, T., Suto, T., Harada, M. *et al*: Four fatal cases of tsutsugamushi disease (scrub typhus) which occurred in Akita and Niigata Prefectures. *Akita J. Med.* **7**:303, 1981 (in Japanese with English abstract).

544. Takahashi, T., Maie, O.: Skin manifestations of tsutsugamushi disease. *Jpn. Med. J.* **2960**:37, 1981 (in Japanese)

545. Suzuki, T., Suto, T.: Observations of a new type tsutsugamushi disease in Akita Prefecture. *J. Jpn. Assoc. Infect. Dis.* **54**:755, 1980 (in Japanese with English abstract).

546. Suto, T.: The up-to-date status of tsutsugamushi disease in Japan and a rapid serological diagnostic method. *Medical Circle* **30**:497, 1985 (in Japanese).

5 Virus infections
5.1 Human papillomavirus infection

547. Howley, P.M.: The human papillomaviruses. *Arch. Pathol. Lab. Med.* **106**:429, 1982.

548. Roseto, A. *et al*: Monoclonal antibodies to the major capsid protein of human papillomavirus type 1. *J. Gen. Virol.* **65**:1319, 1984.

549. Braun, L. *et al*: Immunoperoxidase localization of papillomavirus antigen in cutaneous warts and Bowenoid papulosis. *J. Med. Virol.* **12**:187, 1983.

550. McDougall, J.K. *et al*: Detection of viral DNA and RNA by *in situ* hybridization. *J. Histochem. Cytochem.* **34**:33, 1986.

5.2 Herpesvirus infection

551. Aoyama, Y. *et al*: Viruses. In: *Immunofluorescence in Medical Science.* ed. Kawamura, A. Jr., Aoyama, Y. University of Tokyo Press, p. 101, 1982.

552. Orton, P.W. *et al*: Detection of herpes simplex viral antigen in skin lesions of erythema multiforme. *Ann. Int. Med.* **101**:48, 1984.

553. Kurata, T. *et al*: Detection of viral antigens in formalin-fixed specimens by enzyme treatment. *Ann. New York Acad. Sci.* **420**:192, 1983.

554. Nowinski, R.C. *et al*: Monoclonal antibodies for diagnosis of infectious diseases in humans. *Science.* **219**:637, 1983.

I Tumours
1 Epithelial tumours

555. Weiss, R.A., Eichner, R., Sun, T-T.: Monoclonal antibody analysis of keratin expression in epidermal disease: A 48- and 56-K dalton keratin as molecular marker for hyperproliferative keratinocytes. *J. Cell Biol.* **98**:1397, 1984.

556. Moll, R., Franke, W.W., Schiller, D.L. *et al*: The catalogue of human cytokeratins: Pattern of expression in normal, tumours and cultured cells. *Cell.* **31**:11, 1982.

557. Yoneda, K., Kitajima, Y., Furuta, H. *et al*: The distribution of keratin type intermediate-sized filaments in so-called mixed tumour of the skin. *Br. J. Dermatol.* **109**:393, 1983.

558. Osborn, M.: Intermediate filaments as histologic markers: An overview. *J. Invest. Dermatol.* **81**:104, 1983.

559. Hashimoto, K., Eto, H., Matsumoto, M. *et al*: Anti-keratin monoclonal antibodies: Production specificities and applications. *J. Cutan. Pathol.* **10**:529, 1983.

560. Osborn, M. Weber, K.: Biology of disease: Tumour diagnosis by intermediate filament typing: A novel tool for surgical pathology. *Lab. Invest.* **48**:372, 1983.

561. Shi, S-S., Goodman, M.L., Bhan, A.K., *et al*: Immuno-histochemical study of nasopharyngeal carcinoma using monoclonal keratin antibodies. *Am. J. Pathol.* **117**:53, 1984.

562. Cooper, D., Schermer, A., Sun, T-T.: Biology of disease. Classification of human epithelia and their neoplasms using monoclonal antibodies to keratins: Strategies, application, and limitation. *Lab. Invest.* **52**:243, 1985.

563. Weiss, R.A., Guillet, Y.A., Freedberg, I.M. *et al*: The use of monoclonal antibody to keratin in human epidermal disease: Alterations in immunohistochemical staining pattern. *J. Invest. Dermatol.* **81**:224, 1983.

564. Woodcock-Mitchell, J., Eichner, R., Nelson, W.G., Sun, T-T.: Immuno-localization of keratin polypeptides in human epidermis using monoclonal antibodies. *J. Cell Biol.* **95**:580, 1982.

565. Cown, A.M., Vogel, A.M.: Monoclonal antibodies to intermediate filament proteins of human cells: Unique and cross-reacting antibodies. *J. Cell Biol.* **95**:414, 1982.

2 Paget's disease

566. Lever, W.F., Schaumberg-Lever, G.: *Histopathology of the Skin.* Lippincott, Philadelphia 1985.

567. Paget, J.: On disease of the mammary areola preceding cancer of the mammary gland. *St. Bartholomew Res. Lond.* **10**:87, 1874.

568. Crocker, H.R.: Paget's disease affecting the scrotum and penis. *Trans. Pathol. Soc. Lond.* **40**:187, 1889.

569. Koss, L.G., Brockunier, A.: Ultrastructural aspects of Paget's disease of the vulva. *Arch. Pathol.* **87**:592, 1969.

570. Caputo, R., Califano, A.: Ultrastructural features of extramammary Paget's disease. *Arch. Clin. Exp. Dermatol.* **236**:121, 1970.

571. Medenica, M., Sahihi, T.: Ultrastructural study of a case of extramammary Paget's disease of the vulva. *Arch. Dermatol.* **105**:236, 1972.

572. Penneys, N.S., Nadji, M., McKinney, E.C.: Carcinoembryonic antigen present in human eccrine sweat. *J. Am. Acad. Dermatol.* **4**:401, 1981.

573. Penneys, N.S., Nadji, M., Morales, A.R.: Carcinoembryonic antigen present in benign sweat gland tumours. *Arch. Dermatol.* **118**:225, 1982.

574. Penneys, N.S., Nadji, M., Ziegels-Weissman, J., Katahchi, M., Morales, A.R.: Carcinoembryonic antigen in sweat gland carcinomas. *Cancer.* **50**:1608, 1982.

575. Nadji, M., Morales, A.R., Girtanner, R.E., Ziegels-Weissman, J., Penneys, N.S.: Paget's disease of the skin. A unifying concept of histogenesis. *Cancer.* **50**:2203, 1982.

576. Furue, M., Yamashita, M., Oohara, K., Tamaki, K.: Carcinoembryonic antigen and β_2 microglobulin in genital Paget's disease. *Jpn. J. Dermatol.* **93**:1189, 1983 (in Japanese).

577. Ohji, M., Furue, M., Tamaki, K.: Serum carcinoembryonic antigen level in Paget's disease. *Br. J.*

Dermatol. **110**:211, 1984.

578. Sharon, N., Halina, L.: Lectins: Cell-agglutinating and sugar-specific proteins. *Science.* **177**:949, 1972.
579. Tamaki, K., Hino, H., Oohara, K., Furue, M.: Lectin binding sites in Paget's disease. *Br. J. Dermatol.* **113**:17, 1985.
580. Tamaki, K., Furue, M., Matsukawa, A., Oohara, K., Mizoguchi, M., Hino, H.: Presence and distribution of carcinoembryonic antigen and lectin binding sites in benign apocrine sweat gland tumours. *Br. J. Dermatol.* **113**:565, 1985.
581. Tamaki, F., Furue, M., Seki, Y., Inoue, Y., Tsuchida, T., Kukita, A.: Lectin-binding sites in eccrine sweat gland tumours. *Jpn. J. Dermatol.* **114**:451 (in Japanese).
582. Fuks, A., Banjo, C., Shuster, J., Freedman, S.O., Gold, P.: Carcinoembryonic antigen (CEA): Molecular biology and clinical significance. *Biochem. Biophys. Acta.* **417**: 124, 1974.

3 Malignant melanoma

583. Nakajima, T., Watanabe, S., Sato, Y. *et al*: Immunohistochemical demonstration of S100 protein in malignant melanoma and pigmented nevus and its diagnostic application. *Cancer.* **50**:912, 1982.
584. Dhillon, A.P., Rode, J., Leathein, A.: Neuron specific enolase: An aid to the diagnosis of melanoma and neuroblastoma. *Histopathology.* **6**:81, 1982.
585. Koprowski, H., Steplewski, Z., Herlyn, D. *et al*: Study of antibodies against human melanoma produced by somatic cell hybrids. *Proc. Natl. Acad. Sci. USA.* **75**:3405, 1978.
586. Ruiter, D.J., Bergman, W., Welvaart, K. *et al*: Immunohistochemical analysis of malignant melanomas and nevocellular nevi with monoclonal antibodies to distinct monomorphic determinants of HLA antigens. *Cancer Res.* **44**:3930, 1984.
587. Brocker, E.B., Suter, L., Sorg, C.: HLA-DR antigen expression in primary melanomas of the skin. *J. Invest. Dermatol.* **82**:244, 1984.
588. Miettinen, M., Lehte, V.P., Virtanen, I.: Presence of fibroblast-type intermediate filaments (vimentin) and absence of neurofilaments in pigmented nevi and malignant melanomas. *J. Cutan. Pathol.* **10**:188, 1983.
589. Imai, K., Ng, A-K., Ferrone, S.: Characterization of monoclonal antibodies to human melanoma-associated antigens. *JNCI.* **66**:489, 1980.
590. Kageshita, T., Johno, M., Ono, T. *et al*: Immunohistochemical analysis of anti-melanoma monoclonal antibodies, with special reference to foetal tissue distribution. *J. Invest. Dermatol.* **85**:535, 1985.
591. Ruiter, D.J., Dingjan, G.M., Steijlen, P.M. *et al*: Monoclonal antibodies selected to discriminate between malignant melanomas and nevocellular nevi. *J. Invest. Dermatol.* **85**:4, 1985.
592. Cordell, J.L., Falini, B., Erber, W.N. *et al*: Immunoenzymatic labelling of monoclonal antibodies using immune complexes of alkaline phosphatase and monoclonal anti-alkaline phostphatase. *J. Histochem. Cytochem.* **32**:219, 1984.

4 Nevus cell nevus

593. Nakajima, T., Watanabe, S., Sato, Y. *et al*: Immunohistochemical demonstration of S100 protein in malignant melanoma and pigmented nevus and its diagnostic application. *Cancer.* **50**:912, 1982.
594. Imai, K., Ng, A-K., Ferrone, S.: Characterization of monoclonal antibodies to human melanoma-associated antigens. *JNCI.* **66**:489, 1980.

595. Kageshita, T., Johno, M., Ono, T. *et al*: Immunohistochemical analysis of anti-melanoma monoclonal antibodies, with special reference to foetal tissue distribution. *J. Invest. Dermatol.* **85**:535, 1985.
596. Ruiter, D.J., Bergman, W., Welvaart, K. *et al*: Immunohistochemical analysis of malignant melanomas and nevo-cellular nevi with monoclonal antibodies to distinct monomorphic determinants of HLA antigens. *Cancer Res.* **44**:3930, 1984.

5 Kimura's disease

597. Kawada, A.: Morbus Kimura Darstellung der Rekrankung und ihre differential Diagnose. *Der Hautartzt.* **27**:309, 1976 (in German).
598. Takenaka, T., Okuda, M., Usami, A. *et al*: Histological and immunological studies on eosinophilic granuloma of soft tissue, so-called Kimura's disease. *Clinical Allergy.* **6**:27, 1976.
599. Usami, A.: Clinics of eosinophilic granuloma of soft tissue. *Scope.* **16**:6, 1977 (in Japanese).
600. Sakuma, M., Okuyama, S., Suzuki, M. *et al*: Kimura's disease accompanied with lichen amyloidosis. *Jpn. J. Dermatol.* **94**(3):225, 1984 (in Japanese).
601. Suzuki, M., Kanazawa, K., Yaoita, H. *et al*: Lymph follicles of Kimura's disease. *Acta Dermatol.* Kyoto **779**:75, 1984 (in Japanese).
602. Nagai, T., Nagai, K., Adachi, M. *et al*: *In vitro* production of IgE by human peripheral blood lymphocytes. *Jpn. J. Allergol.* **31**(7):417, 1982 (in Japanese).

6 Lymphoma

603. Lever, W.F.: *Histopathology of the Skin.* Lippincott, Philadelphia (2nd ed.; 1954, 4th ed.; 1967, 5th ed.; 1975).
604. Burg, G. *et al*: Patterns of cutaneous lymphomas. *Dermatologica.* **157**:282, 1978.
605. Souteyrand, P. *et al*: Etude immunocytologique des lymphomas cutanes malins. *Dermatologica.* **157**:269, 1987.
606. Piepkorn, M., Marty, J. *et al*: T cell subset heterogeneity in a series of patients with mycosis fungoides and sezary syndrome. *J. Am. Acad. Dermatol.* **11**:427, 1984.
607. Jimbow, K., Chiba, M., Horikoshi, T.: Electron microscopic identification of Langerhans cells in the dermal infiltrates of mycosis fungoides. *J. Invest. Dermatol.* **78**:102, 1982.
608. Shimoyama, M. *et al*: Immunologic, Clinicopathologic and Prognostic Features of Japanese T cell lymphomas. In: *Leukaemia markers.* Academic Press Inc., pp. 525–528, 1981.

7 Histiocytosis-X

609. Lichtenstein, L.: Histiocytosis-X: Integration of eosinophilic granuloma of bone, 'Letterer-Siwe disease' and 'Schüller-Christian disease' as related manifestation of a single nosological entity. *Arch. Pathol.* **56**:84, 1953.
610. Harrist, T.J. *et al*: Histiocytosis-X: In situ characterization of cutaneous infiltrates with monoclonal antibodies. *Am. J. Clin. Pathol.* **79**:294–300, 1983.
611. Osband, M.E. *et al*: Histiocytosis-X: Demonstration of abnormal immunity, T cell histamine H2-receptor deficiency, and successful treatment with thymic extract. *N. Engl. J. Med.* **304**:146–53, 1981.

612. Hedinger, E.: Zur Frage des plasmacytomas. *Frankfurt Z. Pathol.* **7**:343–350, 1911.

613. Mason, T.E. *et al*: An immunoglobulin-enzyme bridge method for localizing tissue antigens. *J. Histochem. Cytochem.* **17**:563, 1969.

614. George, R.M.: Malignant plasmacytoma cutis. *Arch. Derm.* **101**:59, 1970.

615. Castro, E.B. *et al*: Plasmacytoma of paranasal sinus and nasal cavity. *Arch. Otolaryngol.* **97**:326, 1973.

616. Gromer, R.C. *et al*: Plasmacytoma of the head and neck. *J. Laryngol. Otol.* **97**:326, 1973.

617. Ruhwinkel, B. *et al*: Immunologische Untersuchungen bei extradullaren Plasmacytoma im oberen Respiration-strat. *Laryngol. Rhinol. Otol.* **53**:679–685, 1974.

618. Noorani, M.A.: Plasmacytoma of middle ear and upper respiratory tract. *J. Laryngol. Otol.* **89**:105, 1975.

619. Wiltshaw, E.: The natural history of extramedullary plasmacytoma and its relation to solitary myeloma of bone and myelomatosis. *Medicine.* **55**:217, 1976.

620. Palor, A.L.: Extramedullary plasmacytoma of head and neck, parotid and submandibular salivary glands. *J. Laryngol. Otol.* **91**:241, 1977.

621. Neil, A.M. *et al*: Extramedullary IgM plasmacytoma presenting in skin. *J. Am. Dermatopath.* **3**:79, 1981.

Index

*Page references in **bold** refer to figures; page references prefixed with 't' refer to tables.*

159

160

paucity of fibronectin 58
proteoglycans 54, 64, **64**
psoriasis 108, **109**
– cyclic adenosine 3′,
    5′-monophosphate in **31**
– effect of ultraviolet irradiation 32
– reactivity of deoxyribonuclease I
    32
psoriasis vulgaris, fibronectin in 58,
    59
pustular bacterid, acute generalized
    110
pustulosis palmaris et plantaris 110,
    110

R

renal insufficiency and
    staphylococcal infections 119
reticulin fibres, composition 60
reversed passive Arthus reaction
    100, **101**
ribonuclease A 32, **33**
Rickettsia tsutsugamushi 120, **120**
RNase A 32, **33**
rosette formation on fibroblasts **45**

S

S-100 protein
– in glial cells 48
– as marker for malignant
    melanoma 128
– as marker for sweat glands 40
– in nerve cells 48
– in nevus cell nevus 130, **130**
– staining of nerve fibres 48
scalded skin syndrome,
    staphylococcal 119, **119**
scanning immunoelectron
    microscopy 16-17
scar tissue, hypertrophic,
    distribution of fibronectin 58, **59**
Schönlein-Henoch purpura 93, **93**
schwannoma **49**
scleroderma 82, **83**
– proteoglycan in 64, **64**
scrub typhus 120, **120**
serum anti-nuclear antibodies in
    scleroderma t83
serum immune complexes in
    cutaneous vasculitis 100
SLE sera, anti-nuclear antibodies in
    t78
spiradenoma, eccrine 40
spirochaetal diseases 118
squamous cell carcinoma 124, **125**
– laminin 56

staining methods
– in immunofluorescence techniques
    4-7, **5-7**
– using monoclonal antibodies t19
staphylococcal exotoxin 119
staphylococcal infections 119
subsets of lymphocytes, 50, t50
sweat glands 40, **41**
– reactivities t40
syphilis 118
syringoma **41**
systemic lupus erythematosus 6, **7**
– fibronectin 58
– and pemphigus erythematosus 66
– sera *see* SLE sera
– *see also* lupus erythematosus
systemic manifestations of
    Schönlein-Henoch purpura 93
systemic scleroderma, proteoglycan
    64

T

T cell leukaemia, adult, infiltrates
    51
T cell subsets, predominance in
    dermatoses t50
T cells 50, 104
T4 bacteriophage as marker in
    scanning immunoelectron
    microscopy 16, **17**
technical procedures 4-25
Thy-1 positive dendritic epidermal
    cells 34, **35**
Treponema pallidum 118, **118**
trichilemmoma
– malignant *vs* eccrine
    poroepithelioma 42, **43**
– monoclonal antibodies against,
    specificities t19
Tsutsugamushi disease 120, **120**
tumours *see* neoplasms
Type I collagens 60, **61**
Type III collagens 60, **61**
Type IV collagens 62
Type V collagens 60, **61**
tyrosinase as marker for
    melanocytes 37

U

Ulex europaeus agglutinin I lectin
– in malignant
    haemangioendothelioma **47**
– on vascular endothelial cells 46
ultraviolet irradiation, effect in
    psoriasis 32
urticarial vasculitis 92, **92**

V

varicella-zoster virus infection 122,
    123
vascular endothelial cells 46, t46, **47**
vasculature *see* blood vessels
vasculitis 90-101
vasculitis allergica cutis 94, **94**
vertical observation in
    immunoelectron microscopy in
    pemphigoid 68, **69**
viral hepatitis B vasculitis 96, **97**
viral infections 121-3
visual markers for scanning
    immunoelectron microscopy t16

W

warts 121, **121**
Wegener's granulomatosis 99, **99**